Structural Information Theory

The Simplicity of Visual Form

Structural information theory is a coherent theory about the way the human visual system organizes a raw visual stimulus into objects and object parts. To humans, a visual stimulus usually has one clear interpretation even though, in theory, any stimulus can be interpreted in numerous ways. To explain this, the theory focuses on the nature of perceptual interpretations rather than on underlying process mechanisms, and adopts the simplicity principle, which promotes efficiency of internal resources, rather than the likelihood principle, which promotes veridicality in the external world. This theoretically underpinned starting point gives rise to quantitative models and verifiable predictions for many visual phenomena, including amodal completion, subjective contours, transparency, brightness contrast, brightness assimilation, and neon illusions. It also explains phenomena such as induced temporal order, temporal context effects, and hierarchical dominance effects, and extends to evaluative pattern qualities such as distinctiveness, interestingness, and beauty.

EMANUEL LEEUWENBERG is Emeritus Associate Professor at the Donders Institute for Brain, Cognition and Behaviour at Radboud University Nijmegen, The Netherlands.

PETER A. VAN DER HELM is Assistant Professor at the Donders Institute for Brain, Cognition and Behaviour at Radboud University Nijmegen, The Netherlands.

Structural Information Theory

The Simplicity of Visual Form

Emanuel Leeuwenberg
Peter A. van der Helm

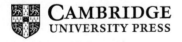
CAMBRIDGE
UNIVERSITY PRESS

CAMBRIDGE
UNIVERSITY PRESS

University Printing House, Cambridge CB2 8BS, United Kingdom

Cambridge University Press is part of the University of Cambridge.

It furthers the University's mission by disseminating knowledge in the pursuit of education, learning and research at the highest international levels of excellence.

www.cambridge.org
Information on this title: www.cambridge.org/9781107531758

© Emanuel Leeuwenberg and Peter A. van der Helm 2013

First published 2013
First paperback edition 2015

A catalogue record for this publication is available from the British Library

Library of Congress Cataloguing in Publication data
Leeuwenberg, E. L. J. (Emanuel Laurens Jan) author.
Structural information theory : the simplicity of visual form /
Emanuel Leeuwenberg, Peter A. van der Helm.
    pages   cm
Includes bibliographical references and index.
ISBN 978-1-107-02960-6 (hardback)
1. Human information processing.   2. Information theory in psychology.
I. Helm, Peter A. van der, author.   II. Title.
QP396.L44   2013
612.8 – dc23   2012020254

ISBN 978-1-107-02960-6 Hardback
ISBN 978-1-107-53175-8 Paperback

Contents

The colour plates are situated between pages 208 and 209.

Figures

Tables

Preface

This book does not provide a comprehensive survey of perception research. Rather, it deals with a specific, some might say idiosyncratic, approach to perception, and to visual form in particular. This approach is called structural information theory (SIT). Basically, SIT is a theory about structures irrespective of whether these structures are perceptual. Historically, however, SIT has been developed within the domain of visual perception research. A fundamental phenomenon in this domain is that, to humans, a visual stimulus usually has one clear interpretation even though any stimulus can, in principle, be interpreted in numerous ways. SIT addresses this phenomenon and aims at producing quantified and falsifiable predictions concerning the human interpretation of visual stimuli.

SIT was initiated, in the 1960s, by Emanuel Leeuwenberg and has been elaborated further by Hans Buffart, Peter van der Helm, and Rob van Lier. It began as a quantitative coding model of visual pattern classification that, in interaction with empirical research, developed into a general theory of perceptual organization. The home of SIT has always been the Radboud University Nijmegen, where it has been tested in collaboration with Harry van Tuijl, Frans Boselie, Rene Collard, Lucas Mens, Hans Mellink, Jantien van der Vegt, Cees van Leeuwen, Jackie Scharroo, Tessa de Wit, Arno Koning, Árpád Csathó, Gert van der Vloed, Matthias Treder, and Vinod Unni. Contributions and applications from elsewhere include those by Frank Restle, Hans-Georg Geissler, Ursula Schuster, Friedhart Klix, Ulrich Scheidereiter, Martina Puffe, Giovanni Adorni, Luigi Burigana, Albina Lucca, Remco Scha, Mehdi Dastani, Rens Bod, and Kasper Souren.

Our goal with this book is to provide an overview of SIT in a way that is accessible to a broad audience. We presuppose no special knowledge in the reader, neither of perception nor of SIT. In the Introduction, we discuss the unique status of perception and the roots of SIT. Then, we discuss SIT, in twelve chapters grouped in three parts. Part I shows how SIT's starting assumptions emerge from attempts to explain visual form phenomena. At the end of this section, an overview is presented of SIT's assumptions and theoretical foundations. Part II begins with a coding manual presenting practical heuristics that can be used to describe various stimulus types. The subsequent chapters report applications of SIT to visual form perception. Part III attends to aspects of visual form beyond the scope of SIT and to applications of SIT beyond the field of visual form. We end the book with an overview and a conclusion. Complementary to this empirically oriented book is a book by Van der Helm (2013) which is focused on SIT assumptions and foundations.

Emanuel Leeuwenberg and Peter A. van der Helm

Introduction

This book is about structural information theory (SIT) and its application to visual form perception. Here, by way of general introduction, we highlight several unique characteristics of perception and we give a sketch of the scientific roots of SIT.

The uniqueness of perception

Almost all textbooks introduce perception by showing visual illusions. Indeed, visual illusions are salient phenomena. The core issues in perception are less salient, however. In fact, they are rather inaccessible and often confusing. This may be illustrated as follows. In every research domain – be it biology, physics, psychology, you name it – perception is the mediating instrument for making observations. The goal is to establish properties of objects. An observation may, for instance, establish that a leaf is green. Notice that this proposition merely deals with the relationship between a leaf and its colour. What is meant by a leaf and by green is supposed to be known. In perception research, however, perception is both mediating instrument and topic of study (Rock, 1983). As a topic of study, perception is the process that starts from an assembly of patches of light at various positions on the retina. This process assesses which patches are grouped together to constitute a leaf, for instance. In other words, the objects we perceive belong to the output of perception and not to the input. The goal of perception is not to establish properties of given objects but to establish objects from properties of the given retinal image.

Hence, in perception research, the two roles of perception (i.e., mediating instrument and topic of study) are virtually opposed to each other. Nevertheless, often, they are hardly distinguished. Usually, only one role is attributed to perception, namely, that of mediating instrument. This role is relevant at the conscious level involved in the everyday human communication of propositions. At this level, there is no sensation of the actual visual input which is an assembly of unstructured patches on the retina. There is also no experience of the perception process. The process

1

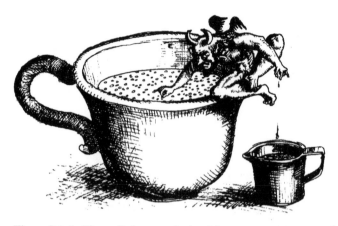

Figure I.1 A Maxwell demon, during his attempt to remove the milk from a milk-coffee mixture. This cumbersome job is similar to that of perception, in that both jobs turn chaos into order. Yet, there is also a crucial difference: to complete the job, the demon needs a lot of time, whereas perception needs only a few milliseconds (Leeuwenberg, 2003a).

is too rapid and too effortless for this. As a consequence, the perceived objects are taken as the actual components of the external scene we look at, even though they are in fact just mental constructs that result from the perception process in our brain.

Perception also exhibits a paradoxical feature, namely, with respect to temporal aspects. Within a few milliseconds, perception turns a mess of unstructured retinal patches into an ordered structure, whereas an analogous physical process from chaos to order may need millions of years. Such a process is illustrated in Figure I.1. It presents a little creature, a so-called Maxwell demon, in his attempt to remove the milk from a milk-coffee mixture. A milk-coffee mixture is obtained within the wink of an eye by pouring milk into black coffee; this is a process from order to chaos. To do the inverse, that is, to go from chaos to order, the Maxwell demon has to pick out the milk molecules one by one.

The above-mentioned confusions and paradoxes are not new. They already inspired Aristotle (350 BC/1957) to make the following, rather pessimistic, prophecy:

In a shorter time more will be known about the most remote world, namely that of the stars, than about the most nearby topic, namely perception.

In our view, Aristotle's prophecy was right on target. Before 1850, perception was hardly acknowledged as a topic of study. Even nowadays, it still has all the features of a young science. It is still approached by numerous independent and loose theories, which are plausible in some respects but untenable in others. Yet, in the mid-twentieth century, there were also developments which triggered the idea that perception should not be merely a topic of psychology and that one should not merely focus on discovering remarkable phenomena (Palmer, 1999). The insight was born that perception research should involve, apart from psychology, also physiology, mathematics, physics, and artificial intelligence. In other words, one realized that only divergent, interdisciplinary, research may lead to a convergent, coherent, understanding of perception as the unconscious process from the unstructured patches on our retina to the structured world we consciously perceive.

Scientific roots of SIT

The first modern approach to perception was given by the Gestalt psychologists (Koffka, 1935; Köhler, 1920; Wertheimer, 1923). SIT stems from their approach and attempts to integrate their findings. To give a gist of this, we first present the basic Gestaltist claims.

The Gestaltists claimed that perception is not a trivial process of copying stimuli but, rather, a complex bottom-up process of grouping retinal stimulus elements into a few stimulus segments. They proposed about 113 grouping cues, the so-called Gestalt laws of perceptual organization (Pomerantz and Kubovy, 1986). An example is the law of proximity. It states that nearby elements in a retinal stimulus tend to be grouped together to constitute one perceived object. Implicit to the application of a grouping cue is that a small change in the stimulus may lead to a dramatic reorganization of the stimulus. Furthermore, the strengths of the grouping cues are not fixed *a priori*. This implies that the perceptual interplay between simultaneously present cues depends on the stimulus at hand. That is, different cues may lead to different segmentations, and one cue may be decisive in one stimulus, but another cue may be decisive in another stimulus.

This stimulus-dependent interplay between cues is expressed by the Gestaltists' claim that 'the whole is different from the sum of its parts'. To specify this 'whole' (i.e., the percept, or Gestalt), they proposed a governing selection principle, namely the so-called law of Prägnanz. It states that the visual system tends to select the stimulus organization that is most 'simple', 'stable', 'balanced', and 'harmonious' (Koffka, 1935). This is reminiscent of the minimum principle in physics, which implies that physical systems tend to settle into stable minimum-energy states.

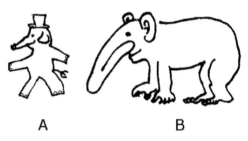

A   B

Figure I.2 Structural versus metrical information. (A) An elephant structure with the metrical proportions of a human. (B) A human structure with the metrical proportions of an elephant (Leeuwenberg, 2003a).

Finally, both the Gestalt cues and the governing principle are claimed to be autonomous and innate, that is, they are not affected by knowledge represented at higher cognitive levels. In line with this is the empirical observation that grouping based on familiarity is actually the weakest Gestalt cue. A general consideration is that perception is an input processor that aims at acquiring knowledge about the structure of the world around us. This perceptually acquired knowledge may, subsequently, be enriched by knowledge represented at higher cognitive levels (e.g., before actions are undertaken), but this is a post-perceptual issue. In this respect, notice that knowledge is a factor external to stimuli whereas, as a rule, the Gestalt cues refer to internal geometrical attributes of stimuli.

Basically, SIT shares the above-mentioned Gestaltist claims. SIT assumes cues for grouping stimulus elements, but instead of 113 cues, it assumes just three cues. These three cues refer to geometrical regularities such as repetition and bilateral symmetry (see Chapter 5 for a theoretical foundation). This restriction is mainly due to SIT's focus on structural rather than metrical pattern aspects. Structural aspects deal with categories such as present versus absent features, whereas metrical aspects refer to quantitative variations within categories. Figure I.2 illustrates the difference. The figure at the left presents an elephant structure with the metrical proportions of a human. The figure at the right presents a human structure with the metrical proportions of an elephant.

SIT's focus on geometrical structures indicates that it shares the Gestaltist claim about the knowledge independence of perception. This claim about the autonomy of perception not only applies to ontogenetic knowledge (i.e., knowledge acquired during one's life), but also to phylogenetic knowledge (i.e., knowledge acquired during the evolution). This contrasts with the Helmholtzian likelihood principle, which assumes that perception is guided by such knowledge. That is, it states that the visual system selects the stimulus organization that agrees most probably with the distal (i.e., actual) object that gave rise to the proximal (i.e., retinal) stimulus. It is true that the likelihood principle is appealing in that it would yield veridical (i.e., truthful) percepts, but it requires probabilties that are hardly quantifiable, if at all (see Chapter 5 for arguments that SIT's approach yields veridical percepts just as well).

The Gestaltists were not concerned with combining grouping cues of different strengths, but SIT is. SIT focuses on stimulus descriptions which specify the contributions of cues to candidate stimulus organizations. Such a description not only represents a stimulus in the form of a reconstruction recipe, but also represents a candidate organization of the stimulus and thereby a class of stimuli with the same structure. This is different from, but yet reminiscent of, Garner's (1962) ground-breaking idea that the visual system, when presented with a stimulus, infers a class of structurally similar stimuli.

Like the Gestalt approach, SIT assumes a governing principle, or criterion, for selecting the perceptually preferred stimulus organization. A difference is that SIT conceives of 'simplicity' as the pivotal concept that includes 'stability', 'balance', and 'harmony'. SIT's simplicity principle agrees with the descriptive minimum principle proposed by Hochberg and McAlister (1953) which, in turn, can be seen as as information-theoretic translation of Koffka's (1935) law of Prägnanz. The simplicity principle implies that the visual system tends to select the stimulus organization that can be described using a minimum of structural information parameters. This structural information load, or complexity, of descriptions can be quantified in a fairly objective way, so that SIT enables falsifiable predictions about perceptually preferred stimulus organizations.

In hindsight, SIT can be seen as a perception-tailored version of the domain-independent mathematical approach called algorithmic information theory (AIT, or the theory of Kolmogorov complexity; see Li and Vitányi, 1997). Historically, however, SIT and AIT developed independently since the 1960s (they interacted only since the 1990s; see Chater, 1996; van der Helm, 2000), and both can be seen as viable alternatives for Shannon's (1948) classical information theory which had been developed in communication theory. Whereas Shannon's approach, just as the above-mentioned likelihood principle, requires probabilities that are often hardly quantifiable, both SIT and AIT resort to descriptive complexities which, as mentioned, can be quantified in a fairly objective way. Furthermore, SIT's simplicity principle corresponds, in AIT, to the so-called minimum description length principle. In fact, both principles can be seen as modern formalizations of William of Occam's (±1290–1349) idea, known as Occam's razor, that the simplest interpretation of data is most likely the best and most favoured one.

There are also crucial differences between SIT and AIT, however. First, SIT makes the perceptually relevant distinction between structural and metrical information (see Figure I.2), whereas AIT does not. Second, SIT encodes for a restricted set of perceptually relevant regularities whereas AIT allows any imaginable regularity. Third, in SIT, the perceptually relevant outcome of an encoding is the stimulus organization induced by a simplest code and this organization establishes the objects we perceive, whereas in AIT, the only relevant outcome is the complexity of a simplest code.

In modern cognitive science, also connectionist and dynamic systems approaches trace their origin back to the Gestaltist ideas (cf. Sundqvist, 2003). In contrast to these approaches, which focus on internal cognitive and neural mechanisms of the perceptual process, SIT focuses on characteristics of the outcomes of this process. In fact, also SIT assumes that the outcome (i.e., the mental representation of a stimulus, or its percept, or its Gestalt) is reflected by a relatively stable cognitive state during an otherwise dynamical neural process. Dynamic systems approaches rightfully focus on the transitions from one neural state to the next, and connectionist approaches rightfully focus on the cognitive mechanisms leading to relatively stable cognitive states, but SIT prefers to focus on the perceptual nature of such relatively stable cognitive states. This may clarify why SIT's selection criterion is not stated in terms of process mechanisms but in terms of process outcomes. A pragmatic reason is that, empirically, these outcomes are better accessible than the internal mechanisms. A more fundamental reason is that, before modeling a process, one should have a clear picture of the outcomes that should result from this process.

The latter indicates that SIT is primarily a theory at what Marr (1982) called the computational level of description, that is, the level at which the goal of information processing systems is described. SIT focuses less on the algorithmic level, at which the method (i.e., the cognitive mechanisms) is described, and even less on the implementational level, at which the means (i.e., the neural mechanisms) are described. Of course, eventually, perception research should arrive at compatible descriptions at all three levels, explaining how the goal is obtained by a method allowed by the means (see Chapter 5 for steps in this direction). The purpose of this book is to give an overview of SIT's contribution to this scientific endeavour.

Part I

Towards a theory of visual form

In Part I, we discuss a number of visual form phenomena. Our intention is to show how structural information theory (SIT) assumptions may emerge step-by step from explanations of these phenomena.

In Chapter 1, the role of the input and output of perception is considered. An extreme position about the role of the input is to assume pure bottom-up effects in the sense that patterns are represented just stimulus analogously. An extreme position about the role of the output is to assume pure top-down effects in the sense that perception is completely guided by acquired knowledge. Both positions are criticized. The conclusion is that there is a stage of pattern interpretation preceding pattern recognition.

In Chapter 2, we deal with the question of which attributes of patterns are described by their representations. These representations are supposed to reveal visual pattern interpretations and segmentations. Four kinds of attributes are considered and compared with each other, namely, dimensions, features, transformations, and Gestalt properties. It is argued that only the latter attributes contribute to candidate pattern representations, and that they require a criterion to select appropriate representations.

Chapter 3 starts from the relevance of Gestalt cues, and focuses on their visual role. To this end, we compare two kinds of criteria for the selection of the actually preferred pattern representation. One kind of criteria applies to the selection process itself and the other kind applies to its output, that is, to the final pattern representation. Arguments are presented against process criteria and in favour of representational criteria.

In Chapter 4, we compare two models that assume representational criteria. One model derives object descriptions from object components, and the other model derives object components from object descriptions. Arguments are presented against the former model. We also contrast two representational selection criteria, namely, the likelihood principle and the simplicity principle. Arguments are presented against the former principle.

In Chapter 5, we summarize the insights that emerge from the preceding chapters, and we present the basic assumptions in SIT's coding model. We further give an overview of the theoretical foundations underlying SIT, regarding the veridicality of simplest codes, regarding the regularities to be extracted in the coding model, and regarding the implementation of the coding process in the brain.

1   Borders of perception

Introduction

Perception can be seen as the process that bridges the gap between incoming stimuli and already stored knowledge. The question here is to what extent perception shares properties of these two ends of the bridge. If it does so to an extreme extent, mental pattern representations are stimulus analogous, or biased by knowledge acquired by earlier observations, or both. In order to arrive at an appropriate global definition of perception, we consider pros and cons of each option separately.

1.1   The stimulus

In favour of stimulus-analogous coding

Reasoning involved in solving riddles is time consuming, requires mental effort, is under conscious control, and can be improved by training. In contrast, perception is rapid, effortless, automatic, and rigid. This multiple contrast may suggest that perception and reasoning are opposed in every respect. This may lead to the conclusion that reasoning is a process of interpretation and classification, whereas perception merely is a registration process that records and stores incoming information the way photographs do. Indeed, seeing is not felt as having to choose, for instance, whether a dark colour stems from a dark paint or from a shadow, or whether two stone parts stem from one stone occluded by a branch or from two separate stones. Chairs, tables, and doors are not experienced as mental constructs but as objects belonging to the external reality the perceiver looks at. After all, they remain present and tangible when closing one's eyes. This introspective argument could be taken to support a stimulus-analogous character of mental representations.

Furthermore, there is the phenomenon that different projections of the same object are not always recognizable as stemming from the same object. Figure 1.1 gives an example. It presents eight views of a tubular

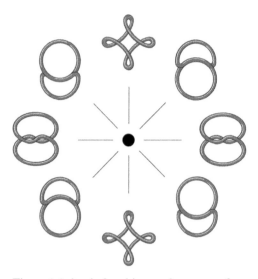

Figure 1.1 A tubular object at the centre of a roundabout, as seen from eight different directions. Even visually trained subjects are unable to infer one view from the other and to infer that views from opposite directions are identical (sculpture by Anneke van Bergen).

object standing at the centre of a roundabout in Beuningen, a Dutch village near Nijmegen. The height, width, and depth of the object are about the same, and the depicted projections agree with the views one gets from different directions; notice that views from opposite directions are identical. The views at the top and at the bottom of Figure 1.1 probably reveal the 3-D structure of the object most perspicuously. With some effort, these views can be inferred from each other. However, even visually trained people are not able to infer the other six views from these views. Also this viewpoint dependency in object recognition could be taken as supporting a stimulus-analogous character of pattern representations (Tarr, 1995).

It is true that less complex objects can usually be recognized viewpoint independently, yet one condition in the experiment by Shepard and Metzler (1971) seems to support that also simple objects are represented stimulus analogously. In each trial, they presented the projections of two objects in different orientations. In terms of not only the perceived 3-D shapes but also the presented 2-D projections, the two objects were either equal or mirrored. The task was to judge whether the two objects are equal or different. For instance, Figure 1.2A depicts a pair of equal objects, being equally handed like two left-hand gloves. Furthermore,

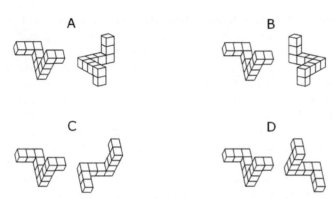

Figure 1.2 Four stimulus pairs in Shepard and Metzler's (1971) experiment. In A and C, the perceived objects are equal, and in B and D they are mirrored. In all pairs, these relationships apply to the perceived 3-D shapes, and only in A and B, they also apply to the presented 2-D projections. The task was to judge whether the two stimuli in a pair are equal or different. Shepard and Metzler found that, in all cases, response time increases linearly with the angle between the two stimuli, and they concluded that handedness discrimination is achieved by way of mental rotation (Shepard and Metzler, 1971).

Figure 1.2B depicts an object and its mirror image, being handed differently like a left-hand and a right-hand glove. The task is therefore said to deal with handedness discrimination. Shepard and Metzler found that the larger the angle between the two objects is, the longer the response time is.

From the linear relation between response time and angular change, as well as from reports by the participants, Shepard and Metzler concluded that handedness discrimination is achieved by way of mental rotation. If mental representations are stimulus analogous, like photographs, then equality can only be established by mentally rotating one representation towards the other and by verifying if this leads to a match. This mental rotation scenario is, in theory, possible in the case of Figures 1.2A and B, so that the finding in this condition agrees with stimulus-analogous representations (cf. Cooper, 1976; Finke, 1980).

Against stimulus-analogous coding

The conclusion above requires further qualification, however. Shepard and Metzler deliberately used equally and differently handed stimuli to prevent that a single feature might be sufficient to perform the discrimination task properly. That is, there is no orientation-free feature that characterizes the difference between an image and its mirror-image (Deutsch, 1955; Hinton and Parsons, 1981; Leeuwenberg and van der Helm, 2000). Precisely for this reason, it is plausible that the representation of handedness is stimulus bound and that, therefore, handedness discrimination is necessarily mediated by mental rotation (see also Chapter 11.2). That handedness is represented in a stimulus-bound fashion does not imply of course that object representations are stimulus bound in all other respects as well. Another point applies to the above statement that the (in)equality of stimulus-analogous representations can only be established by mentally rotating one representation towards the other. It is evident that the reverse is not necessarily true, that is, mental rotation does not require representations to be stimulus analogous.

In this respect, another condition in Shepard and Metzler's experiment is crucial. They again presented the projections of two objects in different orientations, but this time, the two objects were either equal or mirrored only in terms of the perceived 3-D shapes (i.e., not in terms of the presented 2-D projections). Figures 1.2C and D show examples. The task was the same and, surprisingly, their finding was the same as well; that is, response time increased linearly with the angle between the two stimuli. This leads to the conclusion that mental rotation deals with 3-D object interpretations and not with 2-D stimulus-analogous representations. Notice, for instance, that the invisible parts of the objects have to be inferred from the visible parts, before mental rotation can begin.

A finding by Pylyshyn (1973) gives rise to a similar conclusion. He found that pattern regularity and pattern simplicity affect handedness discrimination: response times appeared to be shorter for regular and simple stimuli than for irregular and complex stimuli. For instance, in Figure 1.3, (in)equality is easier to judge for the simple objects in A and B than for the complex objects in C and D. Stimulus-analogous representations do not account for pattern regularity and pattern simplicity; like photographs, they are indifferent to such attributes. In the context of his finding, Pylyshyn also discussed mental rotation as a form of imagery that deals with 3-D object interpretations and not with 2-D stimulus-analogous representations. By the same token, Koning and van Lier (2004) found that mental rotation does not depend on the number of physical stimulus fragments (as would be expected in case of stimulus-analogous representations) but rather on the number of perceived objects in the perceptual interpretation of a stimulus.

A further imagery example against stimulus-analogous coding is given by Moran's (1968) exercise involving an opaque prism (see Figure 1.4). The task is to focus on the view revealing eight edges of the prism and to establish, without using paper and pencil, the number of edges that would

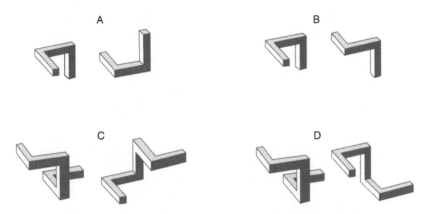

Figure 1.3 The objects in A and B are simpler than the objects in C and D. To judge whether the objects in a pair are equal or different is easier for the simple objects in A and B than for the complex objects in C and D.

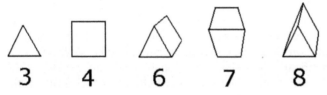

Figure 1.4 The patterns depict five views of an opaque prism. The number of visible edges is indicated below each view. Given the last view with eight edges, one is usually well able to imagine how many edges would be visible from other viewpoints (Leeuwenberg, 2003a).

be visible from other viewpoints. Usually, one is well able to perform this task. This imagery would not be possible if codes are stimulus-analogous, because such codes do not give viewpoint-independent representations.

The foregoing arguments against stimulus-analogous coding could be questioned by arguing that codes of imagined patterns might be different from codes of actually presented stimuli. Kosslyn (1975, 1981), however, found that detection of a briefly presented target pattern is improved if it is preceded by a prime with the same shape, no matter whether this prime is an actually presented stimulus or an imagined pattern. This shows that, in a given task, effects of imagined patterns are similar to those of actual stimuli (see also Moyer, 1973; Petersen, 1975). Further evidence stems from studies involving patients with brain damage and from measurements of regional brain activity (Farah, 1995; Tippett,

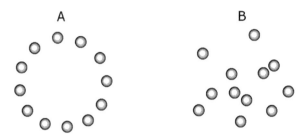

Figure 1.5 Two possible outcomes of throwing twelve billiard balls on a table. The configuration in A is judged to be less likely than the configuration in B. This judgment presupposes that these specific configurations are taken as representatives of classes of similar configurations because, taken as representatives of only themselves, they are equally likely.

1992). These studies suggest that various modality-specific areas, especially in the occipital cortex, are not only used in visual perception but also in imagery. This research corroborates the idea that codes of imagined patterns are functionally equivalent to codes of actually presented stimuli. Hence, it is plausible that representations of imagined and actual patterns are equal with respect to being stimulus analogous or not. That representations of actual patterns are not stimulus analogous is supported by many phenomena (see, e.g., Collard and Buffart, 1983; Hochberg, 1968; Garner, 1974; Neisser, 1967; Palmer, 1977; Restle, 1982; Rock, 1983). Next, we consider two simple phenomena.

First, consider the two configurations of twelve billiard balls in Figure 1.5. One is a circle configuration, and the other is a random configuration. The question is which configuration is the more likely outcome of throwing twelve billiard balls on a table. The common answer is the random configuration. However, if configurations are described by unique stimulus-analogous codes, then this answer is incorrect, that is, then the two configurations are equally likely. Only if each configuration is taken to stand for a class of patterns, the common answer can be taken to be correct. After all, the class of circles is smaller than the class of random patterns. Notice that the common answer arises spontaneously. Hence, pattern classification occurs spontaneously, and it occurs at the level of perception rather than at the level of post-perceptual reasoning. This suggests that perceptual codes are not stimulus-analogous, because stimulus-analogous codes do not give rise to classification.

Second, Gerbino and Salmaso (1987) found that, in Figure 1.6, pattern A is judged to be less related to pattern B than to pattern C. Notice that pattern B shares the physically visible black part of A, whereas pattern C shares the interpretation obtained via so-called amodal

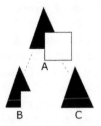

Figure 1.6 A and B share a physically visible stimulus part, and A and C share the interpretation obtained via amodal completion of A. Gerbino and Salmaso (1987) found that A and B are judged to be less related than A and C. This suggests that the perceptual representation of a partly occluded pattern is equivalent to the perceptual representation of the completed pattern (Gerbino and Salmaso, 1987).

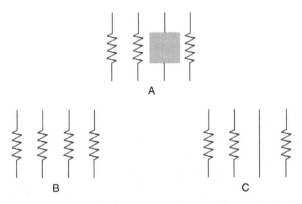

Figure 1.7 The pattern in A can be completed in various ways. Kanizsa (1985) showed that the option in B is a conscious solution and that the option in C a perceptual solution. Hence, not only reasoning but also perception leads to completion. The difference is that B is a globally simple solution, whereas C is a locally simple solution.

completion of A. This supports the idea that codes of amodally completed patterns, which are obviously not stimulus analogous, are functionally equivalent to codes of visible patterns. Furthermore, Sekuler and Palmer (1992) found that such completions are achieved within a time period as brief as 400 milliseconds (ms), that is, at a perceptual level rather than at a post-perceptual level (see also Chapter 8.3).

The claim that amodal completion occurs at a perceptual level has been illustrated well by Kanizsa (1975, 1985). Kanizsa (1985) showed subjects a square surface that partly occludes a series of line patterns (see Figure 1.7A), and posed two questions. First he asked: which series of patterns do you think of as background? The usual answer is given in Figure 1.7B: a completion that is globally simple in that the whole background series is regular. Then he asked: which series of patterns do you see as background? This time, the usual answer is the one given in Figure 1.7C: a completion that is not globally but locally simple in that it comprises good continuation of the visible lines adjacent to the occluding square. This demonstrates two things. First, the outcomes of reasoning and perception are different. Second, not only reasoning but also perception leads to completion, that is, to visual pattern concepts that are obviously not stimulus analogous.

Finally, a theoretical argument against stimulus-analogous codes is that an object can be represented by innumerable stimulus-analogous codes that each capture a different projection of the object. As a consequence, recognition of the object requires that the stimulus is matched with each of the many stimulus-analogous codes stored in memory. An additional problem is the recognition of the object given a novel view. A stimulus-analogous code does not reveal the object to which this view belongs, unless one makes the implausible assumption that all possible stimulus-analogous codes associated with this object have been learned beforehand.

1.2   Knowledge

The view that all knowledge about objects has to be learned stems from Berkeley (1710) and Locke (1690), and is called empiricism. Their assumption was that, at birth, the mind is a *tabula rasa* (blank sheet) without any information content, and that during life, associations established by perception determine further perception. The thus acquired knowledge is called ontogenetic knowledge, that is, knowledge acquired during one's life. This contrasts with so-called phylogenetic knowledge which is supposed to have been acquired during evolution (we go into more detail on this form of knowledge in Chapter 4.2). The extreme position of empiricism hardly has adherents anymore (see Hochberg, 1968 for fundamental criticism on this position), but here, we discuss whether ontogenetic knowledge may yet somehow affect perception.

In favour of knowledge dependence

When discussing the role of knowledge in perception, it is expedient to realize that knowledge comes in many forms. For instance, during the perceptual process of interpreting a given stimulus, visual information in one part of the stimulus affects the visual interpretation of other parts.

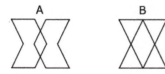

Figure 1.8 Both the pattern in A and the pattern in B comprise two arrows in opposite directions, but these arrows are salient only in A. This shows that perception accounts for relationships between parts within a pattern. In fact, the so-called Gestalt character of perception refers to this intra-pattern information transfer.

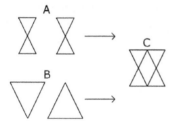

Figure 1.9 If prime A is presented briefly before target C, the latter is preferably seen as a pair of egg-timers, but if prime B is presented briefly before target C, then the latter is rather seen as a pair of triangles. Hence, at the level of the short-term memory, knowledge influences perception.

An illustration is given in Figure 1.8: both patterns comprise two arrows in opposite directions, but these arrows are salient in pattern A whereas they are not salient in pattern B. Good continuation of line segments prevents one from seeing pattern B as two arrows and favours seeing it as a pair of triangles or as a pair of egg timers. In general, the relationships between all parts of a pattern are perceptually relevant, and in fact reflect the so-called Gestalt quality of the pattern. Hence, perceptually, there is obviously an information transfer from one pattern part to the other, and in this sense, perception makes use of the knowledge that is available within a pattern.

Apart from the aforementioned intra-pattern information transfer, there can also be an information transfer from one pattern to another. An illustration is given in Figure 1.9. If pattern A is presented briefly as a prime before target pattern C, the latter is preferably seen as a pair of egg timers. If, however, pattern B is presented briefly as a prime before target pattern C, then the latter is rather seen as a pair of triangles. Hence, the prime patterns affect the visual interpretation and segmentation of the target pattern. The information about the primes probably is stored in

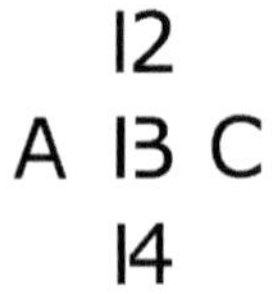

12

A 13 C

14

Figure 1.10 Someone acquainted only with arabic numerals probably sees the centre part as the number 13, whereas someone acquainted only with roman letters probably sees it as the letter B. Hence, also at the level of the long-term memory, knowledge seems to influence perception.

the short-term memory and may still be accessible during the perception of the target pattern. The effect of the primes on the target could be taken to support the influence of knowledge in perception.

Not only information stored in the short-term memory may influence the perception of a target pattern, but also information stored long before in the long-term memory. For instance, imagine one person familiar with roman letters but not with arabic numerals, and another person familiar with arabic numerals but not with roman letters. Suppose that the pattern in Figure 1.10 is presented to these two persons. Then, one person probably recognizes the centre part as the letter B, whereas the other person probably recognizes it as the number 13. This bias is attributed to the so-called familiarity cue which is one of the 113 Gestalt cues in perceptual grouping (Pomerantz and Kubovy, 1986).

Examples like this last one, in particular, give rise to a definition of perception as a process that includes recognition and that is guided by knowledge. This may be illustrated further by referring to face recognition. Within a glance, we identify a face as belonging to a friend, including his name. Within this glance, however, there is no experience of two stages. That is, there is no experience of, first, a stage of visual processing from the retinal stimulus to a specific 3-D structure, and second, a stage of relating this structure to memory content in order to identify it. In other words, the immediate character of face recognition encourages one to include recognition as part of perception.

Finally, another kind of consideration in favour of the influence of knowledge is that perception is part of cognition and is also a form of cognition. At other levels of cognition, at the level of conscious reasoning for instance, the use of knowledge is obvious and usually very fruitful. This knowledge is not only stored in memory but also in libraries, so that it remains accessible to next generations. Why then would knowledge not be used in perception? After all, both perception and conscious reasoning are cognitive processes.

Against knowledge dependence

To perception, knowledge is a context factor, and the arguments above in favour of the influence of knowledge on perception actually are arguments in favour of context effects in perception. Like knowledge, context also comes in many forms.

Often, in empirical situations, context effects are said to occur when the interpretation of a part of a scene (i.e., the target part) is influenced by the rest of the scene (i.e., the context part). Notice that, in such a situation, the empirical task determines which part is the target and, thereby, that the rest is the context of this part. The visual system, however, takes the entire scene as the pattern to be interpreted, and as mentioned earlier, the intra-pattern information transfer from one part to the other reflects the Gestalt quality of the entire scene. Hence, in such a situation, the notion of context is meaningless to the perceptual process, and it becomes meaningful only due to the empirical task which requires a response about the designated part. In other words, if one would argue that this supports the influence of context or knowledge on perception, then one starts from a definition of perception that, in our view, includes non-perceptual factors.

The foregoing spatial context effects differ from the effects of priming and familiarity. The latter are temporal context effects, for which Gottschaldt (1929) already found empirically that there are restrictions. He demonstrated that the interpretation of a target pattern is not necessarily affected by extensive priming (i.e., familiarization) with parts of the target pattern. For instance, extensive priming with the arrows in Figure 1.8A does not imply that they are recognized more easily in the target pattern in Figure 1.8B. It is true that the primes in Figure 1.9A and B affect the interpretation of this target pattern, but these primes differ essentially from Figure 1.8A. In contrast to Figure 1.8A, these primes give perceptually plausible segmentations of the target pattern. Moreover, these segmentations are about equally plausible. Such observations led Rock (1985) to the conclusion that context effects apply only to patterns that give rise to two or more equally plausible interpretations. Such patterns are called phenomenally ambiguous.

Rock's (1985) conclusion reflects further limitations on context effects. Most patterns are not phenomenally ambiguous, and even if they are, only the most salient segmentations may give rise to context effects. All other segmentations do not cause context effects. Notice that the number of possible segmentations of any pattern is a combinatorially explosive function of the number of pattern elements. An illustration, designed by Reed (1972), is presented in Figure 1.11. It shows the so-called

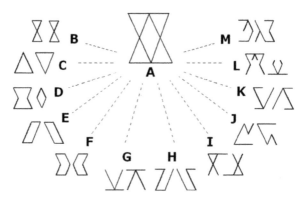

Figure 1.11 Some segmentations of pattern A are presented in B–M (the total number of possible segmentations is infinite). Segmentations B and C are perceptually the most plausible ones and are about equally plausible, so that pattern A is phenomenally ambiguous. The other segmentations all are perceptually implausible, but contribute to the theoretical ambiguity of pattern A (Reed, 1972).

theoretical ambiguity of the pattern in Figure 1.11A. Figures 1.11B–M present some of the possible segmentations, but only the ones in Figures 1.11B and C might be context shapes that affect the perception of Figure 1.11A. In other words, context seems to play a minor role in perception.

As for familiarity, the question is whether its effect really is as visual as the effect of the other Gestalt cues. Familiarity usually is taken to refer to more or less abstract knowledge stored in the long-term memory, whereas the other Gestalt cues are given by geometrical relationships within a pattern at hand. It is therefore still plausible that familiarity may enrich the interpretation of a pattern in a post-perceptual stage, but it is less plausible that it affects the interpretation of a pattern at the perceptual level. Perhaps for this reason, the Gestaltist's empirical conclusion was that familiarity is the least relevant Gestalt cue (Pomerantz and Kubovy, 1986).

Priming usually is taken to occur just before the presentation of a target, and in this sense, its effects are in between the effects of spatial context and the effects of long-term familiarity. Indeed, temporally, there is an upperbound and a lowerbound for priming to be effective. First, it usually is effective if it occurs within 1 or 2 seconds before the presentation of a target. Second, Mens and Leeuwenberg (1988) found that patterns presented subsequently within 20 milliseconds (ms) are processed as if they were simultaneously presented patterns, so that priming effects basically turn into spatial context effects (for more details, see Chapter 9.2). Their experiment was a follow-up study of the experiments by Bachmann and Allik (1976) and Calis *et al.* (1984). The latter studies focused on the microgenesis of perception, to which end they used presentation times and interval times of a few milliseconds. They found interactions at early stages of perception that are to be distinguished from post-perceptual processes at later stages of cognition.

The foregoing discussion shows that knowledge has a very restricted effect on what we define as perception, namely, the perceptual process from stimulus to percept. Perhaps the most direct illustration of knowledge resistance in perception is supplied by visual illusions. Take, for instance, the moon illusion: at the horizon, the moon is perceived as being larger than at the zenith, even though the two moon images are the same size on retinas and photos. The knowledge that they have the same size does not affect the illusion. In the remaining part of this section, we will discuss how this knowledge resistance can be understood by speculating on the functional role of perception from a broader perspective.

The moon illusion is characterized by a psychophysical relationship between the physical size on the retina and the perceived size. In fact, virtually all visual phenomena are characterized by such psychophysical relationships. Usually, visual sensations that deviate from physical measurements are taken to be illusory, because the physical measurements are taken to reflect the true situation. Physical measures, however, are derived starting from observations which, just as visual sensations, are mediated too by perception. So, on the one hand, it seems paradoxical that illusions arise at all. On the other hand, the observations lead to the physical measures by way of conscious reasoning, that is, reasoning based on knowledge. In this sense, the difference between visual sensations and physical measurements reflects the difference between perception and conscious reasoning. The latter difference may be specified further as follows.

As we stated in the Introduction of this book, perception starts from unrelated patches of colour at various positions on the retina. A grouping process divides this retinal input into segments that are supposed to reflect the various objects in a scene, say, 'green leaves'. These objects belong to the output of perception, that is, they are the result of one observation. This output of perception is input of conscious reasoning which deals with various observations and which serves another goal. The goal of conscious reasoning is to relate observations by means of a proposition, say, 'leaves are green'. The question then is no longer what leaves are, but whether they are green. Hence, perception and reasoning are almost opposed. To put it simply, perception establishes objects starting from proximal properties, whereas reasoning establishes properties starting from perceived distal objects. Furthermore, perception establishes objects without assigning truth values to them (see Gibson, 1966), whereas in reasoning, a proposition may be consistent (i.e., logically true) or contradictory (i.e., logically false) with respect to another proposition.

So, in various respects, perception and conscious reasoning are different. It is therefore plausible that also their functional roles are different. In our view, perception provides information about the structure of the world around us; this knowledge results from separate observations which, subsequently, are related by reasoning. In order that such a system is flexible and adaptive to changes in the world, perception is better not influenced by knowledge resulting from reasoning, because such knowledge may lead to observations biased by prejudices. In other words, the output of perception serves as input for reasoning, and to prevent observations biased by prejudices, it would be appropriate that the output of reasoning does not serve as input for perception. It is probably for the same reason that Lady Justice is blindfolded and that knowledge is, in general, not hereditary. Only knowledge of undeniable laws, invariant across different environments, might be useful in perception and might be inborn (Runeson and Frickholm, 1981).

In this section, we discussed the information that might be taken into account in the perceptual interpretation of a stimulus. To put it in terms of Hochberg's (1982) question 'How big is a stimulus?', precise boundaries are hard to give, but it is clear that there are both spatial and temporal boundaries to what constitutes a stimulus. Furthermore, there is abundant empirical evidence indicating an autonomous stage of perception that precedes higher levels of knowing and reasoning (Høffding, 1891) and that is hardly penetrable by information from these higher levels (Fodor, 1983; Pylyshyn, 1999). Of course, one is free to define perception in a broad sense that includes influences by knowledge, attention, action planning, motivations, or even deductive reasoning. But then one tends to equate perception with cognition, and one risks losing sight of the differences between various cognitive functions. We therefore prefer to define perception in the restricted sense of the autonomous process from stimulus to percept, which precedes recognition and other higher-level functions (cf. Ahissar and Hochstein, 2004).

Summary

In the first part of this chapter, we concluded that visual patterns are not represented stimulus analogously, because then, object recognition and object classification would be missions impossible. Instead, perception groups the elements in a retinal stimulus into structured objects that are more easily recognized and classified. In the second part, we concluded that there is an autonomous stage of perception, which is not affected by knowledge represented at higher levels of cognition. Scientifically, it is convenient to define perception in the restricted sense of this autonomous process from stimulus to percept.

Both conclusions are based on converging evidence for a stage of stimulus structuring and classification (the so-called 'Høffding step') that precedes the stage of recognition (Neisser, 1967). Furthermore, both conclusions may be paraphrased as follows. The perceptual process involves a lot of information transfer within a stimulus at hand, but hardly between this stimulus and stimuli that were processed and stored earlier. In Chapters 4 and 5, we continue the discussion on the role of knowledge in perception, by addressing phylogenetic knowledge and the effects of over-learned stimuli.

2 Attributes of visual form

Introduction

In Chapter 1, we investigated the borders within which perception operates. Here, we focus on the visual attributes perception works with, that is, the attributes that are captured in pattern representations. We consider four kinds of attributes, namely, features (Treisman and Gelade, 1980; Tversky, 1977), dimensions (Shepard, 1962a, 1962b), transformations (Leyton, 1992), and Gestalt properties (Koffka, 1935; Köhler, 1920; Wertheimer, 1923). The general question is which attributes are the appropriate ones to represent visual patterns. In this respect, specific questions are whether attributes presuppose pattern segmentations and interpretations, whether they rely on knowledge of pattern sets, and whether they properly represent individual stimuli and classes of patterns.

2.1 Features

In everyday life, one characterizes an object or person by features. Even a single feature may suffice to uniquely identify a specific object. For instance, if all objects under consideration are not red except one, the feature red is sufficient to identify the red object. Features also are useful to indicate classes of objects (Neisser, 1967). In general, the fewer features, the more members the class comprises. For example, the class of 'cars' contains more members than the class of 'blue cars'. Each feature imposes a restriction on class size. For such reasons, the representation by features belongs to the most appealing option in models for technical pattern recognition. Nevertheless, the question is whether features are the appropriate attributes of perceptual representations, and whether they are useful for the recognition of individual patterns and classes of patterns. We attempt to answer this question for two kinds of features, namely, figural and abstract features.

Figural features

A figural feature is supposed to stand for a specific concrete pattern component. For instance, a single feature may stand for a line or a junction. A single feature may even stand for a whole trapezoid or a whole circle. Notice, however, that figural features do not capture their mutual spatial relations (Neisser, 1976), so that a combination of, say, a trapezoid and a circle, still yields an ambiguous representation. After all, the trapezoid may enclose the circle, or the circle may enclose the trapezoid, or the two figures may be adjacent.

An extreme option is to assume a figural feature for any possible stimulus. However, then there should be as many features as there are stimuli. Then feature representations are stimulus analogous. These are useful to represent individual patterns but inappropriate to represent classes of patterns. In fact, the more features are suited to represent individual patterns, the less they are appropriate for representing pattern classes. Besides, the recognition of such a stimulus-analogous pattern representation suffers from all the objections discussed in Chapter 1.

Abstract features

Abstract features, such as 'high', 'red', 'closed', or 'symmetrical' apply to a broad and diverse domain of objects. To uniquely represent individual patterns, the number of features to be considered is an issue. By approximation, the number of imaginable features is about the logarithm of the number of possible patterns, hence less than the number of possible patterns (Shannon, 1948; Wiener, 1948). Nevertheless, the number of features is innumerable. So, a fixed set of abstract features insufficiently specifies a pattern and no set extension resolves its ambiguity. The extreme consequence might be that an ugly duckling will be confounded with a swan (Watanabe, 1969). Only if the set of possible objects is restricted, and if this set is known, may a few abstract features suffice to uniquely identify a specific object. However, the assumption that perception makes use of knowledge is implausible for the reasons presented in Chapter 1.

Commonly, one describes an object by figural features in combination with abstract features, for instance, 'a person with short legs'. Of course, this description still is ambiguous. However, even if a combination of figural and abstract features uniquely fixates an object, there might be a problem. It deals with the imaginary reconstruction of an object from its representation. This reconstruction plays a role in tasks to answer questions about an imagined object when the answers cannot be derived directly from the favoured representation of the object. An instance is the imaginary reconstruction of a prism under varying points of view for the task to indicate their numbers of edges (see Figure 1.4). This task can be performed sufficiently well, but this is not always the case. To illustrate that the imaginary reconstruction of an object can be problematic, we return to Figure 1.11. It presents Figure 1.11A and a few binary segmentations of this pattern. The task is to specify a specific segmentation without having access to these segmentations. The available information is a combination of a figural feature and some abstract features that uniquely fixates the specific target segmentation. This information actually consists of Figure 1.11A and the following three abstract features:

(1) the two subpatterns are equal (except for their orientations);
(2) each subpattern is asymmetrical;
(3) each subpattern is an open figure (it does not comprise closed lines).

We presented this task to seven students, but none was able to find the solution within five minutes. So, the task is not easy. Obviously, the three features are quite unlike pattern reconstruction recipes. They just constrain options. Indeed, the task is easily solvable at recognition level if there is access to Figures 1.11B to M. Then, the strategy is to assess the cross-section of three sets of segmentations. Feature 1 selects (B), (C), (F), (G), (I), (K); feature 2 selects (E), (H), (I), (J), (K), (M); and feature 3 selects patterns (G), (H), (J), (K), (L), (M). The common pattern (K) is the solution.

As has been said earlier, abstract features are appropriate for representing a class of patterns. The question still is whether their pattern classification is compatible with visual classification. For the answer, we assume that the number of features is a plausible measure of the complexity of a feature code. Furthermore, it holds that the more features a code has the fewer patterns there are in the class described by the code (see previous topic on pattern reconstruction). Thus, for feature codes, the relation between complexity and class size is negative (see Figure 2.1A). However, in the visual domain the relation is opposed. We illustrate this for lines and L shapes. Without doubt, lines are visually less complex than L shapes. Furthermore, it holds that the class size of lines is smaller than the class size of L shapes (Garner, 1966). Lines only vary with respect to one length dimension whereas L shapes vary with respect to two length dimensions and one turn dimension. Thus, the class of simple patterns is smaller than the class of complex shapes (see discussion of Figure 1.5).

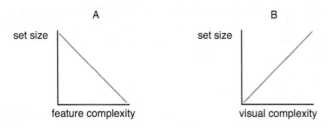

Figure 2.1 If a complex feature code is supposed to deal with many features it represents just a few patterns. So, for a feature code the relation between complexity and class size is negative (see A). However, the relation between visual complexity and class size is positive (see B).

In other words, the relation between visual complexity and class size is positive instead of negative (see Figure 2.1B).

Our overall conclusion is as follows. Figural features appropriately represent individual patterns but not pattern classes. For abstract features the reverse holds. As their application in perception requires knowledge about the set of objects and presumes pattern interpretations, they are inappropriate to visually represent individual patterns unambiguously, and as they merely constrain sets, they are unpractical guidelines for pattern construction. Indeed, abstract features are appropriate for classification but still not for visual classification.

2.2   Dimensions

In many scientific analyses, it is customary to plot data as points in a multidimensional space. This probably inspired Shepard (1962a, 1962b, 1980) to apply multidimensional scaling also in perception research. To this end, one needs to know which figural dimensions are to be assumed. That is, examples of figural dimensions are length, width, orientation, surface size, perimeter, and diameter, but *a priori*, it is not clear which dimensions are appropriate to represent stimuli. This has to be established experimentally, and Shepard developed a mathematical method to establish experimentally the figural dimensions of a given set of stimuli on the basis of their judged dissimilarities (Kruskal's, 1964, well-known analysis is in fact a computer implementation of the method Shepard had developed).

Shepard's method results in a homogeneous multidimensional space, given by a fixed set of figural dimensions. In this space, each stimulus is represented by one point reflecting a unique stimulus description in terms of quantities on various independent figural dimensions. The visual dissimilarity between two stimuli then is taken to be given by the distance between the two related points in this multidimensional space. As we discuss next, Tversky (1977) identified and criticized several properties of such stimulus representations.

Dimensional scaling properties

To verify whether distances in multidimensional space properly reflect visual dissimilarities between stimuli, Tversky (1977) identified various properties of multidimensional stimulus representations. To this end, he used the formal notation $d(A, B)$ to indicate the distance d when going from point A to point B in multidimensional space. In the visual domain, A and B refer to stimuli, and $d(A, B)$ refers to the visual dissimilarity of B with respect to A. The three main properties Tversky identified are the following.

The first property applies to single points or stimuli. It states $d(A, A) = 0$, which simply means that the distance between a point A and itself, or the dissimilarity between a stimulus A and itself, is zero. In other words, it means that a stimulus is represented by only one point in multidimensional space.

The second property applies to two points or stimuli, say, A and B. It states that $d(A, B) = d(B, A)$ which, in multidimensional space, simply means that the distance when going from point A to point B is equal to the distance when going from B to A. For stimuli in the visual domain, this means that stimulus B is as (dis)similar to stimulus A as A is to B. In other words, stimulus similarity is symmetrical.

The third property is the triangle inequality, which applies to three points or stimuli, say, A, B, and C. In multidimensional space, the three points form a triangle, and the triangle inequality then states $d(A, C) \leq d(A, B) + d(B, C)$, which means that the length of one side of the triangle is shorter than or equal to the sum of the lengths of the other two sides. In the visual domain, it means that the dissimilarity between stimuli A and C is less than or equal to the dissimilarity between stimuli A and B plus the dissimilarity between stimuli B and C.

Hence, each of these three formal properties for points in multidimensional space has a specific implication for stimuli in the visual domain. Tversky (1977) criticized these implications in a way that may be sketched as follows (see also Treisman, 1986).

Visual scaling properties

The first property of multidimensional scaling, that a stimulus is represented by only one point, clearly is visually inappropriate in case the

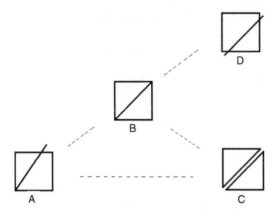

Figure 2.2 The triangle inequality applies to the distances d between the points A, B, and C of a triangle. It states that $d(A, C) \leq d(A, B) + d(B, C)$. In the visual domain, the points stand for figures and d for dissimilarities. Argued is that then $d(A, C) \leq d(A, D)$. However, this inequality is visually implausible.

stimulus is ambiguous. An example of an ambiguous stimulus is given in Figure 2.2B. It is interpreted either as a square plus a line or as a pair of triangles. To assess (dis)similarities with respect to other stimuli, such a stimulus should therefore be represented by two points, one for each of these two interpretations. As we show next, the failing account of visual ambiguity by multidimensional scaling also causes its failure regarding to the other two properties (Leeuwenberg and Buffart, 1983).

The second property $d(A, B) = d(B, A)$ implies, as said, that B is as similar to A as A is to B, that is, it implies that stimulus similarity is symmetrical. However, consider stimuli A and B in Figure 2.3, for which the similarity is not symmetrical. A is unambiguous and is interpretable only as a square plus a line, whereas B is ambiguous and interpretable either as a square plus a line or as a pair of triangles. Because the interpretation of A is one of the two interpretations of B, B is judged to be more like A than A is like B. In other words, when comparing A and B, A is taken to be the prototype and B the non-prototype. This kind of prototyping, which is based on ambiguity, is not the only kind of prototyping (see next subsection), but the literature contains a lot of evidence for its role in pattern classification (see, e.g., Rosch, 1975; Tversky, 1977). A perhaps more common example of this kind of prototyping is given by the colours red and pink. Red is an unambiguous basic colour, whereas pink is a mixture of colours. Therefore, pink is said to be more like red than red is like pink, and red is said to be a prototype for pink.

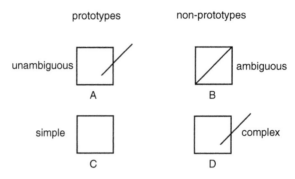

Figure 2.3 Two kinds of prototypes are illustrated each giving rise to an asymmetrical similarity. One is the unambiguous pattern A. Pattern B is ambiguous. It can be interpreted like A but also otherwise. Then it holds that B is more similar to A than A to B. The other prototype is the simple pattern C with respect to its more complex version D. Then it holds that D is more similar to C than C to D.

To assess the visual relevance of the third property, that is, of the triangle inequality, we consider stimuli A, B, C, and D in Figure 2.2. For stimuli A, B, and C, the triangle inequality would imply:

$$d(A, C) \leq d(A, B) + d(B, C)$$

The component $d(B, C)$ stands for the difference between stimuli B and C, and refers to a translation, namely, a translation of a triangle. By the same token, the difference between stimuli B and D is given by $d(B, D)$ which refers to a translation of a line. If we quantify distances by the operations to be performed (here, the translations) rather than by the subpatterns operated on, then $d(B, C) = d(B, D)$ so that the inequality above can be rewritten into:

$$d(A, C) \leq d(A, B) + d(B, D)$$

Furthermore, the distance $d(A, B)$ refers to a rotation of a line and, as said, the distance $d(B, D)$ refers to a translation of a line. The combination of this rotation and this translation corresponds plausibly to the visual difference between A and D. Hence, $d(A, D) = d(A, B) + d(B, D)$, so that the inequality above can now be rewritten into:

$$d(A, C) \leq d(A, D)$$

This expression states that stimuli A and C differ less from each other than do stimuli A and D. However, visually, stimuli A and C are judged to differ more from each other than do stimuli A and D. This shows that, because of visual ambiguity, the triangle inequality from multidimensional scaling does not hold in perception.

Hence, none of the above three properties of multidimensional scaling is valid in perception. As we showed, because of these properties, it cannot account for perceptual phenomena such as visual ambiguity and the asymmetry of stimulus similarity. The underlying cause of this is that multidimensional scaling starts from stimuli instead of stimulus interpretations. Because of this underlying cause, multidimensional scaling also fails to capture the more general perceptual phenomenon of hierarchical relationships between components of stimulus interpretations. This is discussed next in more detail.

Common versus distinctive components

In the previous subsection, we illustrated the asymmetry of stimulus similarity by means of the prototype and non-prototype depicted in Figures 2.3A and B. As indicated, this kind of prototyping is based on ambiguity, where the prototype is given by the common interpretation. Figures 2.3C and D give another illustration, this time by means of a kind of prototyping based on simplicity. The stimuli in C and D are interpreted unambiguously as a square and as a square plus a line, respectively. Because D consists of C (a square) plus an extra component (a line), a simple (i.e., parsimonious) representation of both stimuli together involves an asymmetrical relationship between the common component (the square) and the distinctive component (the line). Precisely because of this asymmetry, D is judged to be more like C than C is like D, so that C is a prototype of D. Hence, here, the prototype is given by the common component. Notice that such an asymmetrical relationship between common and distinctive components is not accounted for by multidimensional scaling.

Further evidence for the latter kind of prototyping comes from Treisman's (1982) visual search experiments. These experiments involved configurations like those depicted in Figure 2.4, each consisting of many identical items (the distracters) and possibly a single deviating item (the target). The task was to respond, as fast as possible, whether the target was present. The results showed that a circle plus a line among circles is detected faster than a circle among circles plus lines (see Figures 2.4A and A′). In this case, the circle is the prototype and the circle plus line is the non-prototype, because the circle is the common component. The results showed further that a C shape among circles is detected faster than a circle among C shapes (see Figures 2.4B and B′). This seems to contrast with the foregoing because, this time, at stimulus level, the

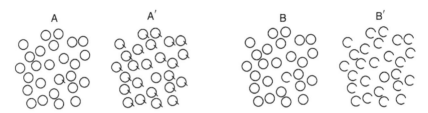

Figure 2.4 Treisman (1982) has shown that distinctive structures are visually more salient than common structures. For instance, a circle plus line among various circles (A) is more salient than a circle among circles plus lines (A'). Also a circle with a gap among circles (B) is more salient than a circle among circles with gaps (B'). The common structure is supposed to be primary, while the distinctive structure, though most salient, is supposed to be secondary.

C shape agrees with the common component. However, the C shape is interpreted as a circle plus a gap, hence, perceptually, the gap plays the same role as the line above so that, this time too, the circle is the proto-type. In other words, the results for all four configurations support the conclusion that a non-prototype is more salient among prototypes than a prototype is among non-prototypes.

This conclusion does not imply that distinctive components are pro-cessed before common components. In fact, it rather implies the reverse. In general, the search for a target in a visual search display is easier as the distracters are more similar to each other and more different from the target (cf. Donderi, 2006; Duncan and Humphreys, 1989). In other words, a target may be a so-called pop-out but only if the distracters allow it to be. Hence, it seems plausible to assume that perception encodes the similarity of the distracters before it encodes a pop-out. This order of encoding would imply that, relative to the distracters, a pop-out is represented higher up in the process hierarchy in the brain. This, in turn, would imply that a pop-out is captured earlier by a top-down deployment of attention (Ahissar and Hochstein, 2004; Hochstein and Ahissar, 2002). Thus, a pop-out does not seem to be a compo-nent that is unconsciously encoded first, but rather a component that is consciously detected first because it is represented high up in the visual hierarchy.

At the phenomenological level, a similar dissociation between com-mon and distinctive components has been demonstrated by Johansson (1975). In an experiment, he presented participants with two moving spots of lights in a dark surrounding. One spot made an ongoing up and down motion, and the other spot made an ongoing circular motion,

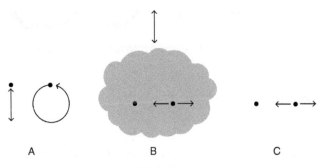

Figure 2.5 A presents two equally rotating lights, but one component is in the viewing plane and the other is in the picture plane. The stimuli give rise to three subsequent impressions (Johansson, 1975; Restle, 1979). The first impression (A) is stimulus like: one component is seen as an up and down motion and the other as a rotation. The second impression (B) deals with an overall common up and down motion of a stationary point and a left-rightward motion. The third impression (C) merely deals with the latter distinctive components. So, the common structure seems to be suppressed in a later stage (Restle, 1979).

in the same phase (see Figure 2.5A). The participants reported to get, successively, three different percepts. The first percept comprised the actually presented motions (see Figure 2.5A). The second percept comprised an overall up and down motion (the common motion component which, in Figure 2.5B, is indicated by a cloud), plus an otherwise stationary spot and an otherwise left and right moving spot (the distinctive motion components in Figure 2.5B). Restle (1979) argued that this second percept reflects the simplest representation with, as before, a hierarchical relationship between common and distinctive components. In this representation, the common component serves as a reference frame, relative to which the distinctive components are encoded. Prolonged viewing may lead to adaptation to this reference frame, that is, as if it becomes the viewer's own reference frame. It may therefore seem to disappear, thus leaving only the distinctive components, which is indeed what some of Johansson's participants reported to get as third percept (see Figure 2.5C).

In sum, the foregoing adds to the earlier evidence against multidimensional scaling. That is, in the previous subsection, we showed that multidimensional scaling has properties which are not valid in perception. Here, in addition, we showed that the hierarchical relationship between common and distinctive components, which is not accounted for by multidimensional scaling, is relevant in perception.

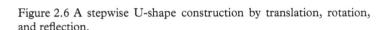

Figure 2.6 A stepwise U-shape construction by translation, rotation, and reflection.

2.3   Transformations

Pattern construction

Digital drawing programs enable us to construe patterns by means of rigid transformations, such as translations, rotations, and reflections, and by means of non-rigid transformations such as stretching and skewing. According to Leyton (1992), such transformations are the proper ingredients of visual pattern representations. They are anyhow suited to construct a pattern. Figure 2.6 presents an illustration.

The construction starts with a point. A horizontal translation of a copy of the point generates a horizontal mini-line of two adjacent points. A translation of a copy of the mini-line generates a horizontal line of four points. A rotation of this line yields a tilted line. A translation of a copy of the horizontal line produces a hook. Finally, a reflection of a copy of the hook about the vertical ends with a U-shape. This series of five construction steps is supposed to present the description of the U-shape. The number of construction steps relates to the complexity of the description. Any pattern can be constructed in many different ways, using different numbers of construction steps. It is therefore almost self-evident that the complexity of the description that uses a minimum number of construction steps is a plausible measure of the complexity of the pattern.

The illustrated description is quite different from a feature representation discussed in section 2.1. It rather is a pattern construction recipe. Besides, it probably does not give rise to the negative correlation between visual complexity and set size of a feature representation. At least, if differences in translation distance and differences in rotation angle are disregarded and not supposed to cause different pattern classes, the correlation between set size and visual complexity is positive and roughly in line with visual pattern classification. Furthermore, the transformational approach does not assume the preferred pattern interpretation. It just aims at the interpretation obtained by a minimum of transformations. Moreover, almost each transformational code reveals the hierarchy that may give rise to asymmetrical dissimilarity, because in most cases, two different transformations are not commutative. For instance, a reflection of a rotated line is not equal to a rotation of a reflected line. In fact, the transformational approach does not suffer from the three troublesome properties of multidimensional scaling (MDS) discussed in section 2.2. Next, we discuss this in more detail.

Dissimilarity assessment

All three properties of MDS deal with the dissimilarity between two pattern interpretations or between two patterns, but before we consider the transformational account, we first make a general comment on dissimilarity from the perspective of perception. In our view, perception aims at pattern representations. It does not aim at assessing pattern complexity, pattern goodness, pattern ambiguity, common features, or distinctive features. These qualities are attributes of pattern representations. Equally, perception does not aim at assessing pattern dissimilarity. Dissimilarity is just an attribute of perception and has to be derived from pattern representations. So, to assess the dissimilarity between two patterns according to the transformational approach, the first step is to efficiently construct the two patterns together. Roughly, this implies the construction of one pattern plus the specification of the transformations needed to change a copy of this pattern into the other. The number of transformations needed to go from one pattern to the other is an adequate shortcut to measure dissimilarity if the two patterns are equally complex. The same holds to measure dissimilarity between two interpretations. Below, in most illustrations of the MDS properties, the two patterns or interpretations are equally complex, and in those cases, we use this shortcut.

Ambiguity MDS does not account for ambiguity because it deals with stimuli. In contrast, the transformational approach deals with stimulus interpretations and can therefore account for ambiguity. For instance, the ambiguous pattern in Figure 2.2B has two interpretations. One interpretation will here be indicated by *B1* and refers to a square plus line. The other will be indicated by *B2* and refers to a pair of triangles. According to the transformational approach, *B1* and *B2* are equally complex, so that it correctly predicts the ambiguity.

Another issue is the internal dissimilarity of an ambiguous stimulus, that is, the dissimilarity between its two interpretations. The transformational approach also accounts for this issue. We illustrate this for the pattern in Figure 2.2B with the two interpretations *B1* and *B2* specified above. In principle, their internal dissimilarity consists of the change of one interpretation to the other. Obviously, this change is less the more the two interpretations share features. However, the two interpretations of Figure 2.2B hardly share features and, in our view, it is not worthwhile to use any information of one interpretation to represent the other. The consequence is that the dissimilarity merely deals with the stimulus construction transformations along the other interpretation. So, if *B1* is the first interpretation, the dissimilarity involves all transformations to construct *B2*. The amount is indicated by $d(B2)$. Equally, if *B2* is the first interpretation, the dissimilarity involves all transformations to construct *B1*. The amount is indicated by $d(B1)$. Hence:

$$d(B1, B2) = d(B2)$$
$$d(B2, B1) = d(B1)$$

Thus, the transformational approach accounts for internal dissimilarity. In fact, internal dissimilarity has a broader scope. It also applies to two unequally complex interpretations of unambiguous stimuli and, because the transformational approach deals with stimulus interpretations, this approach equally accounts for their internal dissimilarities. Notice that, in the example above, the internal dissimilarity between *B1* and *B2* happens to be symmetrical, that is, $d(B1, B2) = d(B2, B1)$ because *B1* and *B2* are equally complex. In general, however, whether two interpretations of an ambiguous or unambiguous pattern are symmetrically or asymmetrically similar is independent of the complexity of the interpretations. This topic is discussed next.

Symmetrical similarity According to MDS, the similarity of two figures *A* and *B* is symmetrical. So, $d(A, B) = d(B, A)$. This means that *B* is equally like *A* as *A* is like *B*. The transformational account of Figures 2.3A and B is different. Pattern *A*, the prototype, is unambiguous and pattern *B*, the non-prototype, is ambiguous. The dissimilarity measure $d(A, B)$ deals with the starting pattern A, being a square plus line, and in this context pattern B is taken as *B1*, also being a square plus line. So, the dissimilarity $d(A, B1)$ is determined by a line translation. Hence:

$$d(A, B) = d(A, B1)$$

In the dissimilarity measure $d(B, A)$, the starting pattern *B* is for 50 per cent taken as a square plus line (*B1*) and for 50 per cent as a pair of triangles (*B2*). So, for 50 per cent the dissimilarity stems from a line translation contributing to $d(B1, A)$ and for 50 per cent the dissimilarity stems from two changes, namely, an interpretation change contributing to $d(B2, B1) = d(B1)$ and a line translation contributing to $d(B1, A)$. Hence:

$$d(B, A) = \tfrac{1}{2}d(B1, A) + \tfrac{1}{2}[d(B1) + d(B1, A)]$$
$$= d(B1, A) + \tfrac{1}{2}d(B1)$$

Because $d(B1, A) = d(A, B1)$, the first dissimilarity $d(A, B)$ is smaller than the second dissimilarity $d(B, A)$. This implies that B is more like A than A is like B. Notice that the decisive difference $\frac{1}{2}d(B1)$ reflects the ambiguity of B and that this ambiguity causes the falsification of symmetrical similarity.

The transformational account of Figures 2.3C and D is as follows. Pattern C presents the prototype, being the common structure, and pattern D presents the non-prototype, being the deviant version. So, according to the shortcut dissimilarity measure, the two figures are symmetrically similar. After all, the line addition in $d(C, D)$ and the line omission in $d(D, C)$ are equivalent. However, as argued, to assess the dissimilarity between two patterns, the first step actually is to efficiently construct the two patterns together. As said, this roughly implies the construction of one pattern plus the specification of the transformations needed to change a copy of this pattern into the other. This can be done either by starting with pattern C as the common part or by starting with pattern D as the common part. For the two patterns together, this yields codes with complexities $d(C) + d(C, D)$ and $d(C) + d(C, D) + d(D, C)$, respectively. The former code involves less transformations and is therefore the simplest code. Hence, assuming that the simplest code is preferred, this code specifies qualitatively that C is the prototype and D the non-prototype, thus revealing the asymmetrical dissimilarity that D is more like C than C is like D.

Triangle inequality According to MDS, the triangle inequality should hold. It states: $d(A, C) \leq d(A, B) + d(B, C)$. The transformational account of Figure 2.2 is different. The left-hand term $d(A, C)$ in the inequality deals with the transformations involved in the construction of pattern C, again, under the assumption that it is not worthwhile to use information of pattern A to construct pattern C. Hence:

$$d(A, C) = d(C)$$

In the right-hand side $d(A, B) + d(B, C)$ of the inequality the term $d(A, B)$ equals $d(A, B1) = 1$ and $d(B, C)$ equals $d(B2, C) + \frac{1}{2}d(B2)$ (see topic on symmetrical similarity), where $d(B2, C) = 1$ while $d(B2)$ is equal to $d(C)$. Hence:

$$d(A, B) + d(B, C) = 2 + \frac{1}{2}d(C)$$

This implies that the inequality $d(A, C) \leq d(A, B) + d(B, C)$ can be rewritten into:

$$d(C) \leq 2 + \frac{1}{2}d(C)$$

This inequality holds only if $d(C) \leq 4$. However, according to any construction recipe, the construction of two triangles requires more than four transformations, so that we conclude that, perceptually correct, the triangle inequality does not hold according to the transformational account.

To summarize, the transformational approach has various attractive properties. First, it completely represents an individual stimulus, namely, by a construction recipe. Second, it implies the visually relevant positive correlation between set size and visual complexity. Third, the approach does not assume pattern interpretations. Instead, it generates them. As a consequence, it accounts for visual ambiguity. Fourth, it explains the asymmetrical dissimilarities between prototypes and non-prototypes. In our view, the complexity measure still is a topic of concern. According to the transformational approach by Leyton (1992), the complexity measure is determined by the transformations in a code and same transformations of different arguments are equivalent. An alternative option is a complexity measure determined by the arguments and not by the transformations. This option is a topic in the next section.

2.4   Gestalt properties

Whereas transformations deal with the steps towards a pattern, as in the theory of Leyton (1992), Gestalt principles depart from a pattern, though in its most primitive appearance. That is, these principles depart from the retinal stimulus. In contrast to features and dimensions, they do not presuppose pattern interpretations. In fact, they deal with the proximal stimulus properties that are supposed to tentatively cue the visual segmentation and interpretation of a pattern (Köhler, 1920; Koffka, 1935; Wertheimer, 1923). However, Gestalt principles do not definitely predict pattern interpretations. Therefore, we rather speak of Gestalt properties or cues instead of Gestalt principles or laws.

About 113 Gestalt cues have been proposed (see Pomerantz and Kubovy, 1986). To give a gist of their perceptual role we refer to a few cues. The so-called 'proximity' cue states that the smaller the distance between two stimulus elements is, the more likely these elements are visually grouped together. A related grouping property, recently proposed by Palmer and Rock (1994), deals with connected stimulus elements with the same texture ('uniform connectedness'). Furthermore, visual grouping applies to stimulus elements that are equal ('similarity'), aligned ('good continuation'), share motion ('common fate'), or mirrored ('symmetry'). Gestalt psychologists not only discovered grouping cues but also visual biases. Some examples are the visual preference for convex instead of concave shapes, for a light source at the top instead of at the bottom, for a viewpoint at the top instead of at the bottom, for interpreting an enclosed stimulus part as foreground and its surround as background. Here, we merely focus on Gestalt cues as they contribute to pattern segmentations and interpretations without presuming them.

In various respects Gestalt cues are diverse. There are cues dealing with single relations and cues dealing with complex relations. For instance, 'proximity' deals with distances between two stimulus elements whereas 'similarity' deals with intra-stimulus relations that may be common to two stimuli. For instance, patterns may be similar because of their common length-width proportions. Also, interactions between Gestalt cues are diverse. For instance, 'proximity' and 'uniform connectedness' partially share features. After all, connectedness is an extreme case of proximity. Nevertheless, these two cues are mainly independent of each other as nearby elements are not necessarily uniform. There are also cues that are completely enclosed by others and therefore less basic than others. For instance, 'good continuation' and 'common fate' can be considered of as versions of the 'similarity' cue. So, cues might be asymmetrically related to each other.

Pattern representation

Without doubt, Gestalt cues are useful anchors of perception but there are still questions about their role in pattern representations. We will answer them by using the fairly independent similarity and symmetry cues in a few demonstrations.

A first question is about the way in which cues can be combined in pattern representations. Figure 2.7A deals with this topic. It presents a series of white and black disks. The first four disks reveal two equal pairs. Their clustering, indicated by the arc in Figure 2.7B, is based on their repeat structure. The last four disks reveal mirrored pairs. Their clustering, indicated by the arc in Figure 2.7C, is based on symmetry. The two clusters are combined in Figure 2.7D. Then, however, they overlap each other and thus give rise to an ambiguous segmentation. Therefore, the repeat and the symmetry in Figure 2.7A are not combinable in one representation.

Another question is which cue information is embedded in a representation to ensure that the stimulus is uniquely fixated. Our answer is as follows. Within the Gestaltist tradition, the main function of cues is to reveal visual segments of patterns. In our view, a pattern representation reveals more. It also reveals the involved kinds of cues. However, this

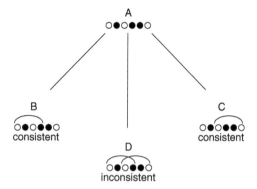

Figure 2.7 The first four disks in A reveal a repeat of pairs. Their clustering is shown by the arc in B. The last four disks in A reveal mirrored pairs. Their clustering is shown by the arc in C. In D the two clusters are combined. However, as they overlap each other they exclude each other. In other words, the repeat and symmetry cannot be combined in one representation of A.

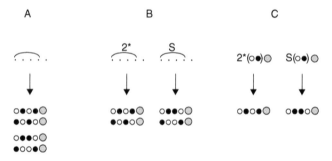

Figure 2.8 A, B, and C illustrate three options for representing series of five disks (two white, two black, one grey). The arc in A clusters the first four disks. This pure segmentation option is quite ambiguous. It does not differentiate the four series below this option. Option B is like option A but with information about the kind of regularity. Repeat is indicated by 2* and symmetry by S. This option is better but still ambiguous. Each version describes two series. Option C deals with an operator (indicated by 2* or S) in combination with an argument. Each representation unambiguously describes just one series.

claim has consequences for the appropriate representation form. To illustrate what is meant we compare three representation options presented in Figures 2.8A, B, and C. The dots in option A are supposed to stand for varying disks. The arc clusters the first four disks either because of the twofold repeat or the symmetry among white and black disks. Obviously, the mere segmentation, indicated by the arc, is ambiguous. It does not differentiate between the four series below this option. Option B is like option A but is combined with information about the kind of regularity. Repeat is indicated by 2^* and symmetry by **S**. This option is better. However, it is still ambiguous as each representation describes two series. Option C deals with an operator applied to an argument. The operator is indicated either by 2^* or **S**. In fact, each operator plays the role of some kind of transformation (see section 2.3). This option is the best for various reasons. First, each representation unambiguously describes just one series. In fact, it is a recipe for the reconstruction of the stimulus pattern. Second, this option seems more complex as it deals with actual disks but it is more parsimonious in other respects. It can do without an explicit index for segmentation (arcs), without the information of the total number of disks, and without the information that there are two white and two black disks. Third, the operator reveals the kind of regularity in the pattern whereas the compactness of the representation reflects both the regularity reduction (two disks) and the remaining irregularity (three disks). The relevance of the compactness of the representation is next considered further.

Interpretation selection

Like a dimension, a Gestalt property is characterized by qualitative and quantitative aspects (MacKay, 1969; van Soest, 1952). Commonly, the name of a Gestalt property is indicated by its quality, for instance 'symmetry' or 'good continuation'. A quantitative aspect of symmetry is, for instance, the number of symmetry axes in the pattern, and a quantitative aspect of good continuation of two subsequent lines is the actual angle in between. If Gestalt cues, purely on the basis of their qualitative aspects, would have a fixed priority order – for instance, if 'proximity' always overrules 'symmetry' and the latter always overrules 'good continuation' – the main issue of form perception would have been solved. Then, Gestalt cues predict the preferred pattern interpretation even for a stimulus in which Gestalt cues evoke conflicting segmentations. However, Gestalt cues do not reveal such a fixed priority rule. Instead, the actual quantitative aspect of a Gestalt property codetermines its strength. So, in case a stimulus deals with two conflicting Gestalt cues, sometimes one cue prevails and sometimes the other. In Figure 2.9 we illustrate this.

In a given pattern code, the operators refer to the qualitative aspects of cues and the arguments refer to the quantitative aspects of cues. As the

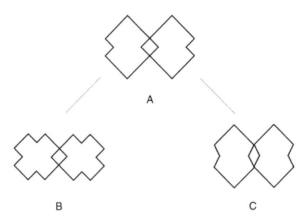

Figure 2.9 A is preferably interpreted as a pair of overlapping parts. Both B and C are preferably interpreted as pairs of mosaic parts, though for different reasons. A and B differ merely with respect to symmetry. Each mosaic part of A has two axes and each mosaic part of B has four axes of symmetry. A and C differ merely with respect to good continuation. Each overlapping part of A has a good continuing contour and each overlapping part of C has a bad continuing contour. Apparently, pattern interpretations depend on the actual strengths of Gestalt cues.

latter aspects codetermine cue strengths, it is plausible to assume that the arguments at the least contribute to complexity. Within the Gestalt approach, but also within SIT, the complexity is even determined solely by the arguments. The operators are assumed to be inborn hardware tools of perception. They aim at reducing the number of arguments in a code so that they can be said to be the carriers of the interpretation, but the informational content of the interpretation is given by the arguments in the code. Therefore, SIT takes the number of remaining arguments in a code as the information load. SIT's official measure is indicated by I and is introduced in Chapter 5.3. A good approximation, however, is given by counting the number of remaining elements in a code; this measure is indicated by I'. For instance, each code at the top of Figure 2.8C comprises three disk elements. So, for each code holds $I' = 3$. Also in the next chapter, this measure I' will be used in illustrations.

Obviously, the latter approach is quite different from the transformational approach. According to the transformational approach, complexity is determined by the number of transformations or the sum of weighted transformations (Leyton, 1992) but not by the arguments. Yet, the transformational approach and Gestalt approach also share features.

Both aim at the representation with a minimum complexity. In other words, code selection is guided by the 'simplicity principle', also called the 'minimum principle' by Hochberg and McAlister (1953). It states that, of all possible codes of a pattern, the simplest code is selected. In fact, this simplicity principle is in line with the so-called Gestalt law of Prägnanz (Koffka, 1935; Wertheimer, 1923). It claims that the most stable and regular pattern representation survives and is visually preferred. The simplicity principle also is the selection criterion promoted within SIT.

Summary

In section 2.1, we discussed that features are useful attributes for the identification of patterns, given knowledge about a restricted set of patterns. However, perception makes no use of knowledge. Besides, it deals with an unrestricted set of patterns. Figural features are distinguished from abstract features. Figural features are appropriate to uniquely represent stimuli but not for pattern classification. Abstract features are appropriate to represent pattern classes but not visual classes. Besides, they neither sufficiently fixate individual patterns nor sufficiently guide the reconstruction of patterns. In fact, abstract features presuppose pattern interpretations.

In section 2.2, we discussed that multi-dimensional scaling is designed to represent stimuli on the basis of their dissimilarity judgments. It is useful for various domains of study but, in our view, not for perception. The scaling deals with stimuli but not with their visual interpretations. As a consequence, dimensional scaling does not account for ambiguity. Because of this failure but also of lacking hierarchy, dimensional scaling is indifferent with respect to the asymmetrical similarity between prototypes and non-prototypes.

In section 2.3, we discussed that the transformational approach provides recipes for the reconstruction of patterns and accounts rather well for visual pattern classification. Besides, it does not assume pattern interpretations but generates them. As a consequence, it accounts for visual ambiguity. As it deals with hierarchical relations, it explains asymmetrical dissimilarities between prototypes and non-prototypes. However, there are questions about the fact that the transformational approach determines complexity by the transformations and not by the arguments.

In section 2.4, we discussed that Gestalt properties also do not presume pattern interpretations. These properties belong to the proximal stimulus and are cues for pattern segmentation. The Gestalt approach and the transformational approach share the assumption that the representation having minimal complexity is the preferred one. There is also a difference. The operators in codes can be seen as the inborn hardware tools of information reduction. Therefore, in the Gestalt approach, not the operators but the remaining arguments are supposed to determine the information load and thereby the complexity.

3   Process versus representation

Introduction

In a model in which the visually preferred pattern representation is supposed to be the simplest of all possible representations, the selection
criterion of simplicity clearly applies to representations. That is, it is a
representation criterion and, as such, it is silent about the underlying
process except that this process should lead to the simplest representation. This seems to require a complex process, so that it is worthwhile
to explore whether a simple process may also be sufficient to arrive at
plausible and visually relevant outcomes. In other words, it is worthwhile
to explore whether simplicity can be used as a process criterion instead
of as a representation criterion. Linear stage models are prototypical of
such simple processes. They propose that the process from stimulus to
representation is a process that involves successive stages without any
feedback loop. In this chapter, we consider four kinds of linear stage
models. Their outcomes are evaluated with respect to their plausibility
and visual relevance. Furthermore, they are compared with the outcomes
of the representation criterion of simplicity.

3.1   Process criteria

Minimal load per stage

We start by discussing a linear stage model suggested by Simon and
Kotovsky (1963). According to their model, the generation of a pattern
code occurs in subsequent stages, such that at each stage the information
load is reduced maximally. In other words, the criterion is minimal load
per stage. In Figures 3.1 and 3.2, various applications are illustrated.
With respect to the coding we refer to Figure 2.8C, and with respect
to information load we refer to the measure I' introduced at the end of
Chapter 2.4.

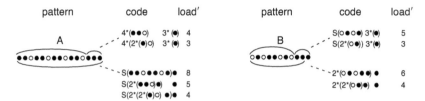

Figure 3.1 The minimal load per stage model states that the coding step that leads to the lowest load should be selected first (the load I' is the number of disks in the code). This model applies to the clusters and codes above each stimulus pattern. The final codes are preferred and are the simplest ones [I'(A) = 3, I'(B) = 3]. The maximal cluster per stage model states that the coding step dealing with the largest cluster should be selected first. This model applies to the clusters and codes below each stimulus pattern. The final codes are not preferred and are not the simplest ones [I'(A) = 4, I'(B) = 4].

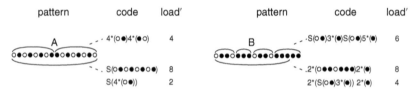

Figure 3.2 Again, the minimal load per stage model applies to the clusters and codes above each stimulus pattern. However, the final codes are not preferred and are not the simplest [I'(A) = 4, I'(B) = 6]. This time, the maximal cluster per stage model, that applies to the clusters and codes below each stimulus pattern, prevails. The final codes are both preferred and the simplest ones [I'(A) = 2, I'(B) = 4].

Figure 3.1 presents two series of white and black disks. Clusters of disks are indicated by arcs above and below each series and are imposed by the codes above and below each series, respectively. The codes above each series are in line with the minimal load per stage criterion. We illustrate this in more detail.

In Figure 3.1A, the operations in the first stage represent the series by a fourfold repeat of three disks (two black, one white) and a threefold repeat of a black disk. The load, I' = 4, stems from the four disks in this code. As it is the lowest possible load that can be obtained in a first stage, the code is in line with the minimal load per stage criterion. This code can be reduced to I' = 3 in a second stage on a deeper hierarchical level, namely, by a twofold repeat operation within the first repeat argument. The resulting code cannot be reduced further. For instance, the coding below the series yields more complex codes at both the first and final stages. In fact, the final code above the series is not only the simplest code possible but it also yields the visually preferred segmentation (van Lier, 1996).

By the same token, in Figure 3.1B, the minimal load per stage criterion yields, at the first stage, a code with load $I' = 5$, and at the second stage, a code with load $I' = 3$. Also this is the simplest code possible and it yields the visually preferred segmentation.

Applied to Figure 3.2, the minimal load per stage criterion fails, however. In Figure 3.2A, the load of the code at the first stage is $I' = 4$. As no further reduction is possible, this first stage also is the final stage. The code below the series, however, may have a more complex code at the first stage, but a more simple code at the final stage, and it also yields the visually preferred segmentation. The same applies to Figure 3.2B. Hence, the minimal load per stage criterion may be successful in some cases (as shown in Figure 3.1) but fails in other cases (as shown in Figure 3.2).

Maximal cluster per stage

In another imaginable linear stage model, the criterion is the maximal cluster per stage. It means that at each stage of coding the regularity with the most extensive cluster is selected. In Figures 3.1 and 3.2, this clustering and coding is indicated below each stimulus pattern.

For instance, in Figure 3.1A, the first stage involves a code that uses the symmetry operation. Its load is $I' = 8$. This code can be reduced in a second stage, namely, by a twofold repeat operation within the symmetry argument, yielding a load $I' = 5$. This code can be reduced once more in a third stage, namely, by a twofold repeat operation. The resulting code cannot be reduced further. Its load of $I' = 4$, however, is still higher than the load of the visually preferred code above the series. Hence, here, the maximal cluster per stage criterion yields neither the simplest code nor the visually preferred segmentation. The same applies to Figure 3.1B.

In Figure 3.2AB, however, the maximal cluster per stage criterion yields final codes that are both simplest ones and that yield the visually preferred segmentations. Hence, whereas the minimal load per stage criterion is successful in Figure 3.1 but fails in Figure 3.2, the maximal cluster per stage criterion is successful in Figure 3.2 but fails in Figure 3.1. This implies that both models are untenable.

Various other imaginable linear stage models are closely related to the two previous models. We briefly characterize four models. Two models are versions of the minimal load per stage model. One aims at a maximum number of clusters per stage, and another aims at a minimum number of hierarchical stages. Both models are more or less supported by Figures 3.1AB but falsified by Figures 3.2AB. Two other models are versions of the maximal cluster per stage model. One aims at a minimum number of clusters per stage, and another aims at a maximum number of hierarchical stages. Both models are supported by Figures 3.2AB but are more or less falsified by Figures 3.1AB. Hence, these four additional models are untenable too.

Global precedence

The previous models presuppose various stages and a same criterion per stage. This is not the case for the 'global precedence' hypothesis of Navon (1977). It deals with one criterion for a first stage and another for a second stage. It assumes a process in early perception that starts with the global shape (like the previous process model that starts with the maximal cluster), and that ends with details. The global shape is the low spatial frequency structure that misses the differentiation of details. It roughly agrees with the pattern seen by squinting eyes. The details are manifest at higher spatial frequency levels. The levels from global to local are formally described by the scale space model of Koenderink and van Doorn (1976).

The global precedence hypothesis is usually tested for 2-D configurations of separate subpatterns (Hoffman, 1975; Navon, 1977). Figures 3.3AA'A'' illustrate such configurations. The first two figures share global shapes whereas the last two figures share subpattern shapes. In support of the hypothesis, the first two figures appear to be visually more related than the last two figures.

Various perception researchers criticized this hypothesis as follows. Martin (1979) looked at size effects and showed that global effects are not categorical but gradual. If the size of subpatterns increases or if their number decreases, the global effect decreases. Figures 3.3BB'B'' present an illustration. The judged similarity of the first two figures, sharing global structures, is hardly more than that of the latter two figures, sharing subpattern shapes.

Beck (1966) looked at the role of colour. He showed that grouping based on common colour overrules almost any grouping based on common shape. An illustration is presented in Figures 3.3CC'C''. The first two figures share a global shape but the last two figures tend to be grouped together due to their common colour.

Kimchi and Palmer (1982) looked at effects of subpattern shape. Figures 3.3DD'D'' give an illustration for closed and open subpatterns. The judged similarity of the first two figures, based on global shapes, is

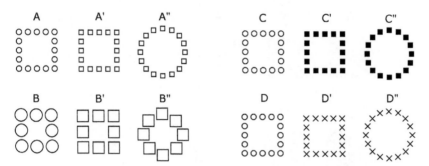

Figure 3.3 AA′ share global structures and A′A″ share subpattern shapes. The global precedence hypothesis (Navon, 1977) correctly predicts that the first two patterns are visually more related than the last two patterns. Also for the other triads, it predicts that the first two patterns are visually more related than the last two patterns, but visually, the last two patterns in these other triads tend to be more related. For BB′B″ this is due to the large size and low number of subpatterns (Martin, 1979), for CC′C″ it is due to colour (Beck, 1982), and for DD′D″ it is due to subpattern shape (Kimchi and Palmer, 1982) (Leeuwenberg, 2003b).

hardly more than the judged similarity of the latter two figures, based on common subpattern shapes.

The application domain of the global precedence hypothesis needs, in our view, some more discussion. As said, most tests of this hypothesis deal with 2-D configurations of separate subpatterns, but if valid, the hypothesis should equally well apply to the shapes in Figure 3.4. The judged similarity of Figures 3.4AA′ is less than that of Figures 3.4A′A″, although the first two figures share more global contours of their envelopes than the last two figures. Also, of Figures 3.4BB′B″, the first two are judged to be less related than the last two, although the first two figures share more contours of their envelopes than the last two figures. Hence, here, the global precedence hypothesis fails.

In our view, it is more plausible that any temporal order from global to local is a suggestive side-effect of stimulus representations. At least, in line with this view are the speed-accuracy studies by de Boer and Keuss (1981) on global and local effects. They drew the conclusion that global effects stem from post-perceptual processes. Furthermore, according to Pomerantz et al. (2003), there is no evidence for a fixed processing order within perception, be it from global to local or from local to global. A similar conclusion has been drawn by Palmer et al. (2003) for Gestalt formation: grouping principles are involved in all stages.

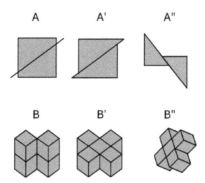

Figure 3.4 According to the global precedence hypothesis (Navon, 1977), the first two patterns of each triad should be visually more related. However, the last two patterns appear visually more related. For AA'A'', it is due to 2-D junctions, and for BB'B'', it is due to 3-D junctions (Leeuwenberg and van der Helm, 1991).

Without doubt, the global precedence hypothesis applies to the domain of art production. Painters and music composers often begin with a global sketch and end with details. This order is efficient as the global configuration consisting of subpattern locations can be indicated, say, by dots, whereas subpatterns cannot be drawn without their locations. If subpatterns are placed at wrong positions, they have to be redrawn later. However, art is opposed to perception. Art deals with the process from code to pattern whereas perception deals with the process from pattern to code.

Orientation precedence

Beck (1982) proposed a special sequence of visual processing stages in case stimuli comprise clusters of randomly positioned subpatterns such that the subpatterns in adjacent clusters either differ with respect to shape or to orientation. He found that the primary visual subdivision of such a configuration seems to be determined by the orientation and not by the shape of subpatterns. An illustration is presented in Figure 3.5.

The configuration consists of three parts: A, A', and A''. The subpatterns of the first two parts have the same orientation but different shapes whereas the subpatterns of the latter two parts have the same shape but different orientations. According to Beck (1982), the first two parts are grouped together in an initial stage of perception on the basis of subpattern orientation.

A   A'   A"

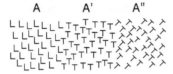

Figure 3.5 Of stimuli that comprise clusters of randomly positioned
subpatterns such that the subpatterns in adjacent clusters either differ
with respect to shape or to orientation, the early visual subdivision
seems to be based on common orientation rather than on common
shape (Beck, 1982). So, in an initial stage of perception, A' is more
related to A than to A".

The proposed sequential order, however, is subject to various restrictions. One restriction is that all subpatterns should be randomly positioned (Beck, 1982). Indeed, if they are not randomly positioned the configurations might be visually grouped according to their global shapes. Further restrictions agree with the aforementioned ones on the global precedence hypothesis, namely, those with respect to the size and number of subpatterns (Kinchla, 1977; Martin, 1979), the colour of subpatterns (Beck, 1982), and the structure of subpatterns (Kimchi and Palmer, 1982).

All in all, the linear stage models, discussed in this section, use process criteria which insufficiently explain visual shape interpretations. So, there is reason to verify whether the final properties of a pattern representation provide better indices for the visually preferred pattern interpretation. This is explored next.

3.2   Representation criteria

Representation selection criteria deal with the goal (i.e., the pattern representation) and not with the method (i.e., the process). Whereas stage models directly lead to a solution without testing alternative routes, models dealing with a representation criterion presume a competition between all possible representations of a pattern (Herbart, 1816; see Figure 1.11). For this reason, such representation models seem unrealistic but, as will be shown in Chapter 5, there is a solution such that all alternatives can be taken into account without considering each of them separately. Therefore, it is worthwhile to explore representation criteria. In fact, we consider two representation criteria. One selects the pattern representation with a minimal structural load. Experimental evidence for its visual relevance is a topic of Chapter 8. The other criterion selects the pattern representation whose hierarchical highest component refers to

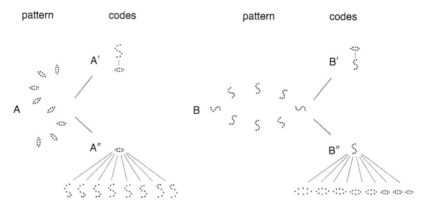

Figure 3.6 A and B present 2-D compound patterns. The code in A′ of pattern A is structurally simpler than the code in A″. Equally, the code in B′ of pattern B is structurally simpler than the code in B″. For this reason, A′ and B′ are predicted to be the visually preferred codes (Leeuwenberg, 2003b).

the largest pattern component. There is visual evidence that the latter criterion merely applies if the first criterion is indecisive.

Structural criterion: complexity

For Figures 3.1 and 3.2, the stage models do not always predict the preferred concepts of serial patterns, whereas the overall simplest codes do. Figures 3.2A and B show that in fact the most complex codes at the first stage lead to the final simplest and preferred codes. So, in order to predict correctly, the minimal load per stage model would have to allow for detours along even the most complex initial coding steps – but then it is no longer a minimal load per stage model. Exploring detours is a well-known strategy in problem solving (Simon, 1969), and it also seems at hand in visual pattern completion where coding goes beyond the directly accessible stimulus information (see Chapter 8). However, perception does not belong to the cognitive level of deliberation and conscious reasoning. Therefore, rather than speaking of detours, we would say that perception automatically explores all possible routes from stimulus to concepts and that it selects the overall simplest concept, that is, the concept with the overall minimal load.

To further explore this minimal load criterion, we attend to stimuli studied by Navon (1977). Two of them are presented in Figures 3.6AB. They consist of configurations of separate subpatterns. For the sake of the demonstration, the number of subpatterns (8) is kept equal to the number of points in each subpattern. Without doubt, of these patterns only the S-patterns and the ellipses are the visually relevant components. Therefore, only codes that represent these components are considered. In fact, in these codes, these components are hierarchically related: one component forms the superstructure and the other component forms the subordinate structure. The superstructure determines the positions of the subordinate structures and, in this case, also their orientations; that is, they have a constant relative orientation with respect to the superstructure. Thus, for each pattern in Figure 3.6, only two codes are considered. One represents an S-pattern of ellipses and the other represents an ellipse of S-patterns.

The hierarchical relationships are reflected by the visualized codes presented in Figure 3.6. In each of them, the upper component stands for the superstructure and the lower component stands for the subordinate structure. The relative orientations of the subordinate structures are not presented in the visualized codes.

In fact, irrespective of how a code is obtained, a code is a recipe for the construction of the pattern. It prescribes this construction in the following steps. The first step deals with the superstructure, the second step with the orientations of the subordinate structures, and the third step with the subordinate structures.

In the code in Figure 3.6A′, the superstructure agrees with an S-pattern and the subordinate structure agrees with a constant ellipse having a constant relative orientation with respect to the superstructure. So, this code merely deals with two constant components. The code in Figure 3.6A″ describes Figure 3.6A as a specific ellipse of S-shapes but, then, all the S-shapes should necessarily be different with, moreover, different relative orientations. So, the upper code is the simplest description. The same holds for Figure 3.6B. The code in Figure 3.6B′ reveals just two constant components whereas the code in Figure 3.6B″ describes a specific S-structure of ellipses with varying sizes (i.e., the inner ellipses are smaller than the outer ellipses) and with, moreover, different relative orientations. So, also this time, the upper code is the simplest description. As the upper codes are the simplest ones, they are predicted to be the visually preferred descriptions. Before we consider their visual relevance, we gather predictions for a few more patterns.

In fact, similar codes also describe the 3-D objects presented in Figures 3.7AB. The simplest code in Figure 3.7A′ presents the first object as an S-shaped superstructure of identical subordinate circles. In fact, this code reflects the way the object surface can be mimicked, namely, by turning a constant circle along an S-shape. The simplest code in Figure 3.7B′ represents the second object as a circular superstructure of identical subordinate S-structures. This code reflects the way the object surface

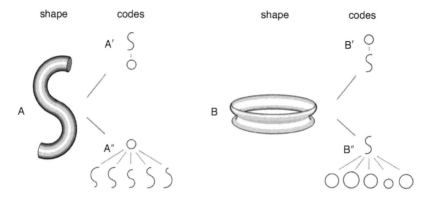

Figure 3.7 A and B present 3-D objects. The code in A′ of pattern A is structurally simpler than the code in A″. Equally, the code in B′ of pattern B is structurally simpler than the code in B″. For this reason, A′ and B′ are predicted to be the visually preferred codes (Leeuwenberg and van der Helm, 1991).

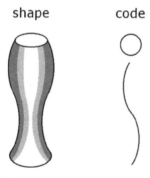

Figure 3.8 The circular superstructure is smaller than the subordinate S-shaped structure. So, the superstructure and the global structure do not coincide (Leeuwenberg, 2003b).

can be mimicked by turning a constant S-shaped wire around a circle. As the alternative codes with reverse hierarchies are more complex, the upper codes are predicted to be the visually preferred descriptions.

Notice that, in Figure 3.7, the orientations of the subordinate structures are 3-D turns. There is a further difference between codes of 2-D patterns and 3-D objects. Of the shapes, shown in Figures 3.6 and 3.7, the superstructures coincide with the global structures, that is, with the most extensive components. This holds for all 2-D configurations, but not for all 3-D objects. Figure 3.8 presents an illustration. The simplest code

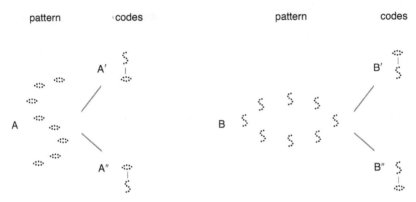

Figure 3.9 The codes of A in A′ and A″ have the same structural information load. The argument to select the hierarchy in A′ is that its
superstructure is larger and therefore visually more prominent than its
subordinate structure. The same holds for the codes in B′ and B″. So,
the codes in A′ and B′ are predicted to be visually preferred.

of the presented object reveals, like the simplest code in Figure 3.7B′, a
circular superstructure and an S-shaped subordinate structure but, this
time, the circle is smaller than the S-shape. So, the superstructure does
not coincide with the global structure.

Metrical criterion: size

Most stimuli used in the experiments by Navon (1977) and Hoffman
(1975) to test the global precedence hypothesis were configurations of
identical subpatterns oriented in parallel. In other words, the global shape
merely specifies the positions of the subpatterns which, independently of
the global shape, have the same absolute orientation. So, this situation
differs from the one considered in the previous subsection. To illustrate the consequences, we attend to Figure 3.9 which presents such
configurations.

Without doubt, Figure 3.9A is preferably represented by the visualized code in Figure 3.9A′ which describes an S-structure of ellipsoidal
subpatterns, and Figure 3.9B is preferably represented by the visualized
code in Figure 3.9B′ which describes an ellipse of S-shaped subpatterns.
So far, the hierarchical relations in these codes seem of the same kind
as those in Figures 3.6A′B′. However, they are quite different. The reason is as follows. If the size of the S-structure in Figure 3.9A is made
sufficiently smaller and the size of its ellipsoidal structures is made sufficiently larger, then Figure 3.9B is obtained. Equally, Figure 3.9A can

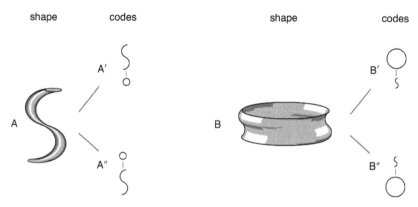

Figure 3.10 The codes of A in A′ and A″ have the same structural information load. The argument to select the hierarchy in A′ is that its superstructure is larger and therefore visually more prominent than its subordinate structure. The same holds for the codes in B′ and B″. So, the codes in A′ and B′ are predicted to be visually preferred.

be derived from Figure 3.9B by just changing the size of its components. The consequence is that the two mentioned codes are structurally equivalent and apply to both patterns. Their opposed hierarchies merely differ in a metrical sense.

So, the code in Figure 3.9A′ is not structurally simpler than the code in Figure 3.9A″ and the code in Figure 3.9B′ is not structurally simpler than the code in Figure 3.9B″. In other words, structurally, these stimuli have an ambiguous hierarchical organization. The perceptual disambiguation is, in our view, caused by metrical factors. That is, the argument to select the hierarchies of Figures 3.9A′B′ is that their superstructures, due to their size, are visually more prominent than their subordinate structures. Here, we resort to the idea that large stimuli evoke higher levels of neural activation and yield more 'weight of evidence' (MacKay, 1969) than small stimuli do. Thus, the codes in Figures 3.9A′B′ are predicted to be visually preferred. For the same metrical arguments, the codes in Figures 3.10A′B′ are predicted to be visually preferred for the 3-D objects in Figures 3.10AB.

Superstructure dominance

For the patterns in the last five figures, we made predictions on their preferred interpretations but we did not yet discuss their visual relevance. For these patterns, the hypothesis of Navon (1977) predicts hierarchical relations with the temporal effect of global precedence. We propose

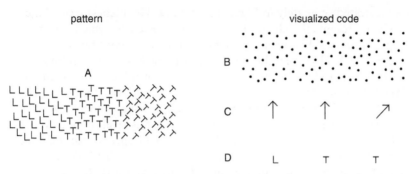

Figure 3.11 Of the description of A, three hierarchical code components are visualized: B presents the global structure of subpattern positions, C presents the subpattern orientations, and D presents the subpattern shapes. B is the highest hierarchical component but misses any grouping cue. C is the next highest component but the highest with a distinctive grouping cue. Hence, the subpattern orientations are the decisive grouping anchors.

alternative hierarchical relations, namely, with the static effect of dominance of the perceived superstructure (Leeuwenberg and van der Helm, 1991). After all, in a code, the superstructure is dominant in that it determines the positions of the subordinate structures, not the other way around. Furthermore, in general, as in Figures 3.6 to 3.8, the perceived superstructure is supposed to be the one in the structurally simplest code. Hence, in general, the predicted dominance is based on structural aspects. Only if there is structural ambiguity, as in Figures 3.9 and 3.10, the perceived superstructure is supposed to be given by the code with the largest superstructure. Hence, only then, the predicted dominance is based on metrical aspects.

Notice that, despite the difference in approach, our predictions on 2-D patterns do not differ from Navon's predictions. After all, as said, the structurally predicted superstructure of 2-D patterns steadily coincides with the most extensive global structure. However, our predictions on 3-D objects differ from Navon's predictions because, as we demonstrated in Figure 3.8, the structurally predicted superstructure of objects does not always coincide with the most extensive global structure. In the next subsection, we refer to arguments for the visual dominance of this superstructure even in cases where it is smaller than the subordinate structure.

In fact, we also invoke the superstructure dominance assumption to oppose the orientation precedence hypothesis of Beck (1982) sketched in section 3.1. This may be illustrated for the compound pattern in Figure 3.11A. Its simplest code consists of three hierarchical levels. These are illustrated separately in Figures 3.11BCD. The highest level (Figure 3.11B) represents the global structure. This structure, which consists of the positions of subpatterns, is the first candidate anchor for segmenting Figure 3.11A. However, this structure just consists of one undifferentiated cloud of random points. Hence, it misses any index for segmentation. Therefore, resort is taken to the next hierarchical level (Figure 3.11C). This level consists of the orientations of subpatterns, namely, two identical vertical ones and another being tilted. So, this level reveals a differentiated subdivision, and this subdivision actually agrees with the visual segmentation of Figure 3.11A. The third level (Figure 3.11D) deals with subpattern shapes. They play a subordinate visual role. So, according to this approach, the perception of random configurations of differently oriented subpatterns is not due to procedural orientation precedence but is due to representational orientation dominance.

Structural before metrical

In the introduction to this section, we claimed that the metrical criterion merely applies if the structural criterion is indecisive. In other words, the metrical criterion is supposed to be subordinate to the structural criterion. Here, for configurations of identical subpatterns, we present direct and indirect visual evidence in favour of this claim.

The direct evidence follows from findings that the superstructure, determined by structural complexity, is visually more dominant than the subordinate structure even if the superstructure is smaller than the subordinate structure (as is the case in Figure 3.8). Evidence for this dominance stems from the experiment by van Bakel (1989). He found that 3-D objects with identical superstructures and different subordinate structures are grouped together more strongly than 3-D objects with identical subordinate structures and different superstructures. Further evidence stems from the primed-matching experiment by van Lier *et al.* (1997). They found that objects are identified better when they are primed by superstructures than when they are primed by subordinate structures. The currently relevant point is that, in both experiments, the predicted superstructures and subordinate structures were based solely on the structural criterion, and that the results were independent of whether the superstructure was smaller or larger than the subordinate structures (for more details on these experiments, see Chapter 10).

The indirect evidence comes from demonstrations that the visual system seems to prefer to encode stimuli such that subordinate structures have a constant orientation relative to the superstructure rather than a constant absolute orientation. The former encoding implies application

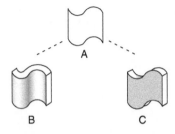

Figure 3.12 Stimulus A gives rise to two options. According to one option, it presents the curved object B described by relatively oriented subordinate structures, and according to the other option it presents the flat object C described by absolutely oriented subordinate structures. The former interpretation is visually preferred.

of the structural criterion, whereas the latter encoding implies application of the metrical criterion (see previous subsections). That is, the visual system seems to avoid the metrical criterion in favour of the structural criterion.

An illustration is given in Figure 3.12. The stimulus in Figure 3.12A gives rise to two equivalent options dealing with S-shape and rectangle components (notice that other components give rise to more complex codes). According to one option (Figure 3.12B), the stimulus is taken as a curved 3-D object described by an S-shaped superstructure and relatively oriented subordinate rectangles. According to the other option (Figure 3.12C), the stimulus is taken as a flat 3-D object described by an S-shaped superstructure and absolutely oriented subordinate rectangles. The former concept involves application of the structural criterion whereas the latter concept involves application of the metrical criterion. Although both concepts are equally complex, the former concept is visually preferred (Hoffman and Richards, 1984), illustrating a preference for relatively oriented subordinate structures and, thereby, for application of the structural criterion.

The reason for this preference seems to lie in the fact that a constant orientation relative to the superstructure yields a more coherent percept than a constant absolute orientation does. This may be illustrated as follows. In case a code describes relative orientations of subordinate structures, a rotation of the superstructure equally applies to the whole object. In other words, this rotation does not change the object. This rotation invariance is illustrated in Figures 3.13AB and A'B'. In contrast, in case a code describes absolute orientations of subordinate structures, a rotation of the superstructure changes the object. This is illustrated in Figures 3.13CD and C'D'.

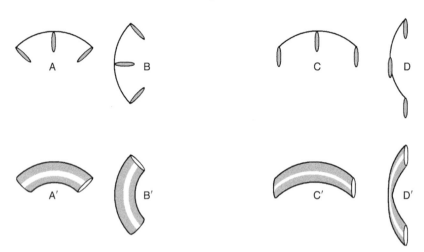

Figure 3.13 The 2-D patterns AB and the 3-D objects A'B' can be described as a curve plus relatively oriented subordinate structures. Then, a rotation of the superstructure implies that the entire pattern or object is rotated and, therefore, remains invariant. The 2-D patterns CD and the 3-D objects C'D' can be described as a curve plus absolutely oriented subordinate structures. Then, a rotation of the superstructure implies that the pattern or object changes.

Another factor relevant to this preference concerns the relation between code and shape components. Shape components which, according to a code, overlap each other in 2-D or in 3-D, actually belong to impossible figures. The so-called 'spatial contiguity' constraint, proposed by van der Helm and Leeuwenberg (1996) excludes such codes (see also Chapters 5 and 7). To show possible and real effects of this constraint, we return to Figure 3.13. If the code of Figure 3.13A would not prescribe three but, say, fifty subordinate ovals, then these ovals would overlap each other. As a 2-D configuration, the figure would be impossible and the code is not spatially contiguous. Only if the ovals are taken as projections of circles in the viewing plane, as shown in Figure 3.13A', and if these circles are described by the code, is the spatial contiguity restored – at least, as long as the circles are not so large that they would cross each other because, then, the code would again cease to be spatially contiguous.

The foregoing shows that the spatial contiguity constraint implies restrictions in case of relatively oriented subordinate structures (which imply application of the structural criterion), but it is even more restrictive in case of absolutely oriented subordinate structures (which imply

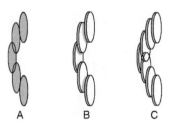

A   B   C

Figure 3.14 The three options ABC deal with the central part of Figure 3.13D. Option A shows overlapping ovals. These ovals are impossible in the picture plane. Option B is possible. It assumes separate circles in the viewing plane. Option C is again impossible. Like option B, it assumes circles but, due to their high number, it includes intertwined circles.

application of the metrical criterion). We illustrate this by way of Figure 3.14. It presents the central part of Figure 3.13D in more detail and with more subordinate shapes. The figure actually presents three options. First, Figure 3.14A shows five 2-D ovals, which overlap each other in the picture plane. So, their representation is not spatially contiguous. As argued earlier, the spatial contiguity of the description can be restored if these ovals are coded as circles in the viewing plane. This option is shown in Figure 3.14B. However, if the number of described circles increases, as in Figure 3.14C, the circles start to overlap each other so that the code is no longer spatially contiguous. The latter would apply to the solid object in Figure 3.13D' if this object is encoded using absolutely oriented subordinate structures. In general, for solid objects, spatial contiguity is violated where the orientation of the superstructure coincides with the absolute orientation of the subordinate structures. Notice that, in such a case, spatial contiguity cannot be restored by changing the size of components.

As a final example, we consider Figure 3.15. Figure 3.15A presents an object that can simply be described by way of relatively oriented triangular subordinate structures. Figure 3.15B presents an object which, equally simple, could be described by way of absolutely oriented triangular subordinate structures. The latter concept, however, implies that its parallel oriented triangular subpatterns are intertwined around the places where the orientation of the curve of the S-shape coincides with the orientation of the triangles. Hence, around these places, this description is not spatially contiguous. In fact, from this perspective, the shape belongs to an impossible figure. As has been argued by Boselie and Leeuwenberg (1986), an impossible figure can still be visually represented, namely,

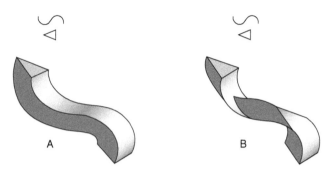

Figure 3.15 Object A can simply be represented by an S-structure and triangles being orientated locally orthogonal to the S-shape. Object B could be represented, equally simple, by an S shape and parallel oriented triangles, but this description is not spatially contiguous (Leeuwenberg and van der Helm, 1991).

as an assembly of parts which, by themselves, are possible. For Figure 3.15B, this implies a description of three parts which, by themselves, are spatially contiguous. This code, however, is more complex than the code of Figure 3.15A, which deals with relative orientations. Notice that Figure 3.15B could be described as an S-shape of relatively oriented triangles, but this code would have an unrealistically high complex load. Similar considerations apply to Figure 3.13D'.

In fact, the description of Figure 3.15B as a single S shape of parallel oriented triangles is a construct invented at the conscious level of problem solving rather than a construct at the level of perception. Our general conclusion therefore is that the visual system tends to avoid codes which imply the application of the metrical criterion, and that it favours codes which imply the application of the structural criterion.

Summary

A comparison is made between models that are guided by a process criterion (section 3.1) and models that use a representation criterion (section 3.2). The main question is which kind of model appropriately predicts visually preferred pattern interpretations.

Section 3.1 tests four simple linear stage models. These models prescribe subsequent stages according to some process criterion. The first model imposes a minimal information load per stage, the second model prescribes a maximal cluster per stage, the third model deals with the global precedence hypothesis of Navon (1977), and the fourth model with the orientation precedence hypothesis of Beck (1982). Illustrations show that these process models do not steadily lead to the visually preferred stimulus interpretations.

Section 3.2 attends to the fact that the simplest codes predict the preferred interpretations of the stimuli used to test the above linear stage models. Special attention is given to codes that reveal hierarchical relationships between superstructures and identical subordinate structures. In case the superstructure determines both the positions and orientations of subordinate components of patterns, the structural criterion is supposed to select the visually preferred code, that is, the simplest code. In case the superstructure merely determines the positions of the subordinate components, the code is as complex as the code with a reverse hierarchy, and then the metrical criterion is supposed to select the visually preferred code, that is, the code whose superstructure agrees with the largest component.

The superstructure is supposed to be visually more dominant than the subordinate structure. This assumption is proposed as an alternative to both the global precedence hypothesis and the orientation precedence hypothesis. Furthermore, the visual system seems to avoid codes which imply application of the metrical criterion. That is, it favours application of the structural criterion, in which case the resulting superstructure is visually more dominant even if it coincides with the smallest pattern component.

4 Models and principles

Introduction

In the previous chapter, we compared several process models (i.e., models which impose a criterion on the process mechanism) to a representation model (i.e., a model which imposes a criterion on the process outcome). In this chapter, we go into more detail on representation models. In the first section, two representation approaches are compared with each other. One is the recognition-by-components model (RBC) proposed by Biederman (1987). It starts from representations of pre-fixed elementary parts, and it assumes that a whole object is perceptually composed of these parts. The other is the structural information theory (SIT) approach. It starts, inversely, from the representation of the whole object, and it assumes that the perceived parts are determined by this representation. The second section deals with representation criteria for selecting the preferred object representation. Two principles are compared with each other. One is the likelihood principle and the other is the simplicity principle. The former is assumed by RBC and the latter by SIT.

4.1 Two representation models

RBC: from parts to wholes

The basic idea of RBC is that visual scenes are composed of components in the way words are composed of letters. For producing words, just twenty-six letters are sufficient. For describing complex objects, Biederman (1987) discerns twenty-four simple geometric components – called 'geons' – such as cones, wedges, blocks, and cylinders. Some exemplars are shown in Figure 4.1.

Any object is assumed to be visually composed of one or more geons, and the borders between geons are supposed to be inferred from local concavities in the stimulus pattern. The geons themselves are supposed to be identified or recognized by specific properties of their projections.

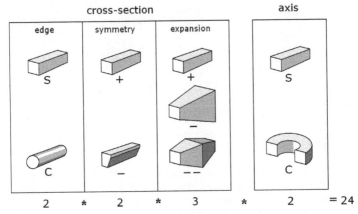

Figure 4.1 The RBC attributes (Biederman, 1987) are illustrated for nine geon objects. The S in column 1 refers to straight edges in the cross-section and the C to curved edges in the cross-section. The + in column 2 refers to a symmetrical cross-section and the − to an asymmetrical cross-section. The + in column 3 refers to a constant cross-section, the − to an increasing cross-section, and the − − to an increasing and decreasing cross-section. The S in column 4 refers to a straight axis and the C to a circular axis. These pre-specified shape attributes give rise to twenty-four different geons (Leeuwenberg and van der Helm, 1991).

These properties are called non-accidental properties (NAPs). Instances are linearity, parallelism, and symmetry (see section 4.2).

Here, we do not consider experiments showing how well geons are visually identified from projections of normal and degraded complex objects. Moreover, we disregard how the actual geon identification process has been elaborated by Biederman (1987) and implemented in an algorithm. We merely consider how objects are classified as geons on the basis of their NAPs. Four variable aspects are supposed to specify a geon. Three aspects apply to the cross-section and one aspect deals with the axis. The axis is orthogonal to the cross-section. The four variable aspects are:

(1) the edges of the cross-section are straight (S) or circular (C);
(2) the cross-section is bilaterally symmetrical (+) or asymmetrical (−);
(3) the course of the cross-section along the axis either is constant (+), or expanding (−), or both expanding and contracting (− −);
(4) the axis is straight (S) or circular (C).

In Figure 4.1, the four aspects are illustrated by nine geons. All combinations of these aspects, each with the given two or three subcategories, give rise to 2 * 2 * 3 * 2 = 24 different geons.

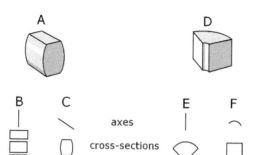

Figure 4.2 A and D are objects that miss a specific longest axis. Then, the geon is chosen whose cross-section is constant or symmetrical. For instance, A gives rise to geon option B or C. The vertical axis of B implies a variable cross-section and the horizontal viewing axis of C implies a constant cross-section. Hence, option C is preferred. Likewise, D gives rise to E or F. Both the straight axis of E and the circular axis of F imply constant cross-sections. However, the cross-section of E reveals less axes of symmetry (1) than the cross-section of F (4). Hence, F is preferred (Leeuwenberg and van der Helm, 1991).

Commonly, the axis agrees with the longest geon component, but there are objects with equally long components. For such objects the axis is determined by structural factors. Namely, the axis is the one for which the cross-section is constant or symmetric or both. Illustrations are presented in Figure 4.2. Of Figure 4.2A, two visualized descriptions are presented in Figures 4.2BC. In these descriptions, the axis is steadily indicated above the cross-section. The description in Figure 4.2B presumes a vertical axis, but then the cross-section is not constant. The description in Figure 4.2C presumes a horizontal axis, and then the cross-section is constant. Therefore, the latter description is preferred by RBC. Of Figure 4.2D, two visualized descriptions are shown in Figures 4.2EF. In both descriptions, constant cross-sections are involved. However, the cross-section in Figure 4.2E is less symmetrical than the one in Figure 4.2F. Therefore, the latter description is preferred by RBC.

A geon presents a solid object, but there is no objection to use geon coding to describe a hole. Figure 4.3 illustrates two applications. One deals with the nut in Figure 4.3A. Its plausible description, $A = B - C$, comprises one positive and one negative geon. Figure 4.3D may stand for the bow of a ship. Along the vertical axis, the cross-section expands in one respect and increments in another respect. So, this bow cannot be described by a single geon. Instead, it can be represented by three geons,

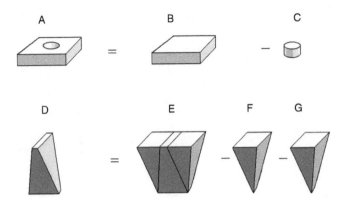

Figure 4.3 The nut shape A cannot be described by a single geon. A plausible solution is to represent the shape by a positive geon for the convex component and by a negative geon for the concave component, namely, by A = B – C. Equally, D cannot be described as a single geon. Its cross-section both expands and increments along the vertical axis. A correct description is D = E – F – G. However, this solution is visually hardly plausible (Leeuwenberg and van der Helm, 1991).

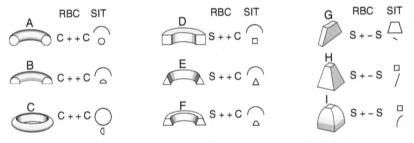

Figure 4.4 Coding according to RBC (discussed in this subsection) and SIT (discussed in next subsection). According to RBC, A, B, and C are three objects with the same geon description. The same holds for the objects D, E, and F and the objects G, H, and I. In contrast, the SIT codes of the nine objects are all different.

namely, by one positive and two negative geons according to D = E – F – G. In our view, however, this complex composition description of the bow is visually hardly plausible.

A strong and appealing property of RBC coding is its classification of objects. However, in some cases, this classification seems too broad. This may be illustrated as follows. The objects in Figures 4.4ABC are all described by similar geons, with circular cross-sections and circular axes. The rule is that the circular property C is attributed to a

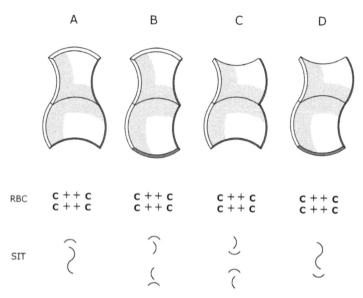

Figure 4.5 According to RBC, all four shapes A to D are composed of pairs of geons with equal geon codes and should therefore look like object pairs. Without doubt this holds for B and C. However, visually, A and D rather are single objects. The account of SIT (see next section) is as follows. B and C are described each by two superstructures and two subordinate structures, that is, as object pairs, whereas A and D are described each by a single superstructure and a single subordinate structure, that is, as single objects.

cross-section or axis if it has at least one circular edge. The consequence is that no differentiation is made between open and closed cross-sections and axes. In our view, however, such differences are not gradual but are categorical. The same holds for the objects in Figures 4.4DEF. All of them are classified as similar geons, characterized by symmetrical straight edge cross-sections and circular axes. Nevertheless, their cross-sections are squares, triangles, and trapezoids. Furthermore, all objects in Figures 4.4GHI are classified as similar geons with expanding rectangular cross-sections and straight axes. However, visually, these objects seem different rather than similar. So, geon classification tends to disregard not only metrical but also structural differences between objects. In the next section, we reconsider these and other objects and we show how SIT describes them.

Figure 4.5 illustrates a similar lack of coding differentiation but, this time, because of a missing account of mutual relations between adjacent object components. The figure presents four objects consisting of two parts. According to the strict rules of RBC, each object is composed of a pair of geons with the same C + + C geon code. This description is plausible for Figures 4.5BC. After all, the discontinuities between their parts facilitate the identification of the two geons within each object. In effect, the axis of the top part of Figure 4.5B is attached to the cross-section of the bottom part, and the cross-section of the top part of Figure 4.5C is attached to the axis of the bottom part. For Figures 4.5AD, the geon-twin descriptions are less obvious. In Figure 4.5A, the two parts share axes, and in Figure 4.5D, the two parts share cross-sections. As a consequence, their top and bottom parts are smoothly connected. Therefore, single geon descriptions seem appropriate. However, in Figure 4.5A, a single geon description implies a horizontal axis which does not agree with the largest component, and in Figure 4.5D, a single geon description implies a vertical axis with the two opposed circular curves of an S-shape. Therefore, the two shapes should still be represented as geon-twins. Apparently, the RBC coding does not differentiate between the duality of Figures 4.5BC and the unity of Figures 4.5AD.

Within RBC, the geon axis is defined as the longest object component but precisely therefore the geon codes of the single geon objects in Figure 4.6 lead to implausible classifications. These codes, presented both in a visualized and in a formal fashion below the objects, are discussed here in more detail. In Figure 4.6A, the longest component is a circular axis and the cross-section is an irregular polygon. The formal geon code is S – + C. The S stems from the straight edges of the cross-section, the – from the asymmetry of the cross-section, the + from the constancy of the cross-section, and the C refers to the circular axis. In Figure 4.6B, the longest component is a straight vertical axis and the cross-section is a variable circle. The formal geon code is C + – – S. The C stems from the circular edges of the cross-section, the + from the symmetry of the cross-section, the – – from the expansion and contraction of the cross-section, and the S refers to the straight vertical axis. In Figure 4.6C, the longest component is a straight line and the cross-section is a variable, partly curved, rectangle. Its formal geon code is also C + – – S. The C stems from two curved edges of the cross-section. Remember, the rule is that C is attributed if the cross-section has at least one circular edge. The + is due to the symmetry of the cross-section, the – – refers to the expansion and contraction of the cross-section, and the S stems from the straight axis.

In effect, the RBC codes of Figures 4.6AB are quite different and those of Figures 4.6BC are similar. However, a judged similarity experiment shows that Figures 4.6AB are visually similar and that Figures 4.6BC

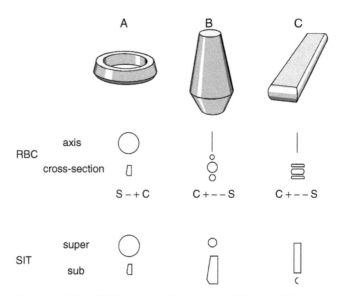

Figure 4.6 The RBC geon codes of A and B are different and those of B and C are similar. In contrast, the SIT codes of A and B are similar and those of B and C are different (for details, see next section). Perceptually, A and B are more similar than B and C.

are quite different (Leeuwenberg *et al.*, 1994). In the next section, we reconsider the objects in the last three figures, and we show how SIT describes them.

SIT: from wholes to parts

In general, SIT differs from RBC as follows. Geons are pre-specified components of objects, so, the components are primary and an object is a derivative. In contrast, in SIT, the simplest code of an object is primary and the object's components are derived from the code. At a more technical level, there are three differences between RBC and SIT. First, the geon attributes of the cross-section and the axis – such as straight versus circular, symmetrical versus asymmetrical, constant versus expanding – are robust categories. In contrast, simplest SIT codes deal with components that may have any shape without any restriction. Furthermore, these codes are pattern construction recipes and, therefore, different for different stimuli. Second, RBC axes are supposed to agree with the largest stimulus component whereas SIT's superstructures are not metrically constrained. These different criteria affect object segmentations. Third, RBC codes represent classes of objects. In contrast, SIT codes describe both classes and individual objects. Under the condition that code elements are taken as variable parameters, the SIT codes describe classes of objects with the same structure, and under the condition that the code elements are taken as the actual stimulus elements, they describe individual objects. Before we elaborate on this topic, we illustrate the first two differences between RBC and SIT.

The first difference is illustrated in Figure 4.4. The RBC codes do not differentiate between the objects in each column. In contrast, the SIT codes, visualized by superstructures above subordinate structures, describe all objects differentially. As said, these codes prescribe the construction of the shapes (see Chapter 3).

The second difference, with respect to object segmentations, is illustrated in Figure 4.5. The RBC codes of Figures 4.5BC each reveal two separate axes. In fact, these axes agree with SIT superstructures. Hence, both figures are predicted to be twin shapes. For the same reason, RBC predicts Figures 4.5AD to be twin shapes. The simplest SIT codes of Figures 4.5AD, however, reveal single superstructures. Remember that SIT's code components may have any size and may refer to any shape. Hence, both figures are predicted to be single shapes. So, in line with the experiments (van Bakel, 1989), SIT predicts that Figures 4.5BC are preferably perceived as dual shapes and Figures 4.5AD as unitary shapes (for more details, see Chapter 10).

The difference with respect to object segmentations is illustrated also in Figure 4.6. In the RBC code of Figure 4.6A, the axis is a circle and the cross-section is an irregular polygon. SIT's superstructure agrees with the RBC axis and SIT's subordinate structure agrees with the RBC cross-section. The arguments to choose these components are different, however. The choice of the circular RBC axis is based on its length whereas the choice of the circular SIT superstructure is based on the simplicity of the code. Precisely for this reason, the RBC and SIT codes of Figure 4.6B differ. The RBC code deals with a straight vertical axis and varying circular cross-sections whereas the SIT code agrees with the code of Figure 4.6A, except for some metrical aspects. Its superstructure does not agree with the axis but with the cross-section of the RBC code. The RBC code of Figure 4.6C formally agrees with the code of Figure 4.6B whereas, this time, the SIT code of Figure 4.6C completely differs from that of Figure 4.6B. Its superstructure is a rectangle and the subordinate structure is a semi-circle. In fact, the SIT codes are in line with judged similarities (Leeuwenberg et al., 1994).

The third difference, with respect to object classification, is introduced as follows. The visualized SIT codes of Figures 4.6AB are similar but still different. So, the question is how their similarity comes across. The clue

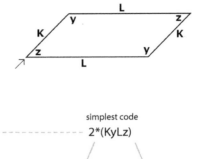

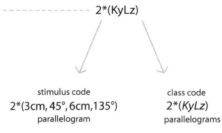

Figure 4.7 The primitive code of the parallelogram is the series of line lengths (K and L) and turns (y and z) along the contour. The maximal account of regularity in the primitive code leads to the simplest SIT code. If its symbols stand for concrete line lengths and turns, the code describes a specific parallelogram, but if its symbols are taken as parameters (italic symbols), the code describes the class of all parallelograms.

is that a code describes both a unique stimulus and a class of shapes with the same structure. To illustrate these two options, we first consider the encoding of the parallelogram in Figure 4.7. To obtain its code, letter symbols are assigned to line segments (K, L) and to turns (y, z) along the contour. Different symbols refer to different contour elements and identical symbols refer to identical contour elements. Then, these symbols are presented serially. Their order agrees with the order of contour scanning, say, clockwise. If the scanning starts at the point indicated by the arrow, the series of symbols will be: KyLzKyLz. This series is called the primitive code. Its information load (I') agrees with the number of symbols. Thus $I' = 8$. The next step is to reduce this load (Leeuwenberg, 1968, 1971). This can be achieved by means of the iteration rule. It transforms the primitive series into the code: 2*(KyLz) having load $I' = 4$. This code cannot be reduced further and is therefore the simplest description. Now, the double role of such a code may be illustrated as follows.

To illustrate that SIT codes describe both unique stimuli and classes of patterns we refer to a mathematical equation, for instance, $Y = aX + b$. It describes a specific line if a and b stand for specific metrical values,

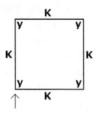

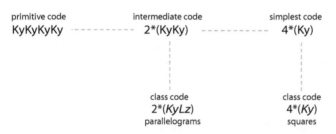

Figure 4.8 A less simple code describes a broader class. An instance is the partly simplified intermediate code of the square. Its parameter version describes the broad class of parallelograms. Only the parameter version of the simplest square code describes the specific class of squares.

and it describes a class of lines if a and b stand for variable parameters. Although this equation imposes a constraint on sets of points and a SIT code is a recipe for the stimulus reconstruction, the two representations share this double role. If the symbols in the $2^*(KyLz)$ code stand for quantified stimulus elements, that is, for actual line lengths and actual degrees of turns, the code describes a unique parallelogram. If the symbols stand for parameters, indicated by bold italic characters, the code is $2^*(\textbf{\textit{KyLz}})$ and describes the class of all parallelograms (under the condition of contour closure). Note that this class includes all simple versions of parallelograms, such as diamonds, rectangles, and squares, but excludes more complex patterns, like trapezoids. In fact, the idea of classes of patterns as being induced by a pattern itself and the idea of set inclusion stems from Garner (1962, 1966, 1970).

Notice that, in contrast to a simplest code, a non-simplest code of a pattern represents a class of more complex patterns. This is demonstrated in Figure 4.8 for a square. Its simplest class code $4^*(\textbf{\textit{Ky}})$ describes all squares and not more complex patterns. A less simple code, however, may describe all parallelograms, for instance. This may be explicated as follows. A less simple code of the square, for instance the intermediate

code 2*(KyKy), actually disregards the identity of the doubly represented Ky pairs of symbols. To express this blindness, all its symbols
are, irrespective of their identity, replaced by different parameters, for
instance, by K, y, L, and z (Collard and Buffart, 1983). This leads
to the class code 2*(**KyLz**), but precisely this inefficient class code of
the square agrees with the simplest class code of a parallelogram (see
Figure 4.7). An instance of an extremely inefficient square code is its
primitive code. The class version describes all regular and irregular
quadrangles.

The latter consideration reveals an interesting property of the simplicity
concept. We have shown that an inefficient or complex code describes a
class of patterns that are more complex than the stimulus pattern itself.
However, such a code would be not only inefficient but also inaccurate as
it would reflect a failure to perceive identical pattern elements. Inversely,
the simplest code, which describes the most concise class of patterns,
stems from the most accurate account of identical pattern elements. In
this sense, simplicity is equivalent to accuracy.

In conclusion, RBC might be suited to represent artificial, man-made,
objects but seems too rigid to describe the varying shapes in nature. In
this respect, SIT seems more appropriate, because it allows for a more
flexible description and classification of objects.

4.2   Two perception principles

In perception research, two general representation principles have been
proposed to deal with the selection of the preferred stimulus representation (see also Chapter 5). One is the likelihood principle. It states that the
preferred stimulus representation agrees with the most probable one in
reality (Gregory, 1980; Rock, 1983; von Helmholtz, 1909/1962). Thus,
its origin is the external reality. The other is the simplicity principle.
It states that the preferred stimulus representation is the simplest of all
possible ones (Hochberg and McAlister, 1953; Koffka, 1935). This principle does not refer to an external reality. Its origin is internal (Goodman,
1972; Sober, 1975).

Within scientific research, likelihood is the obvious selection criterion.
Only if there are two equally veridical theories, the simplest theory is to
be preferred (cf. Hawking, 1988). However, science and perception are
different. As we argued in Chapter 1.2, science deals with reasoning and
aims at establishing propositions, that is, at properties of given objects,
whereas perception aims at objects given retinal properties. Accordingly,
science makes use of knowledge stored in the brain as well as in literature

whereas it is even the question whether perception is anyhow affected by knowledge. So, it is not obvious that the likelihood criterion is appropriate for perception.

Notice that, in this section, we do not compare the simplicity and likelihood principles as such (for this, see Chapter 5). Rather, we focus on verbal claims which have been proposed to be justifiable by the likelihood principle but which, as we argue, actually presuppose the simplicity principle (Leeuwenberg and Boselie, 1988a, 1988b). Whereas the principles as such pertain to the selection of the most simple or most probable distal stimulus, these verbal claims pertain to properties of distal stimuli and, thereby, to categories of distal stimuli.

The likelihood principle

In determining the likelihood of a stimulus representation, two factors play a role. In fact, these factors agree with the two components of the Bayes rule. One factor deals with the conditional probability that a given hypothetical object generates a specific retinal projection. This factor is positively affected by the projective invariance of an object under varying viewpoints and is called the 'view-based likelihood'. The other factor is the prior or unconditional probability. This factor is positively affected by the frequency of occurrence of a given hypothetical object in the real world. This frequency is supposed to be assessed during the evolution of our ancestors and this information is assumed to be hereditary. This factor also is called the 'world-based likelihood'. Next, we discuss two approaches of perception that have been claimed to be justified by the likelihood principle.

Non-accidental properties As we mentioned earlier, Biederman's (1987) RBC makes use of NAPs, and the validity of these NAPs is supposed to be based on the likelihood principle. The argument is as follows. An NAP of an object's projection is a property that is most likely also a property of the object itself. For instance, linearity is an NAP. After all, in virtually any orientation, a straight line object, such as a straight wire or a straight object edge, generates a straight line projection. Under the realistic assumption of a restricted visual resolution, any other 2-D shape, say a hook object, might generate a straight line projection. However, this rarely happens. Therefore, a straight line stimulus probably is the projection of a straight line object. This claim agrees with the so-called general viewpoint assumption which states that an object usually presents itself without the coincidences due to a specific viewpoint.

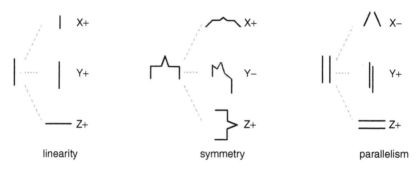

| linearity | symmetry | parallelism |

Figure 4.9 X stands for the horizontal axis, Y for the vertical axis, and Z for the viewing axis being perpendicular to the picture plane. Under all rotations about these axes a linear stick generates a straight line projection. Therefore, linearity is a completely valid non-accidental property (NAP). Symmetry and parallelism are less valid NAPs. A vertical symmetry structure generates a symmetrical projection under all rotations about the X and Z axes but not about the Y axis, and a vertical parallel structure generates a parallel projection under all rotations about the Y and Z axes but not about the X axis.

Not only linearity but also symmetry and parallelism are NAPs. However, the latter two properties are less valid NAPs than linearity. This is illustrated by Figure 4.9. X stands for the horizontal axis in the picture plane, Y for the vertical axis, and Z for the viewing axis being perpendicular to the picture plane. Under all rotations about these axes, a linear line object generates a straight line projection. A vertical symmetry structure generates a symmetrical projection under all rotations about the X and Z axes but not about the Y axis, and a vertical parallel structure generates a parallel projection under all rotations about the Y and Z axes but not about the X axis. In fact, the failures are due to perspective effects. Nevertheless, all mentioned NAPs are of use to infer more or less likely object properties from their projections (Biederman, 1987).

The specific length of a straight line stimulus is not an NAP. The reason is that this stimulus not only might stem from a straight line object viewed orthofrontally but also from slanted line objects with longer lengths. Therefore, quantitative measures are not considered to be NAPs (Biederman, 1987; Leeuwenberg *et al.*, 1994). Notice that the NAP justification, so far, merely deals with the view-based likelihood.

Avoidance of coincidence The aforementioned perceptual tendency to ignore coincidental viewpoints actually is a special case of the

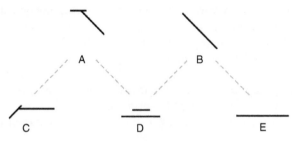

Figure 4.10 A and B are proximal stimuli. C, D and E are supposed to be equally frequent distal objects that merely may rotate clockwise. So, the likelihood that A stems from C is equal to the likelihood that B stems from E. This likelihood is higher than the likelihood that A and B stem from the composition of the two line objects in D. Nevertheless, A is sooner taken as a composition than B is. Rock's (1983) argument would be that a composition is less coincidental for A than for B. This argument is criticized in the next subsection.

'avoidance of coincidence' principle proposed by Rock (1983). Also this principle deals with the view-based likelihood component of the Bayes rule. It applies to any kind of coincidence including, for instance, the simultaneous occurrence of a bang and a light flash. This pair of events is preferably interpreted as a single explosion and not as a coincidental occurrence of a bang from one source and a light flash from another source. Another illustration is presented by Figure 1.5A. It shows twelve billiard balls positioned in a circle. If this configuration is taken as the final result of throwing balls on a billiard table, one tends to assume some kind of magnet underneath the table to explain the regular configuration. In other words, one does not accept coincidences but assumes a common cause that explains coincidences.

Figure 4.10 illustrates Rock's avoidance of coincidence principle of perception. It presents the proximal stimuli A and B and the distal wire objects C, D, and E. Under the condition that these objects are equally frequent options and merely may rotate clockwise, the probability that the T stimulus in Figure 4.10A stems from the T object in Figure 4.10C is equal to the probability that the line stimulus in Figure 4.10B stems from the line object in Figure 4.10E. Furthermore, it is clear that this probability is higher than the probability that the stimuli stem from the combination of the two line objects in Figure 4.10D.

The main focus will be now on Figures 4.10ABD, that is, on the stimuli interpreted as compositions of two line objects. The claim is that the T stimulus consists more probably of two line objects than the single line stimulus. The argument is that the set of two line objects with varying points of attachment and varying turns is larger than the set of two precisely aligned line objects. It is supposed that for this reason the stimulus in Figure 4.10A is taken as a composition of two line objects rather than as the stimulus in Figure 4.10B. In the first stimulus, the two components are weakly attached. In the second stimulus they are strongly attached. After all, the highly improbable coincidence of aligned line objects is avoided by assuming a common cause, namely, their attachment.

In summary, NAPs of stimuli seem to be likely properties of objects, and the avoidance of coincidence principle seems to be a plausible criterion for selecting the visually preferred object components.

The simplicity principle

Above, we argued that the claims about the NAPs, dealing with viewpoints, and about the avoidance of coincidence, dealing with compositions, are justified by the view-based likelihood. According to the Bayes rule, however, this justification is not enough; that is, the justification should also include the world-based likelihood. This is discussed in this section in which we also look at a justification of the claims in terms of the simplicity principle.

On viewpoints In terms of the view-based likelihood component of the Bayes rule, the earlier mentioned NAPs are justifiable. We will illustrate this, once more, as follows for the linearity NAP. A retinal straight line stimulus probably is the projection of a straight line object and not of a non-straight line object because, in virtually any orientation, a straight line object generates a straight line projection, whereas a 2-D non-linear shape, such as a hook object, rarely generates a straight line projection.

As said, this justification not only holds for linearity but also for symmetry and parallelism. In fact, this justification even holds for non-linearity, asymmetry, and non-parallelism, but such NAPs are not taken as geon attributes. This raises the question why RBC uses only NAPs that refer to regularities. That is, in our view, simplicity obviously plays an implicit role in RBC.

Another issue is the role of world-based likelihood in perception. Let us, for the moment, assume that it is assessed in the same way as the view-based likelihood, namely by computational inference. That is, let us assume that it is assessed not on the basis of observations but on the basis of all theoretically possible different cases. For the view-based likelihood, this means that it is assessed on the basis of all theoretically possible orientations of an object. Analogously, we assume that the world-based likelihood is assessed on the basis of all theoretically possible objects. Under the additional assumption of a restricted visual resolution, the consequence for the linearity NAP is as follows.

The linearity NAP reflects the verbal claim that proximal straightness is most likely caused by distal straightness and not by distal non-straightness. To evaluate this NAP, let us consider the category of all possible straight line objects and the category of all possible 2-D non-straight line objects. Given the restricted visual resolution, the number of possible straight line objects with different lengths is limited. Furthermore, the probability that a 2-D non-straight line object generates a straight line projection is small, but not zero. After all, the number of 3-D orientations of a 2-D object also is limited. However, the number of all different 2-D non-straight line objects is countless. These objects vary with respect to their number of line components while each component varies with respect to position, length, and orientation. Thus, countless different 2-D non-straight line objects might generate, each with non-zero probability, a straight line projection. As Leeuwenberg *et al.* (1994) showed, this implies a higher likelihood that a straight line projection stems from a non-straight line object than from a straight line object. In other words, in the virtual world of computational inference, the world-based likelihood overrules the view-based likelihood. This problem does not occur if one starts from the simplicity principle because, then, the linearity NAP can be justified simply on the basis of the relatively low complexity of straight line objects.

Similar considerations apply to the other NAPs shown in Figure 4.9, and it remains to be seen whether the justification in terms of likelihoods does hold in the real world (see also Gigerenzer and Murray, 1987; Pomerantz and Kubovy, 1986). Then, it should deal with the actually existing objects that may generate straight line projections and with the frequencies of these objects. However, the assumption that knowledge about these objects is acquired by learning (Brunswick, 1956) suffers from the objections indicated in Chapter 1. One objection is as follows. Perception is supposed to be a source of knowledge, so, if perception is guided by knowledge, then it actually makes use of its own output and would be involved in a circular loop (Hoffman, 1996; van der Helm, 2000). This objection holds irrespective of whether knowledge is ontogenetic (i.e., acquired during a life span) or phylogenetic (i.e., cumulated over generations during evolution). Moreover, in the latter case knowledge should be hereditary but there is no indication that knowledge is hereditary.

Our tentative conclusion is that the role of NAPs in RBC is justifiable with respect to the view-based likelihood but not with respect to the world-based likelihood. Nevertheless, the likelihood principle and the simplicity principle have the same claims about the visual NAP effects. Both principles attribute linear objects to linear stimuli, and symmetrical objects to symmetrical stimuli.

On compositions Here, we return to Figure 4.10 with the focus on the two proximal stimuli A and B and the distal option D. The claim is that stimulus A is taken as a composition of two straight line objects more quickly than stimulus B. According to the avoidance of coincidence principle (Rock, 1983), presented in the previous subsection, a composition is less coincidental for A than for B. In our view, however, this argument is not sound. Notice that A and B, taken as unique stimuli, are equally probable compositions of two straight line objects. Only if A and B are taken as representatives of classes of stimuli, they are not equally probable compositions of D components. However, where do these classes come from? That is, the conditional likelihood is derived from class size, but then, where are the classes derived from? Though from another perspective, an answer has in fact already been given in section 4.1: because of its irregularity, pattern A is described by a less simple code than pattern B and a less simple code represents a larger class of patterns than a more simple code does. So, classes are derivable from the simplicity of pattern codes. This means that this simplicity is silently presupposed by the above likelihood argument. However, then, the question is why the likelihood argument should make the detour of first assessing codes, then their loads, then their class size, and finally their likelihood, to draw a conclusion which directly stems from the simplicity principle.

Let us finally focus on another triad within Figure 4.10, namely, stimulus B and its two distal options D and E. As said earlier, it is less likely that stimulus B stems from the two straight line objects D than from the single straight line object E, and the conditional likelihood principle favours the same conclusion as the simplicity principle. Another issue concerns the unconditional or world-based likelihood. It deals with the numbers of existing short line objects and long line objects. However, the question is what are objects according to the world-based likelihood? To our knowledge, the world-based likelihood approach does not favour specific stimulus parts over others. In other words, any part of a stimulus can be taken as an object. However, there are more short objects than long objects. After all, long straight line objects consist of many short ones whereas short ones do not consist of long ones. Ultimately, the world-based likelihood would overrule the view-based likelihood in favour of option D with the odd consequence that the single line stimulus B would stem from two line objects rather than from one single line object (Leeuwenberg, 2003).

All in all, NAPs are view invariant properties which are justifiable on the basis of conditional likelihoods. However, they are not justifiable on the basis of unconditional likelihoods. The assessment of the latter likelihood presupposes objects to explain perception whereas perception is supposed to establish objects. Besides, it assumes hereditary knowledge whereas there is no indication for that. For the same reasons, visual compositions cannot be explained on the basis of unconditional likelihoods. These compositions can be explained by conditional likelihoods but only if one presupposes a classification based on descriptive simplicity.

Summary

Section 4.1 compares RBC and SIT representations of objects. The differences are as follows. According to RBC, a complex object is taken as a composition of elementary prefixed object-components, called geons. Each geon is characterized by attributes of its cross-section and axis. According to SIT, there are no pre-specified object-components. The simplest code of a whole object is primary and the object components are derived from this code. In fact, geon attributes are categories with a pre-specified but global content. As a consequence, rather different objects are represented by the same geons. In contrast, SIT codes deal with components that may have any shape. These codes are pattern construction recipes and, therefore, different for different stimuli. Furthermore, the hierarchy in RBC coding is partly determined by metrical shape aspects. The axis of a geon is the longest object component. A SIT code deals with structural hierarchy determined by simplicity of the representation. SIT's superstructure sometimes coincides with the RBC axis, sometimes with the cross-section, and sometimes it does not coincide with any geon component. Finally, SIT codes also describe classes of objects with the same structure, namely, if the code elements are taken as variable parameters.

Section 4.2 deals with the likelihood and the simplicity principles of perception (see also Chapter 5). In most cases, the conditional or view-based component of the likelihood principle explains visual pattern classification. However, to clarify coincidental junctions, this likelihood component assumes pattern classification whereas it is supposed to explain pattern classification. This classification is determined by the simplicity of their representations. The world-based unconditional likelihood is equally circular. Its assumption is that the output of perception is used as its input. Moreover, this likelihood component assumes hereditary knowledge but there is no evidence for that.

5   Assumptions and foundations

Introduction

Structural information theory (SIT) assumes that the visual system selects the simplest organization among all organizations possible for a given stimulus. Thereby, it integrates the notions of phenomenal simplicity and descriptive simplicity (Hatfield and Epstein, 1985). Phenomenal simplicity refers to the idea that the visual system tends to capture a maximum of stimulus regularities – such regularities reflect meaningful invariants in the external world. Descriptive simplicity refers to the idea that the visual system tends to minimize the informational content of mental representations – this implies an efficient usage of internal brain resources. SIT combines these tendencies under the motto: the more regular an organization is, the less information is needed to specify it. Here, we give an overview of this approach, by means of paradigmatic starting points, modeling considerations, and theoretical foundations.

5.1   Visual information processing

Science is an endeavour to capture the reality we experience by means of metaphors that enable us to understand or control this reality. To understand perceptual organization, SIT uses the so-called broad computer metaphor. This metaphor does not imply that the brain is conceived as a computer, but it implies, more generally, that the brain is conceived as an information processing system. Furthermore, in Marr's (1982) terms, SIT is primarily a theory at the computational level of description of information processing systems, that is, not at the algorithmic or implementational levels. It accepts the implementational means (i.e., neural structures) as a source of constraints on the algorithmic method (i.e., cognitive processes), but it focuses on the computational goal (i.e., mental representations). The idea is that insight in characteristics of mental representations forms the basis for insight in principles guiding cognitive

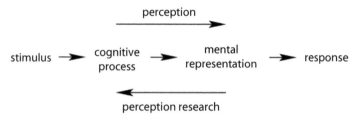

Figure 5.1 Perception and perception research. To understand stimulus-response relations, behaviourism focuses on the responses, and computational approaches like SIT focus on the mental representations. Both are scientifically necessary steps to gain insight into cognitive processes; as philosopher Søren Kierkegaard (1813–55) put it: 'Life can only be understood backward'.

processes (see Figure 5.1). Later in this chapter, we substantiate this idea by discussing what SIT implies with regard to cognitive processing. In this section, we discuss ideas about visual information processing in general.

Cognition and the world

Structure and information are rather vague notions, but generally, structure refers to a configural property and information to the content of messages. SIT combines these terms into the notion of structural information, which refers to the content of codes specifying organizations of distal stimuli that fit a proximal stimulus. The complexity of the organizations is defined by the amount of structural information in the codes, that is, by the amount of information needed to specify the organizations. Different codes may specify different organizations, and the simplest code is assumed to specify the organization humans perceive. In other words, in SIT, simplest codes model the messages the visual system transmits to higher cognitive levels.

Furthermore, as we elaborate later in this chapter, SIT's coding approach to select simplest codes is equivalent to a Bayesian inference model in which higher probabilities are assigned to simpler things. That is, it integrates viewpoint-independent (or prior) complexities and viewpoint-dependent (or conditional) complexities (van der Helm, 2000). For a hypothesized distal stimulus that fits a given proximal stimulus, the prior complexity quantifies the goodness of the hypothesized objects as such; this captures aspects of object perception. Furthermore, the conditional complexity quantifies how well the hypothesized distal stimulus fits the proximal stimulus; this depends on the relative position of hypothesized objects in the proximal stimulus, and it captures aspects of spatial perception. This distinction between priors and conditionals agrees with the functional distinction between the ventral ('what') and dorsal ('where') pathways in the brain (Ungerleider and Mishkin, 1982).

The foregoing view on perception as a communication filter has several implications. First, although Shannon's (1948) ground-breaking work in classical information theory is not directly applicable to perceptual organization, general ideas from communication theory might yet be relevant to perception (see van der Helm, 2000). Second, it implies that perceptual organizations may be enriched at higher cognitive levels by knowledge acquired earlier but are not (or hardly) influenced by such knowledge before entering these higher cognitive levels. Perception thus is conceived as an autonomous source of knowledge about the world. Third, by filtering out a specific organization, perception provides cognition with a specific structure of the world. This structure, either or not enriched by knowledge acquired earlier, determines how we experience the world and how we react to it in recognition tasks or in visual search tasks, for instance (cf. Ahissar and Hochstein, 2004). Thus, conceiving perception as a communication filter may help to answer Koffka's (1935) question: why do things look as they do?

Objects are the output of perception

According to the classical Gestalt motto, the whole is something else than the sum of its parts (Koffka, 1935: 176). Building on this motto, SIT assumes that wholes result from (non-linear) interactions between parts. To be more precise, we assume that perceived wholes (i.e., objects as we experience them) result from interactions between the mental representations of parts. These interactions are assumed to be driven by similarities and differences between parts that may be anything in between perceived wholes and retinal receptive fields. In the next section, we address the question of choosing shape primitives in the empirical practice, but the point here is that we believe perception relies on interactions between things rather than on things as such.

An illustrative effect of such interactions occurs in visual search. The search for a target in a typical visual search display (e.g., a red item among many blue items) is easier as the distracters are more similar to each other and more different from the target (cf. Ahissar and Hochstein, 2004; Donderi, 2006; Duncan and Humphreys, 1989). In other words, a target may be a pop-out but only if the distracters allow it to be.

Therefore, we do not model perception in terms of special-purpose detectors of separate things but, rather, in terms of general-purpose coding rules for the extraction of regularities between things. Perceived wholes then are assumed to be simplest wholes, that is, wholes that result from extracting a maximum of regularity. In other words, the objects we experience do not belong to the input of perception but are the result of perception.

The simplicity principle

The Helmholtzian likelihood principle suggests that perception is guided by veridicality. This would imply that it selects the distal organization with the highest probability of reflecting the true distal stimulus that caused a given proximal stimulus, assuming it has access to such probabilities. In contrast, in the spirit of Occam's razor, the simplicity principle suggests that the visual system selects the simplest distal organization. This is not necessarily the true one, but as we discuss later in this chapter, veridicality yet seems an advantageous emergent side-effect if perception is guided by simplicity.

SIT's simplicity principle is an elaboration of Hochberg and McAlister's (1953) minimum principle, and both are information-theoretic translations of Koffka's (1935) law of Prägnanz. Fellow Gestaltist Wertheimer (1923) had discovered various perceptual grouping tendencies, and Koffka proposed that these tendencies are manifestations of the general tendency of physical systems to settle into relatively stable minimum-energy states. Accordingly, as mentioned in the Introduction, SIT assumes that the outcome of the perceptual organization process (i.e., the mental representation of a stimulus, or its percept, or its Gestalt) is reflected by a relatively stable cognitive state during an otherwise dynamical neural process. As also mentioned in the Introduction, in contrast to connectionist and dynamical systems approaches, SIT focuses on the perceptual nature of such relatively stable cognitive states and models them by simplest codes which are taken to specify perceived organizations. More pragmatic modeling aspects of this approach are discussed next.

5.2   Mental and symbolic codes

In the literature, one may read statements like 'representational approaches assume that the brain performs symbol manipulation'. Such a statement, however, falls in the same category as 'physics assumes that nature applies formulas'. Both statements mistake modeling tools for what is being modeled. Physics uses formulas such as Newton's $F = ma$

and Einstein's $E = mc^2$ to model dependency relationships between things thought to be relevant in nature. Likewise, representational approaches like SIT use symbolic codes to model structural relationships between things thought to be relevant in perception.

In both cases, domain-specific things are labeled with symbols to allow for formal reasonings. Such a labeling is called a semantic mapping and is primarily a conceptualization issue in the domain at hand. For instance, Newton used the symbol F to refer to 'force' which is nothing but a concept that, at the time, seemed practical to understand a natural phenomenon. Likewise, SIT uses symbols to refer to shape primitives that seem practical to understand perceptual organization; the symbolic codes then result from a formal coding model stated in terms of strings of these symbols.

The symbolic codes are meant to capture characteristics of mental representations, and the theoretical foundations in the next section are meant to support this. To ensure that the symbolic codes and the formalizations can indeed be said to be meaningful to perception, we impose two general demands on the semantic mapping. One demand is that codes constitute reconstruction recipes of distal stimuli. The other demand, called spatial contiguity, implies that codes respect the spatial layout of distal stimuli. In Chapter 7, these demands are exemplified extensively by means of concrete applications; here, we discuss the ideas behind these demands.

Codes are construction recipes

SIT assumes that the visual system, when presented with a proximal stimulus, yields a mental representation of a distal stimulus that fits the proximal stimulus. This mental representation is assumed to reflect information that specifies the distal stimulus up to a perceptually appropriate level of precision. Because SIT codes are meant to capture characteristics of such mental representations, these codes are taken to be descriptions from which distal stimuli can be reconstructed. This may be qualified further by the following outline of the coding model's procedure to obtain viewpoint-independent interpretations (see also Figure 5.2).

- First, for a given proximal stimulus, each candidate distal stimulus is represented by symbol strings. Each symbol in such a string refers to a shape primitive in the distal stimulus, such that the string forms a recipe to reconstruct the distal stimulus.
- Then, for each string, a simplest code is determined by applying coding rules that capture regularity in the string. This code specifies a

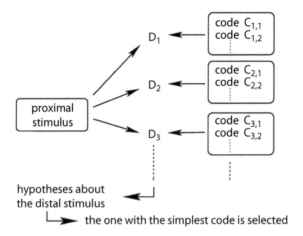

Figure 5.2 The simplicity principle in perceptual organization. Among the distal organizations that might account for a given proximal stimulus, the simplest one is predicted to be perceived.

hierarchical organization of the string and, thereby, also of the distal stimulus represented by the string.

- Finally, the overall simplest code is predicted to specify the perceptually preferred interpretation of the proximal stimulus. The mental representation thus is characterized by a hierarchical organization of a distal stimulus that fits the proximal stimulus.

Hence, SIT codes have more in common with computer codes than with the codes used in the Morse Code and by Shannon (1948), for instance. Whereas the former codes specify the construction of things, the latter codes are just conveniently chosen labels that refer to things without specifying the structure of these things, just as the word 'chair' does not specify how a chair looks like.

In the foregoing outline of the coding model, two modeling questions require further qualification. First, how to ensure that a hierarchical organization of a symbol string pertains to the distal stimulus represented by the symbol string? This question is addressed in the next subsection. Second, what are the shape primitives the symbols refer to? This question is addressed in the remainder of this subsection.

In contrast to, for instance, Biederman's (1987) recognition model, SIT does not start from some set of prefixed primitives but assumes that perceived parts, just as perceived wholes, are the result of the perceptual organization process. In practice, however, formal descriptions can start at an appropriate level of precision, side-stepping lower-level aspects. In

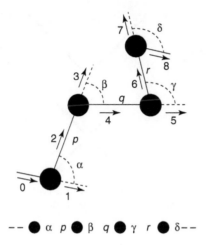

-- ● α p ● β q ● γ r ● δ--

Figure 5.3 Example of a semantic mapping for a random dot stimulus. The string below the stimulus specifies the parameters of a path (the solid line) that scans the stimulus in the order given by the numerals. The arrows indicate the orientation of the scanner. After each dot, two path parameters are needed to specify the relative position of the next dot.

molecular biology, for instance, the 3-D structure of RNA molecules usually can be studied starting from strings of nucleotides, without having to bother about the biochemical process that produced the strings. This is analogous to writing computer algorithms in terms of high-level instructions, without having to bother about the lower-level implementation of these instructions in terms of binary strings.

By the same token, we believe that perceptual phenomena can be studied meaningfully by starting formal descriptions at an empirically appropriate level of precision. For instance, suppose one wants to investigate symmetry detection. Then, it is good empirical practice to use a homogeneous stimulus set, that is, a set consisting of otherwise random symmetrical dot stimuli, for example. The empirically appropriate starting level for a formal description, then, is the level of dots and relative dot positions (see Figure 5.3), because the topic of interest can be assumed to be tractable without having to bother about lower level details (e.g., the pixels the dots are composed of) which, by construction, are not distinctive.

Hence, in general, for a given stimulus set, the semantic mapping can be chosen such that one gets a proper account of the stimulus variation at the level just below the topic of interest. See Chapter 7 for examples that also include the following demand.

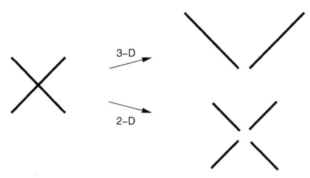

Figure 5.4 Spatial contiguity. The proximal stimulus at the left can, in a 3-D interpretation, be represented by two lines, but in a 2-D interpretation, it has to be represented by four lines.

The spatial contiguity demand

In the previous subsection, we mentioned that a SIT code specifies a hierarchical organization of a symbol string and, thereby, also of the distal stimulus represented by the string. This is not a trivial thing. If one would employ arbitrary coding rules, codes may not specify hierarchical organizations of strings at all, let alone of distal stimuli. Therefore, as we discuss in the next section, SIT demands the usage of so-called hierarchically transparent coding rules, which guarantee that codes specify hierarchical organizations of strings.

This does not yet ensure, however, that a hierarchical organization of a string pertains to the distal stimulus represented by the string. To this end, we require that every substring of the string refers to a spatially contiguous part of the distal stimulus. This simply means that adjacent symbols in the string refer to adjacent primitives in the distal stimulus. Then, segmentations of the string correspond one-to-one to segmentations of the distal stimulus. This, in turn, implies that a hierarchical organization of the string specifies the distal stimulus by a hierarchical organization with properly nested substructures.

The spatial-contiguity demand implements van Tuijl and Leeuwenberg's (1980) object principle, which states that codes should respect the spatial layout of distal stimuli. For instance, it implies that two crossing lines can be represented by one symbol each to describe a 3-D interpretation but not to describe a 2-D interpretation (see Figure 5.4). To be clear, a symbol string does not have to preserve all spatial characteristics of a distal stimulus. A distal stimulus can be represented by many symbol strings and the subsequent encoding process determines which string leads to the simplest organization and, hence, which spatial characteristics are decisive.

The notion of spatial contiguity is also related to Palmer and Rock's (1994) idea that, initially, perception organizes the visual field into uniformly connected regions (i.e., closed regions of homogeneous properties) which, subsequently, may be parsed into subordinate units and grouped into superordinate units. A uniformly connected region is a spatially contiguous region, but spatial contiguity is more general: it applies not only to the units that enter the perceptual organization process but also to the units that result from it. Together, the two notions suggest the perceptual organization process initially locks onto uniformly connected regions and subsequently yields an organization in terms of spatially contiguous regions.

Finally, the spatial-contiguity demand can be seen as an offshoot or extension of SIT's above-mentioned demand that the employed coding rules are hierarchically transparent. As we discuss in the next section, the latter demand ensures that codes specify hierarchical organizations of strings. Hence, together, these two demands ensure that a code specifies a hierarchical organization not only of a symbol string but also of the distal stimulus represented by the symbol string.

5.3   Theoretical foundations

In the previous two sections, we sketched paradigmatic and modeling ideas adhered by SIT. Here, we give an overview of the theoretical foundations of these ideas. A first question concerns the veridicality of the simplicity principle. That is, SIT's implicit assumption is that simplest organizations are sufficiently veridical to guide us through the world – otherwise, such a visual system would probably not have survived during the evolution. A second question, raised by Simon (1972), concerns the details of the coding model. That is, in order that the model's structural descriptions can plausibly be said to reflect mental representations of interpretations, the employed coding rules and complexity metric should have a psychological basis. A third question, raised by Hatfield and Epstein (1985), is the question of how the visual system might select a simplest interpretation from among the huge number of intepretations that are generally possible for a given stimulus. These three fundamental questions have been addressed within SIT, yielding answers that are sketched in the following subsections (for more details on these three answers, see van der Helm, 2000, 2004, 2011, 2012, 2013; van der Helm and Leeuwenberg, 1991, 1996, 1999, 2004).

Veridicality by simplicity

In order that vision is sufficiently veridical to guide us through the world, it seems necessary that vision somehow has knowledge about the world. However, findings from the mathematical domain of algorithmic information theory (AIT, or the theory of Kolmogorov complexity; see Li and Vitányi, 1997) suggest that this is not necessary. Here, we give the gist of this, by contrasting the simplicity principle to the likelihood principle.

The likelihood principle models vision as being a form of hypothesis testing and holds that the visual system selects the interpretation that is most likely true (von Helmholtz, 1909/1962). This implies, by definition, a high degree of veridicality. To this end, it assumes that vision somehow has knowledge about the probabilities of interpretations being correct (e.g., probabilities in terms of frequencies of occurrence in the world). As we discuss next in Bayesian terms, this includes both prior and conditional probabilities.

For an interpretation or hypothesis H, the prior probability $p(H)$ is the probability of H being correct, independently of the actual proximal stimulus. The conditional probability $p(D|H)$ of a hypothesis H is the probability that the proximal stimulus D arises if the distal stimulus is as hypothesized in H. In other words, the prior probability accounts for viewpoint independencies, whereas the conditional probability accounts for viewpoint dependencies. Thus, in terms of the Bayes rule, the likelihood principle states that, for a proximal stimulus D, the visual system selects the interpretation H that maximizes

$$p(H|D) = p(H) * p(D|H)$$

where the posterior probability $p(H|D)$ is the probability that H specifies the actually present distal stimulus (see also Chater, 1996; Li and Vitányi, 1997).

For instance, to decide between the two interpretations in Figure 5.5, one would have to know the prior probabilities of the shapes in B and C, as well as the conditional probabilities that the stimulus in A may arise for each of these two shapes. The conditional probabilities do not seem to pose a big problem: it is fairly obvious that, to obtain the stimulus in A, the arrowlike shape in C would have to assume a more coincidental position with respect to the parallelogram than the shape in B would have to assume. Hence, the conditional probabilities favour the shape in B. However, according to the Bayes rule, also the prior probabilities have to be taken into account, and there seems to be no way of telling which of the two shapes has a higher prior probability.

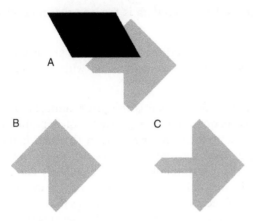

Figure 5.5 Pattern A is readily interpreted as a parallelogram partly occluding the shape in B, rather than the arrow in C. This preference could be claimed to occur either because, unlike shape B, the arrow would have to take a rather coincidental position to yield pattern A, or because shape B is simpler than the arrow. Probably, however, both aspects play a role (van der Helm, 2000).

Hence, although the likelihood principle is appealing, the problem is that it is unclear where, in particular, the prior probabilities come from. That is, it is unclear how vision, or vision research for that matter, might have knowledge about the prior probabilities. Furthermore, notice that the usage of probabilities presupposes not only the interpretations to be judged, but also a categorization of things in the world (see Chapter 4) – the likelihood principle is silent about these issues as well.

These problems do not arise if one starts from the simplicity principle, which holds that the visual system selects the interpretation with the most simple structural description. A structural description implies a categorization (e.g., the simplest description of a square categorizes it as belonging to the set of all theoretically possible squares). The size of these descriptive categories correlates with the complexity of their structural descriptions, and can be used to assign artificial probabilities under the motto: simpler things get higher probabilities. These artificial probabilities, called precisals, may differ from real probabilities in a specific world but which, as elaborated by van der Helm (2000), do suggest a fair degree of veridicality in many worlds.

To give the gist of this, we again distinguish between viewpoint independencies and viewpoint dependencies, but this time, quantified by prior complexities and conditional complexities, respectively. Analogous to the likelihood principle, the simplicity principle models vision as being a form of hypothesis testing, but this time, under the motto:

The best hypothesis to explain given data is the one that minimizes the sum of:

(a) the information needed to describe the hypothesis as such; and
(b) the information needed to describe the data with the help of the hypothesis.

The amount of information in (a) then is the prior complexity $I(H)$ of a hypothesis H, that is, it quantifies the goodness of hypothesis H as such. Furthermore, the amount of information in (b) then is the conditional complexity $I(D|H)$ which quantifies how well hypothesis H fits data D; quantitatively, this conditional complexity $I(D|H)$ corresponds to the number of coincidences one would count intuitively in the relative position of hypothesized objects. Together, this implies that the simplicity principle holds that, for a proximal stimulus D, the visual system selects the interpretation H that minimizes

$$I(H|D) = I(H) + I(D|H)$$

where the posterior complexity $p(H|D)$ is the complexity of interpretation H given proximal stimulus D (see also Chater, 1996; Li and Vitányi, 1997).

Notice that, via $p = 2^{-I}$, this minimization formula is mathematically equivalent to the maximization formula given above for the likelihood principle. Unlike Chater's (1996) suggestion, however, this does not mean at all that the two principles are equivalent – what matters is what each principle puts in the maximization formula. That is, the likelihood principle puts in supposedly real probabilities p based on the size of presupposed categories of things in the world, whereas the simplicity principle puts in precisals 2^{-I} which are artificial probabilities derived from the complexity of individual things (under the motto: simpler things get higher precisals). This does not yet imply that the simplicity principle is veridical, but regarding its veridicality, the following two findings from AIT are relevant.

First, to obtain an ordinal complexity ranking of individual things, it appeared to matter hardly which coding language is used (as opposed to the fact that, in the likelihood paradigm, it does matter which probability distribution is assumed). This was proven mathematically by Solomonoff (1964a, 1964b), Kolmogorov (1965), and Chaitin (1969). In perception, Simon (1972) concluded the same on the basis of an empirical comparison of various perceptual coding models (including SIT).

Second, for an infinite number of probability distributions P, the margin between the real probability p and the artificial probability 2^{-I} was proven to be less than the complexity of the distribution P (for details, see

Li and Vitányi, 1997). This crucial proof means, to vision, that real prior probabilities $p(H)$ may still be quite different from artificial probabilities $2^{-I(H)}$ because, as said, there seems to be no way of telling what the real prior categories and probabilities are. It also suggests, however, that real conditional probabilities $p(D|H)$ might be close to artificial probabilities $2^{-I(D|H)}$ because an object usually gives rise to only a few different view categories, so that the conditional probability distribution is relatively simple. This is corroborated by the work of van Lier on amodal completion (van Lier *et al.*, 1994). That is, van Lier modeled viewpoint dependencies by way of an empirically successful formal quantification of conditional complexities, which agrees well with the conditional probabilities assumed intuitively within the likelihood paradigm. For instance, in Figure 5.5, the conditional complexity of the arrow interpretation corresponds roughly to the number of coincidences one might count in Figure 5.5A assuming that it contains the arrow shape.

Hence, the foregoing is inconclusive about the veridicality of prior precisals, but suggests that conditional precisals are fairly veridical in many worlds (i.e., under many different real conditional probability distributions). This is relevant to the everyday perception by a moving observer who, while moving, gets different views of a same distal scene. These subsequent views imply different conditionals (be they artificial precisals or real probabilities), and allow a continuing update of the observer's percept. This update process can be modeled by way of a recursive application of the Bayes rule. During this recursive process, the effect of the first priors fades away as the priors are updated continuously on the basis of the conditionals which then become the decisive entities. Because the simplicity-based artificial conditional probabilities seem to be close to the real conditional probabilities, simplicity seems to provide sufficient veridicality in such everyday situations. In other words, a visual system that focuses on internal efficiency seems to yield external veridicality as side-effect, fairly independent of the real prior probabilities in the world.

Thus, whereas the likelihood principle suggests that the visual system is a special-purpose system in that it yields a high degree of veridicality in this world, the simplicity principle suggests that the visual system is a general-purpose system in that it promises to yield a fair degree of veridicality in many worlds, possibly including this world. This qualifies Mach's (1886) idea that simplicity and likelihood are different sides of the same coin. It also qualifies the idea of Occam's razor, that the simplest interpretation of data is most likely the best one, that is, the one that is most likely true (see also Perkins, 1976; Sober, 1975). Finally, notice that the distinction and integration of viewpoint independencies and viewpoint dependencies can be said to model the distinction and interaction between the ventral ('what') and dorsal ('where') streams in the brain (Ungerleider and Mishkin, 1982). This interaction can in fact be said to yield a first, still perceptual, enrichment from percepts of objects as such to percepts of objects arranged in space, on the road to further enrichment by knowledge stored at higher cognitive levels.

Transparent holographic regularity

The veridicality finding discussed above is based on the complexity of simplest codes and holds virtually independently of which specific regularities are chosen to be extracted to obtain simplest codes. Curiously, in the 1960s, the finding that simplicity is fairly independent of the chosen coding language boosted the rise of AIT in mathematics, whereas Simon's (1972) empirical version of this finding led, albeit temporarily, to a decreased interest in perceptual coding approaches like SIT. The only thing Simon concluded, however, was that the employed coding language should have a psychological basis. After all, the primary purpose of simplest codes in vision is to yield perceptual organizations, and in this respect it is crucial to extract regularities that are visually relevant. Within SIT, this issue has been taken up as follows.

To meet Simon's demand, we first developed a mathematical formalization which established the unique formal status of the so-called hierarchically transparent and holographic nature of the regularities SIT employs to arrive at simplest structural descriptions (van der Helm and Leeuwenberg, 1991). Then, we provided empirical evidence that this hierarchically transparent and holographic nature is indeed decisive with respect to the role of these regularities in vision (this empirical line of research started with van der Helm and Leeuwenberg, 1996). To give a gist of this, we contrast this so-called holographic approach to the traditionally considered transformational approach which, in perception, has been promoted most prominently by Garner (1974) and Palmer (1983).

As with the holographic approach, the transformational approach provides a formalization of visual regularity, but by way of another characterization. As a result, the two approaches yield slightly different sets of regularities. Here, we focus on the characterization of symmetry and repetition, which are generally considered to be relevant in perception, and which are included in both approaches. Furthermore, the transformational formalization was stated originally in terms of 3-D objects and the holographic formalization is stated in terms of 1-D symbol strings, but here, we discuss them in terms of 2-D stimuli, which is pre-eminently the domain of empirical research on visual regularity.

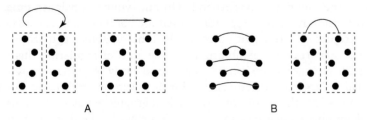

A   B

Figure 5.6A The transformational approach characterizes symmetry by
a 3-D rotation about the symmetry axis (which matches the symmetry
halves) and repetition by a translation (which matches the repeats); thus,
transformationally, both symmetry and repetition get a block structure. Figure 5.6B The holographic approach characterizes symmetry
as composed of identity relationships between elements, and repetition as composed of identity relationships between repeats; thus, holographically, symmetry gets a point structure and repetition gets a block
structure.

The transformational approach characterizes visual regularity as a
property that is invariant under motion. Transformationally, a regularity is defined as a configuration that, if present in an object, yields
image invariance under rigid translations or rotations of the object. For
instance, as illustrated in Figure 5.6A, symmetry is characterized by a 3-
D rotation about the symmetry axis, because the image remains invariant
under this transformation. Similarly, repetition is characterized by lon-
gitudinal translations the size of one or more repeats, again because the
image remains invariant under such a transformation (the image actually
remains invariant only if it extends beyond the visual field, but this is a
detail we do not quibble about).

Transformational invariance clearly captures a functional property of
visual regularity. Transformationally invariant objects look the same from
various viewpoints, so that such objects can be recognized fairly independently of viewpoint (cf. Enquist and Arak, 1994). However, we do not
feel that transformational invariance captures the intrinsic nature of visual
regularity. It capitalizes on a consequence of regularity rather than on a
property of regularity as such. Furthermore, it may be useful to recognize
or classify objects, but it leaves open how they are perceived preceding
recognition or classification. Finally, it does not explain empirically found
detectability differences, among which is the well-known phenomenon
that symmetry is better detectable than repetition.

Therefore, we developed the holographic approach which characterizes visual regularity as a property that is invariant under growth. For
instance, as illustrated in Figure 5.6B, a symmetry remains a symmetry

when the configuration is expanded by one symmetry pair at a time, while a repetition remains a repetition when the configuration is expanded by one repeat at a time. In other words, a holographic regularity is made up of substructures exhibiting the same kind of regularity; this implies that its representation can be constructed easily by going step-wise from small to large substructures. As shown in van der Helm and Leeuwenberg (1991), there are only twenty holographic regularities. This set of holographic regularities was restricted further by the demand that a regularity should be describable by a hierarchically transparent coding rule. This means that, if a regularity is described by a coding rule which allows for the description of additional hierarchically nested regularity, then this additional regularity should also be describable separately (i.e., independently of this coding rule); this ensures that codes specify hierarchical organizations with properly nested segments. Only three kinds of regularity are both holographic and hierarchically transparent, namely, bilateral symmetry (mirror and broken symmetry), repetition (i.e., juxtaposed repeats), and alternation (i.e., non-juxtaposed repeats). Therefore, only these regularities are proposed to be the ones to be described by a visual coding model.

In terms of symbol strings, this description is done by way of coding rules which can be applied to any substring of an input string, while a code of the entire input string consists of a string of symbols and encoded substrings, such that decoding these encoded substrings yields the input string. In formal terms, this implies the following definition:

SIT's coding language: *a code $\overline{X}$ of a string X is a string $t_1 t_2 \ldots t_m$ of code terms t_i such that $X = D(t_1) \ldots D(t_m)$, where the decoding function $D : t \rightarrow D(t)$ takes one of the following forms:*

I-form:	$n * (\overline{y})$	$\rightarrow \quad yyy \ldots y$	(n times y; $n \geq 2$)
S-form:	$S\left[\overline{(x_1)}\,\overline{(x_2)} \ldots \overline{(x_n)}, (\overline{p}) \right]$	$\rightarrow \quad x_1 x_2 \ldots x_n p x_n \ldots x_2 x_1$	($n \geq 1$)
A-form:	$\langle (\overline{y}) \rangle / \left\langle \overline{(x_1)}\,\overline{(x_2)} \ldots \overline{(x_n)} \right\rangle$	$\rightarrow \quad y x_1 y x_2 \ldots y x_n$	($n \geq 2$)
A-form:	$\left\langle \overline{(x_1)}\,\overline{(x_2)} \ldots \overline{(x_n)} \right\rangle / \langle (\overline{y}) \rangle$	$\rightarrow \quad x_1 y x_2 \ldots x_n y$	($n \geq 2$)
Otherwise:	$D(t) = t$		

for strings y, p, and x_i ($i = 1, 2, \ldots, n$). The code parts $(\overline{y})$, $(\overline{p})$, and $(\overline{x_i})$ are called chunks; the chunk $(\overline{y})$ in an I-form or an A-form is called a repeat; the chunk $(\overline{p})$ in an S-form is called a pivot which, as a limit case, may be empty; the chunk string $(\overline{x_1})\,(\overline{x_2}) \ldots (\overline{x_n})$ in an S-form is called an S-argument consisting of S-chunks $(\overline{x_i})$, and in an A-form it is called an A-argument consisting of A-chunks $(\overline{x_i})$.

In this definition, an overlined string stands for a code of this string. Hence, a code may involve not only recursive encodings of strings inside chunks, that is, from (y) into $(\overline{y})$, but also hierarchically recursive encodings of S-arguments or A-arguments $(\overline{x_1})\,(\overline{x_2})\dots(\overline{x_n})$ into $\overline{(x_1)}\,\overline{(x_2)}\dots\overline{(x_n)}$. For instance, below, a string is encoded in two ways, and for each code, the resulting hierarchically transparent organization of the string is given.

String:	$X = a\,b\,a\,c\,d\,a\,c\,d\,a\,b\,a\,b\,a\,c\,d\,a\,c\,d\,a\,b$
Code 1:	$\overline{X} = ab2 * (acd)\,S\,[(a)\,(b)\,,\,(a)]\,2 * (cda)\,b$
Organization:	$a\,b\,(acd)(acd)\,(a)(b)(a)(b)(a)\,(cda)(cda)\,b$
Code 2:	$\overline{X} = 2 * (\langle\langle(a)\rangle\,/\,\langle S\,[((b))\,((cd))]\rangle\rangle)$
Organization:	$(((a)(b))\,((a)(cd))\,((a)(cd))\,((a)(b)))\,(((a)(b))\,((a)(cd))\,((a)(cd))\,((a)(b)))$

Code 1 does not involve recursive encodings, but Code 2 does. That is, Code 2 is an I-form with a repeat that has been encoded into an A-form with an A-argument that has been encoded into an S-form. These examples may also illustrate that a string generally has many codes which have to be considered all in order to select a simplest code (this computational problem is addressed in the next subsection).

The foregoing also gave rise to an improved complexity metric. This metric implies that the complexity of a code is judged by the number of different constituents it specifies in the resulting hierarchical organization. We think this is the appropriate way to measure the informational content of codes, because hierarchical organizations are the messages the visual system transmits to higher cognitive levels. The following formal definition of this metric may seem somewhat ad hoc, but it accurately reflects the aforementioned idea in a form that can be applied directly to codes.

SIT's complexity metric: let $\overline{X}$ *be a code of symbol string* $s_1 s_2 \dots s_N$. *The structural information load I (or I-load) of* $\overline{X}$ *in structural information parameters (or sip) is given by the sum of, first, the number of remaining symbols and, second, the number of chunks* $(\overline{y})$ *in which y is neither one symbol nor one S-chunk.*

Thus, for instance, Code 1 above, that is, $\overline{X} = ab2 * (acd)\,S\,[(a)\,(b)\,,\,(a)]\,2 * (cda)\,b$, gets an I-load of $I = 14$ sip, because it contains twelve symbols and two chunks that contain neither one symbol nor one S-chunk, namely, the chunks (acd) and (cda). Furthermore Code 2 above, that is, $\overline{X} = 2 * (\langle\langle(a)\rangle\,/\,\langle S\,[((b))\,((cd))]\rangle\rangle)$, gets an I-load of $I = 8$ sip, because it contains four symbols and four chunks that contain neither one symbol nor one S-chunk, namely, the chunks (cd), $((b))$, $((cd))$, and the repeat of the I-form.

The foregoing indicates how the holographic approach led to SIT's current set of coding rules and SIT's current complexity metric. This ensemble was tested positively in empirical studies on pattern segmentation (van der Helm, 1994; van der Helm et al., 1992), and it is also the standard in the empirical studies reported later in this book. To test the hierarchically transparent holographic nature of the individual regularities more directly, we engaged in a separate line of research which started with van der Helm and Leeuwenberg (1996). As we sketch next, this line of research focused on the detectability of single and combined regularities, whether or not perturbed by noise.

As illustrated in Figure 5.6A, the transformational approach characterizes symmetry by a transformation that matches the symmetry halves, and it characterizes repetition by a transformation that matches the repeats. This implies that, transformationally, both symmetry and repetition can be said to have a block structure. In contrast, as illustrated in Figure 5.6B, the holographic approach can be said to assign a point structure to symmetry (given by the symmetry pairs) and a block structure to repetition (given by the repeats). Unlike the transformational structure, this holographic structure explains the basic phenomenon that symmetry is generally better detectable than repetition (see, e.g., Barlow and Reeves, 1979; Mach, 1886). That is, holographically, a repetition is sustained by only a few identity relationships between repeats, whereas a symmetry is generally sustained by many identity relationships between individual elements.

The latter observation led to a quantitative model in which the detectability of a regularity is measured by $W = E/n$ (van der Helm and Leeuwenberg, 1996). This is a sort of weight-of-evidence measure (cf. MacKay, 1969), in which E is the number of holographic identity relationships a regularity is composed of, while n is the total number of elements in the configuration. For instance, for a perfect mirror symmetry, $E = n/2$, so that its detectability is quantified by $W = 0.5$. Likewise, for a perfect twofold repetition (i.e., with two repeats), $E = 1$, so that its detectability is quantified by $W = 1/n$. This quantitative model not only explains that symmetry generally is better detectable than repetition, but it also predicts that the detectability of repetition depends on the total number of elements in the configuration, whereas the detectability of symmetry does not. This prediction has been tested and confirmed by Csathó et al. (2003).

This quantitative detectability model also gave rise to a qualitative detection model involving so-called holographic bootstrapping (van der Helm and Leeuwenberg, 1999). This model is a modification of the original bootstrap model proposed by Wagemans *et al.* (1991, 1993), and it implies that symmetry is detected via an exponential propagation process, whereas repetition is detected via a linear propagation process (see also Baylis and Driver, 1994). This processing difference not only agrees well with the aforementioned number effect in repetition but not in symmetry, but it also predicts that salient blobs (which are presumably processed first) hinder the detection of symmetry but help the detection of repetition. Also this prediction has been tested and confirmed by Csathó *et al.* (2003).

These are just a few of the regularity-detection phenomena (some were already known in the literature, others were newly predicted) that can be explained by the holographic approach to visual regularity. For further corroborating evidence concerning topics such as perturbed regularity and nested regularities, we refer the reader to Csathó *et al.* (2004), Nucci and Wagemans (2007), Treder and van der Helm (2007), Treder *et al.* (2011), van der Helm (2010), van der Helm and Leeuwenberg (2004), van der Helm and Treder (2009), van der Vloed *et al.* (2005), Wenderoth and Welsh (1998).

All in all, this line of research can be said to have yielded sufficient theoretical and empirical evidence to conclude that the hierarchically transparent holographic nature of SIT's regularities is indeed decisive with respect to their role in vision. This, in turn, implies that SIT's coding scheme yields structural descriptions that can indeed plausibly be said to reflect characteristics of mental representations of interpretations.

Transparallel processing

The foregoing subsection established a psychological basis for the coding scheme SIT proposes to arrive at simplest interpretations, but this does not yet answer the question of how the visual system might arrive at simplest interpretations. This issue has been raised by Hatfield and Epstein (1985), who argued that it is unrealistic to assume that each and every candidate interpretation is judged separately before a simplest one is selected. After all, any stimulus gives rise to a combinatorially explosive number of candidate interpretations, and judging them all separately could easily take more time than is available in this universe.

To give a gist of how SIT met this challenge, we first sketch the encoding algorithm PISA (P-load, Iteration, Symmetry, Alternation) which computes guaranteed simplest codes of symbol strings. Then, we discuss how subprocesses in PISA relate to subprocesses which, in neuroscience, are thought to take place in the visual hierarchy in the brain.

In the encoding algorithm PISA, three intertwined subprocesses can be distinguished, namely, feature extraction, feature binding, and feature selection. Feature extraction involves the search for hierarchically transparent holographic regularities in an input string. The search for separate regularities is computationally fairly simple, but because regularities also have to be recoded hierarchically recursively, this search yields so many features that a superexponential number of different codes for the entire string become possible. To be more precise, for a string of length N, the number of candidate codes is in the order of magnitude of $2^{N \cdot \log N}$, or in mathematical notation, $O(2^{N \cdot \log N})$. Clearly, it would be unrealistic to assume that each and every candidate code is judged separately before a simplest one is selected. As we sketch next, the solution to this problem lies in the binding of similar features.

Before regularities are hierarchically recoded, similar regularities can be gathered (or bound) in distributed representations. Such a distributed representation requires only $O(N^2)$ computing time to be constructed, and it is special in that it represents $O(2^N)$ similar regularities which can be hierarchically recoded as if only one regularity were concerned. That is, the regularities do not have to be recoded in a serial fashion (i.e., one after the other by one or more processors), nor in a parallel fashion (i.e., simultaneously by many processors), but they can be recoded in what we call a transparallel fashion (i.e., simultaneously by one processor). These special distributed representations are therefore called hyperstrings; for the full formal details on transparallel processing by hyperstrings, we refer the reader to van der Helm (2004), but the following example may give an idea of what transparallel processing entails.

Imagine that, for some odd reason, the longest pencil is to be selected from a number of pencils (see Figure 5.7A). Then, one or many persons could measure the lengths of the pencils in a serial or parallel fashion (see Figure 5.7B), after which the longest pencil could be selected by comparing the measurements. A much smarter method, however, would be if one person gathers all pencils in one bundle and places the bundle upright on a table (see Figure 5.7C), so that the longest pencil can be selected in a glance. This smart method does not judge the pencils in a serial or parallel fashion, but in what we call a transparallel fashion.

The binding role of the bundle in this example is analogous to the binding role of hyperstrings in SIT's encoding algorithm PISA. Hyperstrings serve a more intricate purpose (namely, hierarchical recoding) but this example shows that, sometimes, a set of similar items can be dealt with as if only one item were concerned.

In PISA, the binding of similar regularities into hyperstrings, and the subsequent hierarchically recursive recoding of these hyperstrings yields,

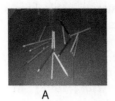
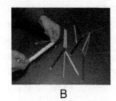
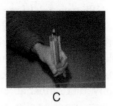

A   B   C

Figure 5.7A Suppose the longest pencil is to be selected from among many pencils. Figure 5.7B Then, one or many persons could measure the lengths of the pencils in a serial or parallel fashion, after which the longest pencil can be selected by comparing the measurements. Figure 5.7C A smarter method would be if one person gathers all pencils in one bundle and places the bundle upright on a table, so that the longest pencil can be selected in a glance; thus, the pencils are not judged separately in a serial or parallel fashion, but in what we call a transparallel fashion.

in total, a hierarchical tree of hyperstrings, from which a simplest code for the input string has to be selected. This selection is done by applying, to each (hyper)string, Dijkstra's (1959) shortest path method. This method exploits the fact that $O(2^N)$ candidate codes of a (hyper)string can be represented by $O(N^2)$ code parts, and it requires only $O(N^2)$ computing time to select a simplest code from among the $O(2^N)$ candidate codes.

Hence, PISA implements three intertwined subprocesses which, by the methods discussed above, together yield a tractable total process, that is, a process that can be performed in a realistic amount of work and time. Notice that, in PISA, such a hierarchical tree of hyperstrings is input-dependent; that is, it is a hierarchical distributed representation which represents all possible outputs for only the input at hand. This contrasts with standard connectionist modeling, in which one pre-defined distributed representation is taken to represent all possible outputs for all possible inputs. That is, standard connectionist modeling takes (the construction of) the output space for granted, and it only selects an output for a given input. The connectionist selection method, by the way, is computationally comparable to Dijkstra's (1959) shortest path method as used in PISA – both selection methods can be expressed, if you will, in terms of activation spreading through a network.

In other words, in contrast to connectionist models, SIT assumes that such a hierarchical tree of hyperstrings is transient in nature, that is, it reflects a momentary state of the brain. This brings us to the subprocesses which, in neuroscience, are thought to take place in the visual hierarchy in the brain, and from there, to a concrete picture of cognitive architecture.

The visual hierarchy comprises a dozen or so distinguishable hierarchical levels, with feedforward and recurrent connections between these levels, and with horizontal connections between areas within these levels (Felleman and van Essen, 1991). These three types of connections are thought to be responsible for three intertwined but functionally distinguishable subprocesses (see, e.g., Lamme *et al.*, 1998). In fact, functionally, these three neural subprocesses correspond one-to-one to the three subprocesses implemented in SIT's encoding algorithm PISA, namely, feature extraction, feature binding, and feature selection. First, feedforward connections seem responsible for a fast bottom-up processing of incoming stimuli. This so-called feedforward sweep seems to involve an increasingly more intricate encoding of features. Second, horizontal connections seem responsible for the integration (say, binding) of similar features encoded within an area, that is, for the encoding of regularities. Third, recurrent connections seem responsible for the selection and integration of different features into a percept.

Hence, SIT's encoding algorithm PISA can be said to provide a model that is neurally plausible in that it incorporates those intertwined but functionally distinguishable subprocesses. In fact, inversely, PISA's transparellel processing by hyperstrings may give a computational explanation of the intriguing phenomenon of neuronal synchronization. This is the phenomenon that neurons, in transient assemblies, tend to synchronize their activity (Milner, 1974; Singer and Gray, 1995; von der Malsburg, 1981). Such transient assemblies may arise when neurons shift their allegiance to different groups by altering connection strengths (Edelman, 1987). Both theoretically and empirically, neuronal synchronization has been associated with cognitive processing, but thus far, it did not find a concrete computational explanation (for reviews, see Finkel *et al.*, 1998; Gray, 1999).

Neuronal synchronization has been studied most extensively in vision (see, e.g., van Leeuwen *et al.*, 1997). The horizontal connections in the visual hierarchy, in particular, have been implicated in this phenomenon (see Gilbert, 1992). That is, temporarily synchronized neural assemblies seem to be constituted by horizontal connections which, as indicated above, also seem responsible for the binding of similar features encoded within a visual area. In other words, these transient horizontal assemblies can be seen as the neural counterparts of the transient hyperstrings in SIT's encoding algorithm PISA. Furthermore, neuronal synchronization is a special dynamical event in an otherwise parallel distributed processing neural network (cf. van Leeuwen, 2007). That is, it seems to reflect a form of processing that is more than just parallel distributed processing, and functionally, it might well reflect transparallel processing as characterized within SIT (van der Helm, 2012, 2013).

Finally, Fodor and Pylyshyn (1988) argued that connectionism may provide, at best, an account of the neural architecture in which classical (i.e., representational) cognitive architecture is implemented. Our account above seems to confirm this. That is, it suggests a picture of cognition as being mediated by transient neural assemblies forming flexible, input-dependent, hierarchies of hyperstring-like networks within the fixed neural network of the brain. These transient networks can be conceived of as cognitive information processors which, in a transparallel fashion, deal with many similar features in order to get, eventually, a structured representation of the input. They signal their presence by synchronization of the neurons involved, and this synchronization can be seen as the neural signature of transparallel processing. Hence, SIT's encoding algorithm PISA leads to a neurally plausible picture of cognitive architecture as being constituted by temporarily synchronized neural assemblies. Notice that a flexible architecture constituted by hyperstring-like networks involved in transparallel processing would do justice to both the high combinatorial capacity and the high speed of the perceptual organization process.

Summary

SIT models perceptual organization as a form of information processing that relies on interactions between things. These interactions are assumed to be driven by regularities, and the simplest (i.e., most regular) distal organization that fits a proximal stimulus is predicted to be perceived. To make predictions, SIT represents each candidate distal stimulus by symbol strings that, subsequently, enter an encoding and selection process. To ensure that the result of this process is perceptually meaningful, SIT demands that (a) symbol strings are reconstruction recipes of distal stimuli, and (b) substrings refer to spatially contiguous parts of distal stimuli. These demands imply that spatial characteristics of the distal stimuli are preserved in the symbol strings. SIT's coding approach is supported by theoretical foundations which focus on three aspects. First, findings in the mathematical domain of algorithmic information theory suggest that SIT's integration of viewpoint independencies and viewpoint dependencies yields sufficient veridicality to guide us through the world. Second, a mathematical formalization of regularity established that the regularities, which SIT uses to determine simplest codes, have a unique hierarchically transparent holographic nature, the perceptual relevance of which is supported by empirical evidence concerning the detectability of these regularities. Third, the encoding algorithm developed within SIT to compute simplest codes was shown to provide a neurally plausible model of perceptual organization. It puts its central mechanism of transparallel processing by hyperstrings forward as computational explanation of the neuroscientific phenomenon of synchronization in transient neural assemblies.

Part II

Applications to visual form

This part is concerned with the application of structural information theory (SIT) to visual form perception.

Chapter 6 provides the formal rules for establishing SIT codes of symbol strings. First, the kinds of regularity described by codes are specified. Then, the structural information load of codes is specified and demonstrated. Finally, three code attributes are introduced. These are supposed to predict dominance relations within or between patterns.

Chapter 7 provides pragmatic guidelines for the application of SIT coding to visual shapes, such as line drawings, surfaces, and solid objects. In order to assess perceptually preferred representations of such stimuli, these guidelines aim at representing them, in a psychologically plausible way, by primitive codes (which then can be coded by means of the formal rules discussed in Chapter 6). This means that, rather than being fixed rules that hold for any stimulus in any context, these guidelines take the experimental context of stimuli into account.

Chapter 8 tests the preference strength of simplest pattern interpretations with respect to alternative competing interpretations. Its visual relevance is demonstrated for occluding layers dealing with pattern completion and subjective contours, and for translucent layers revealed by line drawings, visual transparency, neon illusions, and assimilation versus contrast. Finally, we present evidence suggesting that the preferred code emerges from a competition between codes.

Chapter 9 deals with the simplest interpretations of pattern pairs consisting of prototypes and non-prototypes. The hierarchical relationship between their codes is argued to give rise to temporal effects. In one case, simultaneously presented patterns induce the perception of temporal order. In another case, subsequently presented patterns induce the perception of simultaneously presented patterns.

Chapter 10 focuses on the hierarchy within the simplest code of a pattern. This hierarchy specifies superstructures and subordinate structures. It is assumed that the former dominate the latter. This assumption is tested directly by way of unity and duality judgments and primed object matching, and indirectly by way of mental rotation tasks to match mirrored objects. An additional section deals with the role of reference frames in pattern interpretations.

6 Formal coding model

Introduction

This chapter deals with the formal rules of the structural information theory (SIT) coding of symbol strings. The symbols we use are letters, but precisely because we used them as symbols, the alphabetical order of the letters and the shape of individual letters are irrelevant. This implies, for instance, that the strings KBBK and ATTA have exactly the same (symmetrical) structure. In this chapter, such symbol strings are taken as patterns in themselves, whereas in all subsequent chapters, they are mostly taken as primitive codes of visual patterns, each symbol referring to a visual pattern element.

In section 6.1, three kinds of regularity are introduced that share the properties of holographic regularity and transparent hierarchy (see Chapter 5). By means of coding operations which are based on these kinds of regularity, a symbol string can be simplified. Furthermore, we discuss structural information load as a measure of complexity of encoded strings. It is assumed that this simplest code reveals the preferred structure plus the class of strings with the same structure (commonly, we use 'the code' to refer to the simplest code). In section 6.2, three simplest-code attributes are introduced which are supposed to predict dominance relations within or between patterns, namely, preference strength, hierarchical dominance, and figural goodness.

6.1 Structural information

Kinds of regularity

As pointed out in Chapter 5, SIT makes use of three kinds of regularity, that is iteration, symmetry, and alternation (van der Helm, 1988; van der Helm and Leeuwenberg, 1991). Figure 6.1 illustrates what they entail and in which form they are denoted.

	strings		codes
iteration	AAAAAA	<=	6*(A)
	ABABAB	<=	3*(AB)
symmetry	ABCCBA	<=	S[(A)(B)(C)]
	ABCBA	<=	S[(A)(B),(C)]
	ABCAB	<=	S[(AB),(C)]
	ABCDAB	<=	S[(AB),(CD)]
alternation	ABACAD	<=	<(A)>/<(B)(C)(D)>
	ADBDCD	<=	<(A)(B)(C)>/<(D)>
	ABCABD	<=	<(AB)>/<(C)(D)>
	ACDBCD	<=	<(A)(B)>/<(CD)>

Figure 6.1 A few symbol strings with codes to illustrate how the three kinds of regularity (iteration, symmetry, and alternation) are formally represented. The arrows point left to indicate that a code represents just one pattern whereas a pattern can be represented by various codes.

A general issue is that, in Figure 6.1, the mapping between patterns and codes is indicated by backward arrows. This way it is made clear that a code describes only one unique pattern whereas a pattern can be described by various codes. Each pair of parentheses in the codes refers to a chunk which contains a string of one or more elements (symbols or chunks). A symmetry code with only chunks of single symbols represents a mirror symmetry, whereas a symmetry code which also contains chunks of more symbols represents a so-called broken symmetry (cf. Weyl, 1952). The square brackets in a symmetry code enclose the whole cluster of symmetry chunks. The second part in a symmetry code (i.e., the part after the comma) is called the pivot of the symmetry. An alternation code shows two components, each enclosed by arrow brackets. One component consists of just one chunk, and the other consists of two or more chunks. In this way, the alternation code compactly describes one repeated chunk in between various other chunks. The repeat either is at the left side, as in <(A)>/<(B)(C)>, or at the right side, as in <(A)(B)>/<(C)>.

Notice that both chunks and clusters determine the perceptual segmentation of patterns, albeit in different ways. A chunk is a substructure of a represented regularity, whereas a cluster comprises all parts involved in this regularity. For instance, in the code 2*(AB) of ABAB, the term

(AB) is the chunk and [ABAB] is the cluster. Likewise, in the code S[(A)(B)] of ABBA, (A) and (B) are the chunks and [ABBA] is the cluster. As we discuss later on, chunks play a role in assessing the structural information load of a code, whereas clusters do not.

To illustrate the role of regularities in the representation of patterns we consider the string AAAAAA. Taken as a pattern, one of course sees that all symbols are identical, but these identity relationships are not yet described explicitly. That is, taken as a code, it is still a primitive code because it does not reveal any reduction towards simplicity. An instance of a reduced code is 4*(A) 2*(A). This description reflects more about the actual equality of the symbols than the primitive code does. As a consequence, it contains fewer symbols. However, it is not optimal. The most optimal representation with a minimum of symbols is 6*(A). Only this code explicitly describes all the identity relationships between the symbols.

The quality of these bad, mediocre, and good descriptions of the string can be illustrated by considering the classes of patterns that are represented by each description. As the first code AAAAAA ignores the identity of all its symbols, it is actually equivalent to a string of arbitrary symbols. So, as a class-code it also characterizes patterns whose elements are different. This class can be indicated by the parameter string **BCDEFG** in which each parameter stands for an arbitrary symbol (Collard and Buffart, 1983). So, this class contains all strings consisting of six symbols. The mediocre description 4*(A) 2*(A) is better than the previous one, but it still ignores that the first four symbols are equal to the last two symbols. Thus, according to this description, the pattern belongs to the class specified by the parameter string **BBBBCC**. This class is smaller than the class given above by **BCDEFG**. The description 6*(A) characterizes the class **BBBBBB**. This class merely contains all strings of six identical symbols, so that it forms the smallest possible class. Because it does not ignore any identity relationship, it can be conceived of as the most accurate description of the pattern. So, in this sense simplicity corresponds to accuracy (see Chapter 4).

Information load

For a string, a code specifies a hierarchical organization composed of symbols and chunks and consisting of various hierarchical levels. According to the code, some of these elements (i.e., these symbols and chunks at all levels) are identical, and some are different. The structural information load of a code now corresponds to the number of these different elements in the hierarchical organization. From this conceptual definition of information load the following pragmatic definition can be derived (for the precise definition, see Chapter 5):

The structural information load, or I-load, of a code equals the number of symbols plus the number of chunks in the code. There are two exceptions. If the content of a chunk is just one symbol or one symmetry chunk, then the chunk does not contribute to the I-load.

We illustrate this definition for a few codes.

- The code $3^*(K)$ comprises one symbol $(I = 1)$. The chunk (K) does not count as its content K is just one symbol. So, the total load is: $I = 1$.
- The code $S[(A)(B)]$ comprises two symbols $(I = 2)$. The two chunks (A) and (B) do not count as they contain just one symbol each. So, the total load is: $I = 2$.
- The code $2^*(AB)$ comprises two symbols $(I = 2)$. The content AB of the chunk (AB) is neither one symbol nor a symmetry chunk. Therefore, this chunk (AB) counts $(I = 1)$. So, the total load is: $I = 3$.
- The code $<(2^*(A))>/<(B)(C)>$ of the string AABAAC contains three symbols $(I = 3)$. The chunks (A), (B), and (C) contain just one symbol each, so they do not count. The content $2^*(A)$ of the chunk $(2^*(A))$, however, is neither a single symbol nor a symmetry chunk, so this chunk counts $(I = 1)$. Hence, the total load is: $I = 4$.
- The code $<(A)>/<2^*((B))(C)>$ of the intermediate code $<(A)>/<(B)(B)(C)]>$ of the string ABABAC contains three symbols $(I = 3)$. The chunks (A), (B), and (C) contain just one symbol each, so they do not count. The content (B) of the chunk $((B))$, however, is neither a single symbol nor a symmetry chunk, so this chunk counts $(I = 1)$. Hence, the total load is: $I = 4$.
- The code $S[S[((AB)),((C))]]$ of the intermediate code $S[(AB)(C)(AB)]$ of the string ABCABABCAB contains three symbols $(I = 3)$. The content AB of the chunk (AB) is neither a single symbol nor a symmetry chunk, so this chunk counts $(I = 1)$. The content (AB) of the chunk $((AB))$, however, is a symmetry chunk, so this chunk does not count $(I = 0)$. Furthermore, the content of chunk (C) is one symbol, and the content of chunk $((C))$ is a symmetry chunk, so neither chunk counts. Hence, the total load is: $I = 4$.
- The code $<(A)>/<S[((B))((C))]>$ of the intermediate code $<(A)>/<(B)(C)(C)(B)]>$ of the string ABACACAB contains three symbols $(I = 3)$. The chunks (A), (B), and (C) contain just one symbol each, so they do not count. The content (B) of chunk $((B))$ and the content (C) of chunk $((C))$ are neither single symbols nor symmetry chunks, so they count $(I = 2)$. Hence, the total load is: $I = 5$.

6.2 Attributes of simplest codes

Structural information load is an intra-pattern measure which differentiates between interpretations of a pattern, that is, not between patterns. The measure is appropriate to establish the simplest of all possible interpretations of a pattern. This subsection discusses three attributes of simplest codes. They are supposed to predict dominance relations within or between patterns. The three attributes are preference strength, hierarchy, and figural goodness. The visual relevance of preference strength is sustained in Chapters 8 and 9, and the visual relevance of hierarchy is sustained in Chapter 10. The application of the attribute of figural goodness lies outside the scope of this book, and for evidence sustaining it, we refer the reader to van der Helm and Leeuwenberg (1996, 1999, 2004).

Preference strength

The preference strength of a code is supposed to reflect the visual prominence of this target code with respect to the prominence of an alternative code. The measure of preference strength is defined as the load of the alternative code divided by the load of the target code. In most applications, the simplest code is chosen to serve as target code. Generally, the alternative code is a description of the stimulus that represents a concept that contrasts semantically to the concept described by the target code. For all stimuli involved in the experiments reported in Chapter 8, the target and the alternative patterns concepts are induced by the task. In some cases, the experiments deal with a forced choice task and the two contrasting interpretations are given explicitly. In most cases, a property of the target interpretation is tested. Then, the interpretation that misses this property is the obvious alternative option. An instance is the occlusion interpretation. Then, the mosaic interpretation is the alternative option. Also, in studies of subjective contours, transparency, and neon illusions, the mosaic interpretations are the alternative options. In some cases, the target describes the stimulus as a single whole and the alternative represents an assembly of parts, or the target describes a quite regular structure whereas the alternative represents a quite irregular structure.

Sometimes, the contrasting interpretations are given by the experimental task, but in the past, suggestions have been made in case they are not given. For instance, for the stimuli used by Mens (1988), the second-best code appeared to be an adequate alternative of the simplest code.

For other stimuli, however, these two codes are not quite appropriate. This is illustrated by way of the next example:

ABABAB	<=	3* (AB)	I = 3	simplest code
ABABAB	<=	A S[(B)(A), (B)]	I = 4	second-best code

The second-best code is just one information unit more complex than the simplest code, with the consequence that the preference strength does not reveal the outstanding prominence of the above completely regular pattern. Notice that, generally, any completely regular pattern has a description which is just one information unit more complex than the simplest code.

An alternative has been suggested by Collard and Buffart (1983) who contrasted the so-called 'complementary code' with the simplest code. The complementary code is the simplest description which establishes all identities not established by the simplest code. If there are no identities left over, the complementary code agrees with the primitive code. As a consequence, the simplest code and the complementary code together fixate the unique structure of the stimulus pattern. An illustration is follows:

ABABB	<=	S [(A),(B)] 2*(B)	I = 3	simplest code
ABABB	<=	2*(AB) B	I = 4	complementary code

The simplest code describes the class **ABACC**. It ignores the identity of the first and second B symbols. The complementary code describes the class **ABABC**. It ignores the identity of the second and third B symbols. The common class, constrained by both classes, reveals the **ABABB** structure of the stimulus. The preference strength of the simplest code is 4/3.

The latter suggestion is useful for certain stimuli, especially for serial patterns that have just one complementary code. Hence, completely regular patterns, such as ABABAB or ABCCBA, are excluded as they do not have complementary codes. Also excluded are patterns that require two or more complementary codes to establish all identities not established by the simplest code.

Hierarchical dominance

For a shape whose simplest code has a hierarchical structure, the least nested level is called the superstructure and the more nested level is called the subordinate structure. The claim is that, perceptually, the superstructure is more dominant than the subordinate structure (Leeuwenberg and van der Helm, 1991). The argument for this so-called superstructure dominance hypothesis is that the superstructure specifies features of the subordinate structure and not the other way around.

In serial patterns, the cluster of the superstructure regularity includes the clusters of the subordinate regularity. Two illustrations are as follows:

ATTA ATTA ATTA	<=	3*(ATTA)	<= 3*(S[(A)(T)])
ATATAT TATATA	<=	S[(A)(T)(A)(T)(A)(T)]	<= S[3*((A)(T))]

The first string is described by a repeat superstructure with a symmetry subordinate structure. The second string is described by a symmetry superstructure with a repeat subordinate structure. For 1-D and 2-D patterns, the superstructure agrees with the global or most extended pattern part, but as we argued in Chapter 3.2, for 3-D objects the superstructure might be smaller than the subordinate structure. That is, the size just is an accidental and not an intrinsic feature of the super-structure. For this reason, the experiments in Chapter 10, which were set up to test the superstructure dominance hypothesis, deal with 3-D objects.

The hierarchy between the superstructure and the subordinate struc-ture might suggest that the process from pattern to code occurs in steps starting with the superstructure and ending with the subordinate structure. This suggestion, however, is incorrect. The hierarchy is just a (static) property of the code which is selected on the basis of its over-all simplicity, that is, not on the basis of a specific temporal order in subsequent processing steps (see Chapter 3). It is true that the inverse process, that is, from code to pattern, might start with the superstruc-ture and end with the subordinate structure (like in the creative pro-cess from concept to composition), but the perceptual process from pattern to code is actually more likely to start with subordinate details in order to end with more-dominant superstructures (Hochstein and Ahissar, 2002).

Figural goodness

Both preference strength and representational hierarchy apply to intra-pattern aspects. In contrast, figural goodness is a measure that enables comparisons between patterns. Like the other two attributes, figural goodness is an attribute of the simplest code. It is different from simplicity and therefore also different from the figural goodness measure introduced by Garner (1970). After all, Garner's concept is almost equivalent to

No	string	simplest code	W = E/N

| | 1: (ABPQT)(ABPQT) | 2*(ABPQT) | 0.1 |

iteration

| | 2: ((A)(A)(A)(A)T) ((A)(A)(A)(A)T) | 2*(4*(A)T) | 0.7 |

| | 3: (A)(B)(P)(Q)(T)(T)(Q)(P)(B)(A) | S[(A)(B)(P)(Q)(T)| | 0.5 |

symmetry

| | 4: ((A))((A))((A))((A))(T)(T)((A))((A))((A))((A)) | S[4*((A))(T)| | 0.8 |

| | 5: (A)(B)(A)(P)(A)(Q)(A)(T)(A)(U) | <(A)>/<(B)(P)(Q)(T)(U)> | 0.4 |

alternation

| | 6: ((A)(B))((A)(B))((A)(B))(A)(C)(A)(D) | <(A)>/<3*((B)) (C)(D)> | 0.6 |

Figure 6.2 Of six strings of ten symbols, the simplest codes are presented. The arcs relate pairs of chunks that are specified as being identical by the codes. The arcs above the strings belong to superstructures
and the arcs below the strings belong to subordinate structures. The W
stands for the measure of figural goodness (van der Helm and Leeuwenberg, 1996). E is the number of non-redundant identity relationships
(indicated by the arcs) specified by the simplest code and N is the
number of symbols in each series.

simplicity. Figural goodness, as discussed here, refers to the detectability of a regularity in a pattern, and the measure we discuss exploits the
concept of weight of evidence (MacKay, 1969).

According to a proposal by van der Helm and Leeuwenberg (1996),
the weight of evidence (W) for a regularity in a pattern is given by $W = E/N$, where N is the number of pattern elements, while E is the number
of non-redundant identity relationships specified by the simplest code.
This weight of evidence W then is taken to quantify the goodness, or
detectability, of the regularity in the pattern. In Figure 6.2, the value of
W is specified for each string. For all strings holds that $N = 10$, while

E is equal to the number of the arcs which indicate the non-redundant identity relationships specified by the simplest code.

The W measure has various interesting characteristics. One deals with the difference between the plain twofold repeat structure of string 1 and the plain symmetry structure of string 3 in Figure 6.2. These plain structures reveal first order global regularities without additional nested regularities. For string 1, $W = 0.1$, and for string 3, $W = 0.5$. So, the repetition (given by only one identity relationship) has a low W value, and the symmetry (given by five identity relationships) has a high W value. This agrees with the observations by Mach (1886) and Julesz (1971) that plain twofold iteration is less detectable than plain symmetry. Furthermore, considering that identity relationships reflect visual binding, the foregoing supports the findings by Corballis and Roldan (1974) and Treder and van der Helm (2007) that twofold repetition is a cue for the presence of two objects, whereas symmetry is a cue for the presence of one object.

Another characteristic of the W measure is that iteration is predicted to be more vulnerable to noise than symmetry is. Iteration is composed of identity relationships between chunks of generally several symbols and has, therefore, a block structure, whereas (mirror) symmetry is composed of identity relationships between single symbols so that it has a point structure (van der Helm and Leeuwenberg, 1996). So, even the slightest perturbation may destroy an iteration, but if symmetrical elements are combined with some asymmetrical elements, the symmetry of the whole configuration is only gradually weakened (which agrees with Barlow and Reeves, 1979). This contrasts with the transformational approach (see Chapter 2), according to which both iteration and symmetry have block structures so that they are predicted to be equally vulnerable to noise.

If twofold iteration and symmetry are enriched with the same additional regularity on a deeper level, an opposed effect emerges. Then the W value of twofold iteration is affected more positively than the W value of symmetry. Figure 6.2 illustrates this. For the iteration string 1 to string 2, W increases from 0.1 to 0.7, whereas for the symmetry string 3 to string 4, W increases from 0.5 to 0.8. Hence, additional regularity is predicted to help iteration detection more than it helps symmetry detection. This agrees with Corballis and Roldan's (1974) finding that the repeat in the pattern $>>$ is as salient as the symmetry in the pattern $<>$ is.

More evidence for the figural goodness measure can be found in Csathó (2004), Csathó et al. (2003, 2004), van der Helm and Leeuwenberg (1996, 1999, 2004), van der Vloed (2005), and van der Vloed et al. (2005).

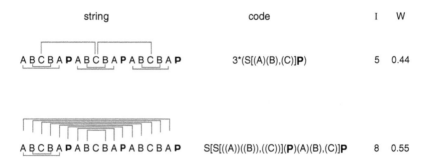

string	code	I	W
A B C B A P A B C B A P A B C B A P	3*(S[(A)(B),(C)]**P**)	5	0.44
A B C B A P A B C B A P A B C B A P	S[S[((A))((B)),((C))](**P**)(A)(B),(C)]**P**	8	0.55

Figure 6.3 Simplicity (I) and figural goodness (W) seem related but are different. The upper pattern is simpler than the bottom pattern but its figural goodness is lower. Simplicity is used as the selection criterion of the preferred pattern representation whereas figural goodness is the property of the simplest code that refers to the ease of detecting the perceived object's structure.

Finally, we return to the fact that figural goodness is an attribute of the simplest code and that it differs from simplicity. As said, the simplest code specifies the preferred interpretation of a pattern, and the W value specifies the weight of evidence of a regularity in this preferred interpretation. For instance, code 3*(A) of AAA and the code 6*(A) of AAAAAA have the same complexity (I = 1), but the iteration in the former code has a W value of W = 2/3, whereas the more redundantly present iteration in the latter code has a higher W value of W = 5/6. Furthermore, as illustrated in Figure 6.3, a simpler code may have a lower W value than a more complex code. This also illustrates that, in general, complexity I and weight of evidence W are not correlated, and that W is not meant to be used to predict preferred interpretations.

Summary

Section 6.1, on structural information, illustrates the three kinds of regularity that share the properties of holographic regularity and transparent hierarchy (see Chapter 5). These kinds of regularity are iteration, symmetry, and alternation. Their description contributes to the load reduction of representations. The structural information load of a code corresponds to the number of different elements (symbols and chunks) in the hierarchical organization specified by the code.

Section 6.2 introduces three dominance attributes of simplest codes, namely, preference strength, hierarchical dominance, and figural goodness. The preference strength of a target code (usually the simplest code) is defined as the load of a perceptually contrasting alternative code divided by the load of the target code. Hierarchical dominance refers to the claim that, perceptually, the superstructure is more dominant than the subordinate structure. The least nested level in a code corresponds to the superstructure and the more nested level to the subordinate structure. Figural goodness is specified by $W = E/N$, where N is the number of pattern elements, while E is the number of non-redundant identity relationships determined by the simplest code. The W measure refers to weight of evidence and is taken to quantify the detectability of the regularity in a pattern. It accounts for various perceptually evident detectability differences between iteration and symmetry patterns.

7   A perceptual coding manual

Introduction

This chapter deals with the practical rules for applying structural information theory (SIT) to visual shapes. The coding of visual shapes involves the coding of symbol strings (see Chapter 6) but, then, preceded by the so-called semantic mapping. This mapping implies that a primitive code is provided for each of the candidate distal stimuli that fit the proximal stimulus, that is, a symbol string which can be read as a construction recipe for such a distal stimulus. The simplest code over all these primitive codes then is taken to represent the preferred interpretation of the proximal stimulus. In this chapter, we go into more detail on the semantic mapping, and we give examples of predictions involving attributes of simplest codes.

Papers on SIT, published in the past, may have given the impression that the semantic mapping is part of SIT and that it deals with fixed rules that uniquely transform stimuli into symbol strings. This impression is incorrect. The semantic mapping is not part of SIT but is part of the application of SIT in the empirical practice. The semantic mapping rules rather are sort of perceptually plausible guidelines to obtain preferred interpretations of visual shapes. These rules are not hard and fast rules which we demand to be applied in any context, but rather suggestions of how the semantic mapping might be performed in several different contexts. For instance, experiments usually use a set of stimuli which are homogeneous just below the level of interest in an experiment. This implies that the semantic mapping can disregard the common features by starting at this homogeneity level, in order to focus on the distinctive features which are relevant in the experiment.

In general, a candidate interpretation of a proximal stimulus describes a distal stimulus as consisting of one or more hypothesized objects (with parts that may or may not be assumed to be connected physically). Each hypothesized object is described by a so-called unified code, and if the candidate interpretation involves two or more hypothesized objects, it is represented by a so-called dissociated code. A dissociated code describes the hypothesized objects by way of separate unified codes, and it takes the complexity of their spatial relations into account.

7.1   Line drawings

We first consider unified representations of stimuli, that is, codes reflecting interpretations which involve only one perceived object. Then, we consider dissociated representations reflecting interpretations which involve several perceived objects in a certain spatial arrangement.

Unified representations

As a rule, we propose to represent line patterns by their subsequent line segments and turns. These line segments and turns are supposed to be the primitive stimulus elements and are represented each by one symbol. A line segment is the line part in between junctions or ends. A turn stands for the angle between the preceding and the next line segment. In other words, the turn represents the angular deviation from linear continuation, that is, the outside and not the inside angle. As linear continuation, which corresponds to a zero turn, does not stand for an angular deviation it is not represented by a symbol. Note that neither the position nor the orientation of a pattern is represented by symbols. In other words, a pattern code is a viewpoint-independent description.

The line segments are indicated by capitals (e.g., **KLM**). The turns or angles are indicated by small letters (e.g., **abc**). If the pattern elements are visually different, the symbols should be different, and if the pattern elements are equal, that is, if their difference is not noticeable, the symbols should be equal. The order of the symbols agrees with the order of scanning the pattern elements. In general, we start the tracing at the left of the pattern. To avoid confusion, we often present an arrow in the figure to indicate the starting point. An illustration is presented in Figure 7.1A. Its primitive code is:

K a L b M

Figure 7.1B presents a pattern with a branch. In the representation, a branch is a sub-element of the pattern and is enclosed by brackets. The primitive code is:

K {c P} a L b M

The orientation of **K** is the reference frame both of turn **c** of the branch and of turn **a** of the subsequent trunk. The two brackets in {**c P**} actually

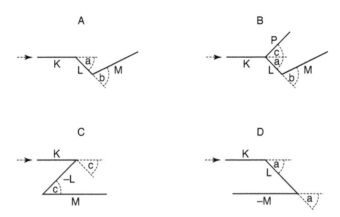

Figure 7.1 Simple line patterns. The convention is to build their primitive codes by scanning the subsequent line lengths (**KLM**) and turns
(**abc**). A is a common serial pattern. B is a branching pattern. C and
D reveal parallel lines. Their coding makes use of serial backward
scanning.

are semantic instruction symbols for the introduction and closure of the
branching subseries.

In Figure 7.1C the lines **K** and **M** are in parallel. To understand its
representation it is helpful to imagine a scanning that is achieved by
driving a car. Turns in the pattern are supposed to agree with turns
of the steering-wheel. The driving is supposed to be both forward and
backward. The pattern scanning is as follows. It starts with the forward
tracing **K** from left to right. At its end the car stops. Then, the wheel
makes a right turn **c**. Thereafter, the car drives backward along **-L** while
the wheel is returned into the neutral standard orientation. At the end
the car stops and the wheel makes again a right turn **c**. Thereafter, the car
drives forward along **M** while the wheel returns into the neutral standard
orientation. In the code, forward and backward scanning is indicated by
positive and negative values, respectively. The parallel structure can be
described by symmetry. The primitive code is:

K c - L c M

Figure 7.1D shows another kind of parallel structure. It can be
described analogous to the way the previous figure is described, namely,
by serial scanning which is partly backward. The primitive code is:

K a L a - M

This code can be simplified by the alternation rule.

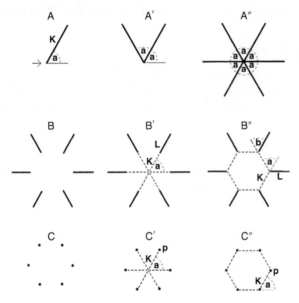

Figure 7.2 AA′A″ stepwise show the branching coding of a radiation pattern. The radiation pattern B can be represented either from its centre (B′) or from a hexagon (B″). B′ is simpler than B″. The dot pattern C can be represented either from its centre (C′) or from a hexagon (C″). This time C″ is as simple as C′.

A series of angles, for instance **aaaaaa**, represents a point of diverging directions and is useful to describe a radiation pattern. Its construction is illustrated stepwise in Figures 7.2AA′A″ for **a** = 72°. The code, with I = 3, is:

6 * (**a** {**K**})

The **a** components belong to the superstructure and the branching line segments {**K**} belong to the subordinate structure.

Underlining is an index to make an angle or a line element invisible. It enables us to describe the radiation pattern of separated lines shown in Figure 7.2B. There are two descriptions of this figure. One is illustrated in Figure 7.2B′. It is characterized by the branching superstructure 6*(**a**). This superstructure is completely underlined and the subordinate structure is partly underlined. The code, with I = 4, is:

6 * (**a̲** {**K̲** L})

The other code is illustrated in Figure 7.2B″. It is characterized by the serial superstructure 6*(**a̲** **K̲**), being an invisible regular hexagon.

The subordinate structure is a branching turn plus line. The code, with I = 5, is:

6 * (**a K** {**b L**})

So, the branching code is simpler than the serial code. Also, for describing Figure 7.2C, either a branching or a serial superstructure code is an option. The branching code illustrated in Figure 7.2C', with I = 4, is as follows:

6 * (**a** {**K** P})

Also, in the serial contour code, illustrated in Figure 7.2C'', each dot is represented by the symbol **P**. The code, with I = 4, is:

6 * (**a K** P)

So, this time, the branching code is as complex as the serial code.

Somewhat similar to this serial code, the following code, with I = 3, describes a regular polygon, such as an equilateral triangle, a square, or a regular pentagon (each under appropriately chosen parameters):

N * (**a K**)

This code even describes a circle. That is, a circle is described as an extreme version of a regular polygon, involving a large number of pairs of small turns and small lines.

Dissociated representations

As discussed above, a unified representation describes a stimulus as one object. In contrast, a dissociated representation, introduced by van Lier (1996), interprets a stimulus as an assembly of independent objects. To clarify how the two representations are related we attend to Figure 7.3. It presents four configurations. Each configuration can be taken either as one object, to be described by a unified representation, or as a combination of two objects, say, two sticks, to be described by a dissociated representation. (In the figure and in most following figures, turns are, just for practical reasons, indicated at inside angles.)

We first consider the single object interpretations of the four configurations as described by unified representations. In Figure 7.3A, the two stick components have an irregular spatial relation. In the next figures the spatial relations between the two stick components are gradually more regular. Hence, due to the increasing regularity of the junctions, the loads of Figures 7.3A to D gradually decrease. Of all the relations between the parts, the linear continuation in the last pattern is the regularity that

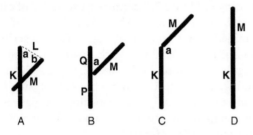

Figure 7.3 Four combinations of two sticks. A unified representation takes each pattern as one object, for which the increasing regularity from A to D contributes to simplicity (Iu). A dissociated representation takes the two components as two arbitrarily positioned objects (van Lier *et al.*, 1994). Then, the increasing regularity from A to D reflects an increasing amount of coincidences contributing to complexity (Id) (van Lier *et al.*, 1994).

maximally contributes to simplicity. So, from the perspective of the unified interpretation, Figure 7.3D is the simplest one and can, therefore, be conceived of as the prototype of the series.

The dissociated representation assumes that the stimulus presents two independent stick objects. Hence, there is no reason to expect that these objects have a regular spatial relation. In fact, their most likely spatial relation, as perceived from the so-called 'general viewpoint' (Binford, 1981), rather is quite irregular. So, this time, Figure 7.3A is the prototype of the series and Figure 7.3D is the most coincidental and therefore the most unlikely configuration of the series (Rock, 1983). Hence, regularity in the spatial relation between parts simplifies the unified representation but contributes to the complexity of the dissociated representation.

To arrive at a quantification of the load of a dissociated representation, van Lier *et al.* (1994) distinguished between two structures. One is the 'internal structure', which deals with the separate view-independent stimulus components described in the dissociated representation. For instance, in Figure 7.3, the two sticks are the two components of the internal structure. The load of this structure is indicated by I-int and is quantified by the sum of the unified complexities Iu of the separate components. The other is the 'external structure', which deals with the view-dependent spatial relation between those components. The load of this structure is indicated by I-ext (we illustrate its quantification in a moment). The total load of the dissociated representation, indicated by Id, just is the sum of loads of the two structures:

$$Id = I\text{-}int + I\text{-}ext$$

Because all four patterns in Figure 7.3 comprise two sticks of different lengths, for all of them holds I-int = 2. The quantification of I-ext is illustrated next. The unified representation of Figure 7.3A describes two sticks in the actual dissociated position, which yields Iu(actual) = 5. Likewise, the more regular positions in Figures 7.3B, C, and D yield Iu(actual) = 4, 3, and 2, respectively. Then, the complexity I-ext is quantified by subtracting the Iu(actual) of the positions in Figures 7.3A, B, C, and D from the maximal Iu(actual), that is, the Iu(actual) of the dissociated position in Figure 7.3A. Hence:

$$\text{I-ext} = \text{Iu(maximal)} - \text{Iu(actual)}$$

In other words, this complexity I-ext reflects the effort needed to bring the components in their actual proximal position starting from a dissociated position of these objects, that is, from a position for which the perceiver can be said to be in a general viewpoint position. This yields the following quantitative schema:

Figure	Iu(maximal) − Iu(actual) = I-ext	I-int + I-ext = Id
7.3A	5−5 = 0	2 + 0 = 2
7.3B	5−4 = 1	2 + 1 = 3
7.3C	5−3 = 2	2 + 2 = 4
7.3D	5−2 = 3	2 + 3 = 5

Hence, for a dissociated representation, the internal view-independent structure of the components can be said to be enriched by the external view-dependent structure which deals with the actual proximal position of the components.

Notice that, in general, components may meet at several junctions. At each of these junctions, edges are 'glued' perceptually in ways like those shown in Figure 7.3. Van Lier et al. (1994) now argued that, to perceptually dissociate components, their edges should be dissociated at each of these junctions separately. That is, by the method above, each junction can be assigned its own local I-ext, and van Lier et al. (1994) argued that their sum yields the global I-ext for the entire dissociated interpretation (this is illustrated later on; see Figures 7.8 to 7.11).

Finally, we make a comment on line drawings. The stimuli, discussed in this section, are line drawings but are supposed to stand for objects, say, sticks or wires. This is the claim of the 'object principle' introduced by van Tuijl (1979). His argument is that our world is not an art gallery of drawings. As has been argued in Chapter 5, this principle is an offshoot of the spatial contiguity principle, and constrains the two interpretations of the X-shaped cross. Remember, taken as two crossing lines, the stimulus stands for two independent straight wire segments which, of necessity, are on two planes and which, like Figure 7.3A, are described by a dissociated representation with $I = 2$. Notice that, taken as four regularly diverging lines in one plane, the pattern is appropriately described by a unified representation like Figure 7.2A″, with $I = 3$. In this case, the latter code is more complex than the former but, in another visual context, it may be the other way around (as usual, this depends on how this part is embedded in the simplest code that includes the visual context).

7.2 Surfaces

Single layers

Here, we start with discussing the coding of monochromatic surfaces on one plane. In our view, the contour of a surface reveals to a great extent the regularity of the surface. Therefore, we have the convention to represent a surface by its contour. The contour is described by a series of line segments and turns along the contour. The order of the line segments and turns agrees with the order of the contour scanning. It should be clear, however, that regularity among line segments and turns merely contributes to code simplicity if the contour correctly reflects the regularity within the surface (see later in this chapter).

The contour of a surface can be represented visually by a closed 2-D line pattern which is supposed to be enriched with a one-tailed colour filling-in within the contour (Blum and Nagel, 1978; Buffart and Leeuwenberg, 1983). In this sense, the filling-in can be considered as subordinate to the contour which, in turn, is comparable to a superstructure. Therefore, when coding such stimuli, we usually focus on the contour and we disregard the hardly distinctive colour filling-in. Obviously, the filling-in takes place within the area of convex turns and outside the area of concave turns. So, if a code does not represent all turns of a contour, it describes a contour that is not closed. Therefore, a surface code should describe all turns of the contour. In other words, the contour elements are represented in a cyclic fashion. Notice that there is no *a priori* fixed starting point of the code. In principle, during the coding, all possible starting points are to be considered, and then the overall simplest code is to be selected.

The colour filling-in also restricts the scanning order that is supposed to be involved in coding. As is said, the scanning order of a line pattern that stands for a wire object is arbitrary. However, the scanning order of a surface contour is not arbitrary. The reason is that the filling-in has two

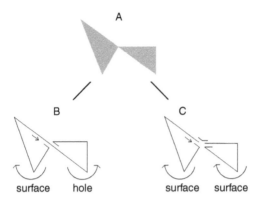

Figure 7.4 Stimulus A gives rise to two coding options. B is simple but inappropriate. If the left contour is scanned clockwise and describes a surface, the right contour is scanned anti-clockwise and describes a hole. The code suggested by C describes two adjacent surfaces and is correct.

options. For a scanner it is either leftward or rightward. So, a choice has to be made. Our choice is a rightward filling-in. This implies that, for the standard forward scanning, only the clockwise scanning is appropriate to represent a surface and the anti-clockwise scanning is appropriate to represent a hole.

Figure 7.4 illustrates a consequence for coding a surface. It depicts an incorrect and a correct unified representation of Figure 7.4A. According to the first representation, which is presented in Figure 7.4B in an exaggerated fashion, the contour of the left part is scanned clockwise and includes a surface. The contour of the right part, however, is scanned anti-clockwise. Hence, it surrounds a hole. So, this code incorrectly describes the stimulus. The second representation, which is presented in Figure 7.4C in an exaggerated fashion, is correct. The scanning is completely clockwise and leads to a unified representation of two adjacent surfaces.

Figure 7.5A shows a stimulus where the turn in the centre visually coincides with the baseline. Also, this figure gives rise to two unified codes. The first code, illustrated in Figure 7.5B, takes the stimulus as a single surface. The whole baseline **K** is one of its sides. The second code, illustrated in Figure 7.5C, takes the stimulus as two separate adjacent surfaces. Line **L** belongs to one and line **M** belongs to the other surface. To find out whether these options are visually acceptable we resort to a heuristic for segmenting surfaces, as proposed by Blum and Nagel

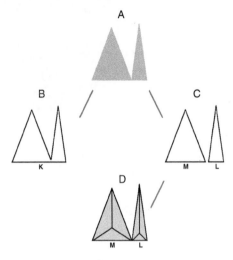

Figure 7.5 Stimulus A gives rise to two coding options. B assumes a single surface and C assumes two adjacent surfaces. The latter option is compatible with the grass fire segmentation shown in D (Blum and Nagel, 1978). This segmentation divides the baseline into the two separate line elements of option C.

(1978). Their heuristic guarantees spatial contiguous surface-contour relations. They assume, as we do, a contour filling-in, but their filling-in is analogous to grass fires that simultaneously start from all points of the contour. The points where these fires meet each other form the axes, and are shown in Figure 7.5D. These axes give rise to a subdivision of the pattern into surface segments and only the sides of these surface segments are supposed to be the contour elements of the pattern. So, for Figure 7.5A, the grass fire segmentation divides the baseline into two contour segments **L** and **M**, implying that only the second option, shown in Figure 7.5C, is correct. This constraint on the semantic mapping was overlooked by Hulleman and Boselie (1999) in their studies of randomly positioned equilateral polygons.

The latter figures illustrated how surface properties impose restrictions on the contour elements to which symbols are attributed. It is also possible that a surface property imposes a restriction on the coding of the symbols that are attributed to contour elements (Boselie, 1988). An illustration will be given. The contours of Figures 7.6AB seem to give rise to equally complex representations of bilateral symmetry. Indeed, Figure 7.6A reveals parts that are spatially symmetrical, namely, around the vertical (Figure 7.6A′ presents these parts explicitly). Therefore, its

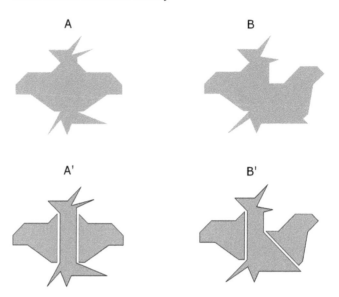

Figure 7.6 The contour codes of A and B give rise to representing both patterns as symmetrical structures. The surface of A reveals symmetry. Therefore, the symmetry code correctly describes A. However, the surface of B does not reveal symmetry. Therefore, the symmetry code inappropriately represents B.

bilateral symmetry can properly be described by its contour code. However, this does not hold for Figure 7.6B. Indeed, the symbols attributed to its contour elements reveal bilateral symmetry but, even without using grass-fire tools, it is clear that this symmetry is not a property of the surface. Therefore, the bilateral symmetry coding is not an option. In fact, the figure reveals glide symmetry that can be described by a repeat of one part and a 3-D reflection of the other part, but this description is highly complex and merely efficient if the glide symmetry is sufficiently redundant (Figure 7.6B′ presents these parts explicitly).

Homogeneous surface stimuli give rise to another pitfall. An illustration follows for the stimulus in Figure 7.7A. Its single surface interpretation, shown in Figure 7.7B, reveals equal line segments. Therefore, this option might seem to yield the simplest code ($I = 16$). The alternative interpretation, illustrated in Figure 7.7C, does not optimally reveal equal line segments. It assumes an isosceles triangle and a parallelogram in one plane, and a trapezoid in another plane. So, these subpatterns are on different planes and are independent of each other. However, they can be described by a dissociated representation whose

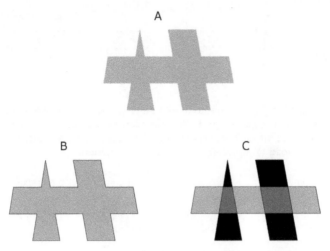

Figure 7.7 Stimulus A gives rise to two coding options. The one in B assumes a single surface with equal contour segments. Therefore, its unified contour code seems to be the simplest solution. However, the stimulus also gives rise to a dissociated representation of three independent surfaces on two planes shown in C. This dissociated code still is simpler than the unified code of B.

load ($I = 4 + 5 + 5 = 14$) is yet simpler than that of the previous option (see also next subsection). Also this fact has often been overlooked by Hulleman and Boselie (1999).

Double layers

Here we attend to dissociated representations of surfaces that might be on two layers. Like the external load (I-ext) specifications for the junctions in Figure 7.3, those for surface pairs are specified by means of the earlier mentioned formula: I-ext = Iu(maximal) – Iu(actual). Without details, we present their outcomes in Figure 7.8 by small circles. Each circle refers to a unit of I-ext and agrees with an independent coincidental relation between two surface components.

Figure 7.9 illustrates the load assessments for three transparency patterns. Of the patterns in column 1, the mosaic interpretations are shown in column 2. These interpretations are efficiently described by unified representations. Their loads are indicated by Iu. The components often can be attached to each other without extra loads for connections. Column 3 shows the transparency interpretations which, of necessity, should be described by dissociated representations. Their loads are

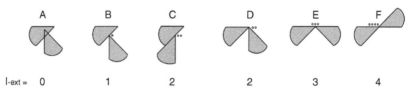

Figure 7.8 Each mini-circle in a pattern refers to a single coincidental aspect of two surface parts. As coincidences go against the assumption of independent surface parts, the number of mini-circles, I-ext, contributes to the load of dissociated pattern representations.

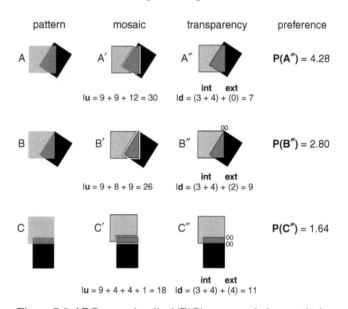

Figure 7.9 ABC are stimuli. A′B′C′ present their mosaic interpretations, described by unified representations, and A″B″C″ present transparency interpretations, described by dissociated representations. The number of mini-circles around the patterns is I-ext. The preference strength (P) applies to the transparency interpretation.

indicated by Id. The small circles around the patterns refer to I-ext. The contribution to I-ext only stems from Y or T-junctions between the contours of two surfaces. Steadily, the target of the preference strength (P) is the transparency interpretation. Though, for each pattern, the transparency interpretation is predicted to be preferred, P shows that there are yet differences in preference strength.

As has been argued earlier, the external structure is a viewpoint-dependent pattern component of a dissociated representation. In case

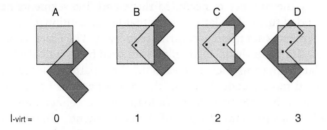

Figure 7.10 Each black mini-square in a pattern refers to a contour element in the occluded area. The contour elements comprise occluded turns and line segments between occluded turns. Their number, I-virt, contributes to the load of the dissociated occlusion representation.

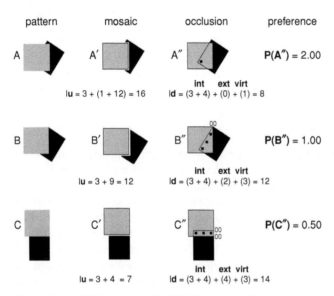

Figure 7.11 ABC are stimuli. A'B'C' present their mosaic interpretations described by unified representations, and A"B"C" present occlusion interpretations described by dissociated representations. The number of mini-circles around the patterns is I-ext and the number of mini-squares within the occluded areas is I-virt. The preference strength (P) applies to the occlusion interpretation.

of occluding surfaces, there is, according to van Lier (1996), a second viewpoint-dependent pattern component, namely, the 'virtual structure'. It deals with the invisible contour elements in the occluded surface part. These elements have to be imagined. The load, indicated by 'I-virt', is specified by the number of occluded turns and line segments between these occluded turns. The latter means that linear continuation of a visible line segment is not taken to contribute to I-virt. The I-virt is illustrated in Figure 7.10. Each virtual load unit is indicated by a small black square.

A similar coding approach applies to the three patterns in Figure 7.11. Each unified mosaic code describes the components as being pair-wise attached to each other without extra load for the connections. So, the total load equals the sum of loads of the components. The only exception is the number 1 in the Iu specification of the mosaic interpretation in Figure 7.11A′. This number refers to a 180° return to ensure that the second subpattern is equally scanned clockwise as the first subpattern. The small circles around the junctions refer to I-ext, and the small black squares within the occluded areas refer to I-virt of the dissociated representations. Notice that this time, in contrast to Figure 7.9, the occlusion interpretation is not always preferred. This is also reflected in the preference strength P. There is one case where P = 1, which refers to pattern ambiguity, and there is another case where P < 1, which means that the mosaic interpretation is supposed to prevail over the occlusion interpretation.

7.3   Objects

Representing 3-D objects by symbol strings involves rules with a rather technical character (somewhat like rules to make carpentry). Therefore, readers are free to skip this section which serves no other goal than to justify the codes used in Chapter 10. In this section, we start with fairly simple examples and we end with an account of the 3-D bias which Rock (1983) observed for complex line patterns (see Figure 7.17).

As a leg up to coding objects, we consider the surface stimuli shown in Figure 7.12. These stimuli give rise to two interpretations each. The stimuli are taken either as the given surfaces in the picture plane, or as slanted surfaces revealed by their projections.

Figure 7.12A is a stimulus and Figure 7.12A′ presents it literally. The load is: $I = 12$. Figure 7.12A″ presents the same stimulus as the projection of a slanted L shape. The load of the L shape is: $I = 7$. For the slant we count: $I = 2$ (later on we give the argument for this; see Figure 7.14). So, the total load is: $I = 9$. The latter L shape plus slant is the simplest concept of Figure 7.12A. A similar calculation reveals that Figure 7.12B is almost ambiguous and that Figure 7.12C is predicted to be interpreted literally as a pattern in the picture plane. Thus, in principle, both the literal and the slanted projection options of each stimulus have to be considered to establish the simplest interpretation.

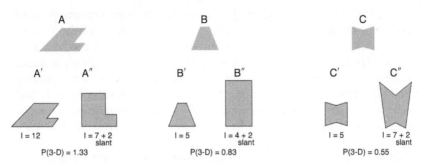

Figure 7.12 Of each of the stimuli A, B, and C, two concepts are illustrated. One concept is 2-D and presented in A′, B′, and C′. They just stand for the given surfaces in the picture plane. The other concept is 3-D and presented in A″, B″, and C″. They present projections of slanted surfaces. For any slant holds: $I = 2$ (see text). The 2-D load divided by the 3-D load is the preference strength (P) of the slant concept.

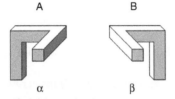

Figure 7.13 AB present stylized screws. They are the main building blocks of 3-D turns in view-independent object descriptions. A is called an α screw and agrees with a left-turn corkscrew. B is called a β screw and agrees with the common right-turn corkscrew.

3-d turns

In the following illustrations, surfaces are mostly supposed to be slanted and codes are supposed to represent the hypothetically simplest objects irrespective of viewpoint. To introduce these codes we focus on two stylized screws each standing for a basic 3-D turn. Figure 7.13A is called an α screw. Scanned from top to bottom, it consists of a 90° left-turn in the floor plane and a 90° left turn in the picture plane. Figure 7.13B is called a β screw and agrees with the common corkscrew for opening bottles. Scanned from top to bottom, it consists of a 90° right turn in the floor plane and a 90° right turn in the picture plane. Any single change of turns changes the screw. For instance, if the downward leg in Figure 7.13A is replaced by an upward leg, the shape agrees with a β screw.

Pairs of terms like the ones we just used and which are commonly used to describe shapes, namely, left vs. right, upwards vs. downwards, forward vs. backward, horizontal vs. vertical, may seem to be suitable to represent objects. However, by such terms even each screw give rise to, at least, twelve quite different descriptions, namely, of the screw from varying points of view. In fact, also these terms are viewpoint dependent, and because we aim at view-independent object representations, we avoid these terms. Instead, we will use the screws themselves as 3-D turn components (Leeuwenberg, 1971).

To show how we employ them for representing objects we attend to Figure 7.14. The top circle in Figure 7.14A is taken as superstructure and is supposed to be scanned clockwise. The subordinate structure is introduced by an α screw anchored at some point of the superstructure in line with the scanning direction. The last leg of the screw indicates the orientation of the screw within the plane determined by the last two legs. The convention is to use $\alpha(0°)$ for a 90° outward turn within the superstructure plane. In Figure 7.14A, the actual orientation $\alpha(90°)$ is downwards. Then, the upwards orientation is $\alpha(-90°)$. Figure 7.14B illustrates an application of the α turn. It shows an $\alpha(45°)$ turn, anchored at various equally distant points of a circle. This turn fixates the orientation of a straight wire length (K). So, the subordinate wire structure is described by $\alpha(45°)$ K.

Figure 7.14C presents α' being an additional screw. This screw shares the two last legs of the preceding α screw taken in a positive sense. This means that, even if the preceding screw α has a negative orientation $(-x°)$ the leg with the opposed orientation $(x°)$ is assigned to the subsequent α' screw. This measure guarantees a consistent pointing direction of α'. In Figure 7.14C this direction steadily is from right to left. The α' plane is determined by its two last legs. An $\alpha\alpha'$ combination $(I = 2)$ is appropriate to represent flanking object surfaces (see Figure 7.17) or to represent slanted surfaces (see Figure 7.12). Besides, an $\alpha\alpha'$ combination specifies any orientation in 3-D. An application of this combination is illustrated in Figure 7.14D. It presents again an $\alpha(45°)$ turn which is anchored at equidistant points on a circle and which fixates the orientation of a straight wire length (K). The subsequent turn $\alpha'(90°)$ determines the orientation of a subsequent straight wire length (L). So, the subordinate structure is described by $\alpha(45°)$ K $\alpha'(90°)$ L.

Figure 7.14E presents a third turn. It is determined by a β screw. The way this turn is anchored to the previous α' is similar to the way α' is anchored to α. By means of a β turn any plane in 3-D can be fixated. The β turn is especially suitable to specify the bottom plane of an object (see Figure 7.17). Besides, it plays a crucial role for the mass filling-in within

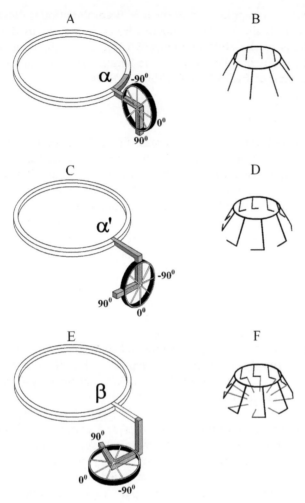

Figure 7.14 A shows an α(90°) screw anchored at some point of a circle. This turn, and any other screw turn, agrees with the orientation of the last leg in the plane determined by the last two legs. B illustrates an application. It shows sub-wires comprising an α(45°) turn and a line. C shows an α(90°) turn extended by an α'(90°) screw. The two screws share two legs. D illustrates an application. It shows sub-wires comprising an α(45°), a line, an α'(90°), and a line. E shows an α(90°)α'(90°) combination extended by a β(90°) screw. F illustrates an application. It shows sub-wires comprising an α(45°), a line, an α'(90°), a line, β(90°), and a line.

an object surface. An application of the α α′ β combination is illustrated by Figure 7.14F. It shows a subordinate wire code that for its first part has all elements of the code of Figure 7.14D. The remaining part is introduced by a β turn followed by a line length (M). The subordinate structure is described by: α(45°) K α′(90°) L β(90°) M.

Superstructures

For coding solid objects we assume a mass filling-in operation which, in various respects, is similar to the 2-D filling-in for coding surfaces. For surface filling-in, we used the clockwise scanning as standard. Then, anti-clockwise scanning generates a 2-D hole. A similar consequence applies to mass filling-in. The standard clockwise scanning of the superstructure in a hierarchical solid object code implies that a positive β turn is consistently oriented towards the object's centre and is appropriate for the mass filling-in. An anti-clockwise scanning of the superstructure implies that a positive β turn generates a 3-D hole.

Obviously, the contour is the reference frame of surface filling-in. Similarly, the object's surface is reference frame of mass filling-in. So, the content of filling-in is subordinate to these frames and does not belong to these frames. It is like the relation between subordinate structure and superstructure. Besides, it is plausible that all such hierarchical relations are reflected by the stages in the reconstruction of a stimulus from its code. That is, these stages occur from superstructure to subordinate structure, or from frame to surface or mass. There is still another feature of superstructures and frames. They are, like coordinates, conceptual components whereas subordinate structures and contents of filling-in, such as surface and mass, stand for the material aspects of shapes.

To illustrate the mentioned superstructure and frame features, Figure 7.15 will be introduced. The presented objects are accompanied with visualized codes and we first repeat a few conventions about their form. One is that the superstructure is indicated at the top of the visualized code. In most examples, this superstructure also agrees with the top component of the stimulus object. The subordinate structure is indicated at the bottom of the visualized code. This structure steadily agrees with the left subordinate component of the stimulus object. The 2-D or 3-D turns, which relate subordinate structures to superstructures, are not indicated in the visualized codes. Also, the 2-D surface and 3-D mass filling-in are not indicated in the visualized codes.

The object in Figure 7.15A can be represented by a so-called 'double code'. Such a code consists of two subcodes each representing one of the two parts of the object. Both subcodes deal with clockwise (+)

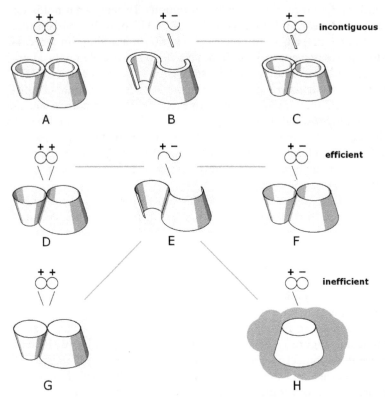

Figure 7.15 A, D, and G can be described each by a 'double code'. Such a code consists of two subcodes that represent two object parts separately. Both subcodes deal with clockwise scanned superstructures (+ +) and different subordinate structures. The codes of B and E are single codes. Their meandering superstructures are first scanned clockwise (+) and thereafter anticlockwise (−). Also C, F, and H are described each by such a single code. For C this code is not spatially contiguous, for F this code is efficient, and for H this code is inefficient.

scanned superstructures but they describe different subordinate structures. In contrast, the object in Figure 7.15B can be described by one superstructure and one subordinate surface structure. The scanning of its superstructure from left to right is first clockwise (+) and thereafter anticlockwise (−). A similar single code, presented in Figure 7.15C, seems an appropriate and efficient representation of the object in Figure 7.15A. However, this code describes the slightly different object presented in Figure 7.15C. Besides, it describes the mass in the central intersection twice and is, therefore, not spatially contiguous. In fact, what holds for Figures 7.15AB also holds for Figures 7.15DE. The only difference is that the first figures present solid objects presuming mass filling-in whereas the latter figures present surface shapes made up by wire elements. However, what holds for Figure 7.15C does not equally hold for Figure 7.15F. The single superstructure of the latter figure is an 8-shape with a beginning and an end that are not adjacent to each other but that are adjacent to the wire part through the central point (hence, no gap). In our view, for this reason, the object in Figure 7.15F approximates the object in Figure 7.15D so closely that their difference is negligible. Instead, their codes are not equally complex. The single code in Figure 7.15F most efficiently describes both objects.

The visualized code for Figure 7.15D can be interpreted otherwise and can be used to represent the solid object in Figure 7.15G. According to this interpretation, this solid object can be reconstructed from the code by the following four reconstruction stages. The first stage is the fixation of the superstructure. The second stage is the fixation of the subordinate structure. The third stage deals with the surface filling-in of the superstructure and the subordinate structure (see next subsection). The fourth step is the 3-D mass filling-in within all surfaces.

The single code in Figure 7.15H, being analogous to the single code of the object in Figure 7.15E, might seem to be appropriate and efficient to represent the object in Figure 7.15G. However, as the first circle is scanned clockwise and the second anti-clockwise, the surface filling-in of the first circle is within the circle and that of the second circle is outside the circle. As a result, the whole surface filling-in generates a hole within an indefinitely extended surface and the subsequent mass filling-in generates a hole within an indefinitely extended mass. So, the single code in Figure 7.15H merely describes one 3-D hole in a rather inefficient way.

Subordinate structures

A closed object surface is needed to obtain an appropriate mass filling-in. For the circular superstructure we have used so far, this requirement seems sufficiently satisfied. At least, a vase object suggested by turning a constant S-shaped wire around a circle reveals a closed object surface (see Chapter 3). Here, the motion, being a conceptual object component, refers to the superstructure, and the S-shaped wire, being a material object component, refers to the subordinate structure. However, the static reconstruction of the same object from its code, namely, by attaching S-shapes at all points of a circle, does not convincingly end with

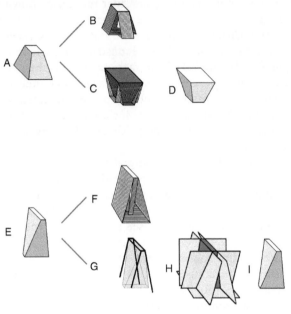

Figure 7.16 B illustrates the failing reconstruction of A from its code where its small top square is superstructure and a fixed hook is subordinate structure. C illustrates the initial reconstruction of A from its code with the large square as superstructure. The object D is the outcome of a cut-off operation. It presupposes an indefinitely extended mass and eliminates all the mass beyond the planes. E misses a larger superstructure. The reconstruction recipe of using the top rectangle as superstructure and a hook as subordinate structure generates F instead of E. To represent E, an alternative option is to extend the top superstructure with subordinate components that represent the flanking and floor planes. The final object I is the proper outcome of a cut-off operation.

a closed object surface. Moreover, we represent a circle as an extreme exemplar of a regular polygon such as a square (see Chapter 7). This implies that a tenable static object reconstruction from a circular superstructure has to agree with a tenable static object reconstruction from a square superstructure. To find an appropriate construction recipe that applies to both shapes we make use of the illustrations in Figure 7.16.

Figure 7.16A presents an object characterized by a square superstructure. Figure 7.16B shows an object reconstruction by attaching some subordinate hooks at all points of the small top square. Obviously, the hooks only partly represent the flanking surfaces and the floor plane. In other words, this reconstruction does not reveal a closed object surface. An alternative approach is to consider the upside down version of the object in Figure 7.16A and to use the large square as superstructure. The object reconstruction, illustrated in Figure 7.16C, seems more promising. At least, the surfaces of the reconstruction include the complete target version in Figure 7.16D. In fact, object D is the outcome of a cut-off operation. This operation presupposes an indefinitely extended mass and eliminates all the mass beyond the planes indicated by Figure 7.16C, that is, beyond the superstructure surface at the top of the object and beyond the subordinate planes comprising the flanking surfaces and the floor surface.

The object in Figure 7.16E, which is equal to its upside down version, misses a largest superstructure. So, the question is: what is the recipe for this object? Figure 7.16F illustrates the reconstruction from the code with the rectangle as superstructure and hooks as subordinate structures. This reconstruction, however, is not closed and disagrees with the target object in Figure 7.16E. Yet, there is a solution that actually applies for all cases. Its basic information is illustrated in Figure 7.16G and deals with a rectangular superstructure. Each long side is extended with a line component described by $\alpha(60°)K\{\alpha'\}120°\{\alpha'\}$, $I = 4$, and each short side is extended with a line component described by $\alpha(120°)\{\alpha'\}$, $I = 2$. All the subcomponents $\{\alpha'\}$ fixate the indefinitely extended flanking planes and the floor plane indicated in Figure 7.16H. Finally, it is assumed that the mass included by these planes and the superstructure is obtained by a mass cut-off of the mass beyond all planes from an arbitrary extended mass. The result, shown in Figure 7.16I, agrees with the target in Figure 7.16E. In fact, such a cut-off recipe is usually applied by a carpenter if he uses a saw or a chisel to fabricate a shape from a piece of wood.

Figure 7.17 shows an application of the cut-off recipe. Figure 7.17A presents an irregular line pattern and it was demonstrated by Rock (1983) that its 3-D interpretation is visually preferred over its 2-D interpretation. Besides, Rock (1983) claimed that the 3-D concept is more complex than the 2-D concept. So, this order of complexity disagrees with the order of preference. According to our approach, the order of complexity is reverse, as we show next.

The assessment of the 2-D concept of Figure 7.17A is simple. As illustrated by Figure 7.17B, this concept is minimally fixated by fourteen different line segments and eleven different 2-D turns. So, the total load is $I = 25$. The assessment of the 3-D concept is less obvious. Its coding can be shown in three steps. The first accounts for a skeleton illustrated in Figure 7.17C. This skeleton comprises a 2-D top quadrangle that has four lengths and four turns. So, $I = 8$. Furthermore, each turn of the quadrangle is extended with a pair of 3-D turns: $\alpha\{\alpha'\}$. So, $I = 8$. One of

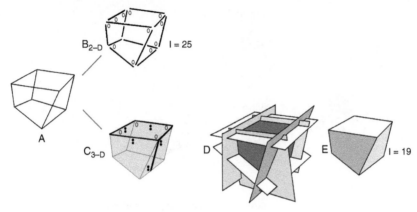

Figure 7.17 Stimulus A gives rise to two interpretations. One is the 2-D concept in B. Its load, I = 25, stems from fourteen line segments and eleven turns (open disks). The other interpretation is the 3-D cube concept. The recipe of its code prescribes three steps. The first is shown in C. It comprises the fixation of the quadrangular superstructure, I = 8, the fixation of four pairs of 3-D turns attached to each corner of the quadrangle, I = 8, and the extension of one pair with a line length plus two 3-D turns, I = 3. The second step deals with surface filling-in. The resulting six surfaces are shown in D. The third step deals with the mass cut-off operation. E shows the space enclosed by all surfaces. The total load is I = 19.

the pairs is extended with a line towards the floor described by $\mathbf{K} \, \alpha' \{\beta\}$. So, I = 3. The $\{\alpha'\}$ components fixate the flanking planes and the $\{\beta\}$ component fixates the floor plane of the cube. The second step deals with the surface filling-in of the superstructure and the planes. The result is illustrated in Figure 7.17D. The third step is the mass cut-off operation that selects the object in Figure 7.17E. The load (I = 19) of this 3-D concept is lower than the load (I = 25) of the 2-D concept.

The mass cut-off operation suffices for convex shapes but not for shapes with one or more concavities. We will illustrate this by Figure 7.18A which presents an object with one concavity. The superstructure and subordinate structures of its code fixate all six indefinitely extended surfaces of the target object. The four lines in the disk presented by Figure 7.18B refer to the indefinitely extended flanking surfaces of the target object. The cut-off operation presumes an indefinitely extended mass, indicated by grey. The latter figure shows the result of this operation, namely, a grey pattern that disagrees with the superstructure of Figure 7.18A.

A solution is based on the following two rules. One is that mass cut-off, which presumes an indefinitely extended mass, is appropriate for convex

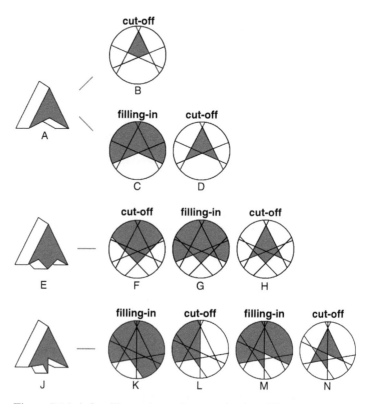

Figure 7.18 A few illustrations of mass selection. The lines within the disks refer to extensions of the flanking object surfaces. Grey stands for present mass and white stands for absent mass. The mass cut-off, which presumes an unlimited mass, leaves the dark grey pattern in B but not the superstructure of A. The reason is that cut-off merely applies to convex parts and filling-in to concave parts. Moreover, the order of these operations should be from most nested to least nested parts. According to these rules, object A is obtained by a mass filling-in within concave surfaces (C) and a subsequent cut-off of mass beyond convex surfaces (D). For the more complex objects J and N the mass selection operations are applied according to the same rules.

parts and mass filling-in, which presumes empty space, is appropriate for concave parts. As has been noticed, mass cut-off is usually applied by a carpenter if he uses a saw to fabricate a shape from a piece of wood. The mass filling-in is applied by a founder who casts a mould to fabricate a shape. The second rule states that the order of filling operations occurs from the most nested to the least nested parts.

As the most nested part in Figure 7.18A is concave, the first operation deals with mass filling-in. This operation assumes empty space indicated by white. The filling-in is shown in Figure 7.18C. The remaining part is convex. Hence, the next operation deals with mass cut-off. The result is presented in Figure 7.18D and reveals the pattern of mass that agrees with the superstructure of the target object. To give some more illustrations of the above rules, the mass selection operations are shown for the slightly more complex objects in Figures 7.18E and J.

All in all, we tend to conclude that hierarchical codes of solid objects comprise sufficient information to take them as correct object construction recipes. These recipes assume a mass cut-off operation to eliminate mass beyond convex object surfaces and a mass filling-in operation to fill mass within concave object surfaces under the condition that the order of operations occurs from most nested to least nested parts.

Summary

Section 7.1 is on line drawings. It starts with the distinction between unified and dissociated representations. A unified representation describes connected elements of a pattern in relation to each other and is a stimulus construction recipe. The primitive code consists of the subsequent line and turn elements. The scanning either is serial or bifurcating. Besides, the scanning either is forward or backward. Zero turns are only needed if an undivided line is yet described by sub-lines and if an undivided angle is yet described by sub-angles. A line stimulus, interpreted as an assembly of independent components, is described by a dissociated representation. Its load equals the sum of loads of the components (internal structure) plus the sum of coincidences between components at local junctions (external structure).

Section 7.2 is on surfaces. The code of a surface only describes its contour but presupposes a coloured surface filling-in operation. To ensure an unambiguous filling-in, the contour should be described in a cyclic fashion, that is, by all its subsequent lines and turns. For the same reason, one kind of scanning, say, clockwise, is used to represent a surface, and then anti-clockwise scanning is used to represent a hole. The regularity of a contour is not always properly reflected by the enclosed surface. So, the surface constrains codes. Likewise, the spatial contiguity principle constrains codes. Commonly, a mosaic interpretation is efficiently described by a unified representation and a transparency or occlusion interpretation is efficiently described by a dissociated representation. In case of occluding layers, also the virtual structure load, that is, the number of occluded elements, contributes to the load of the code.

Section 7.3 is on objects. A simple object is commonly represented by a 2-D superstructure and a 2-D subordinate structure whose relation is specified by a 3-D turn. This turn is fixated by one or more screws. It is specified by the orientation in the plane of the last two legs of the last screw. Two screws determine any direction and three screws determine any plane. The object surface, being the frame for mass selection operations, is sufficiently fixated by the indefinitely extended surfaces that include the surfaces of the object. To represent a solid object the mass cut-off operation is used to eliminate mass beyond convex object surfaces and the mass filling-in operation is used to fill mass within concave object surfaces. The order of operations occurs from most nested to least nested parts. So, hierarchical object codes sufficiently prescribe the reconstruction of objects.

8   Preference effects

Introduction

This chapter reviews published experiments with stimuli that can be interpreted as consisting of overlapping layers. In most cases, this double-layer interpretation corresponds with an optic illusion. As the overlapping layers are supposed to be independent of each other, they are appropriately described by a dissociated representation. The alternative, more literal, 2-D stimulus concept often deals with one layer consisting of juxtaposed mosaic parts and is efficiently described by a unified representation. Steadily, the preference strength of the illusory concept is the target of study. Its measure is specified by the load of the alternative concept divided by the load of the target concept. Furthermore, we do not use the information load metric applied in those published experiments, but we re-evaluate the stimuli using the metric proposed more recently by van der Helm *et al.* (1992) and van Lier *et al.* (1994).

Section 8.1 deals with occlusion patterns and shows how our global simplicity approach contrasts to local cue approaches. It is demonstrated further that subjective contours are pattern occlusion effects and that the preference measure accounts for the brightness effects within subjective contours.

Section 8.2 is concerned with translucent double layers which do not hide any of their structures. We start discussing simple line patterns and their favoured segmentations. Further studies deal with visual and auditory transparency, neon effects, and brightness assimilation versus contrast. These phenomena have been topics of earlier research but mostly with respect to their metrical aspects. Here, attention is focused on their form.

Section 8.3 focuses on the supposition underlying the preference strength measure, namely, that a stimulus not only activates the simplest interpretation but also less simple rivaling interpretations. Evidence for this supposition is shown both for occluding and translucent layers.

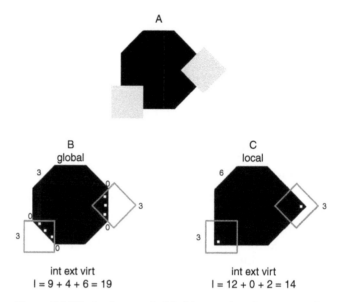

Figure 8.1 The background of A either can be taken as a regular polygon (see B) or as an irregular polygon (see C). The dissociated representation, proposed by van Lier *et al.* (1994), explains the preference for C in line with the simplicity principle. The load of C is lower than that of B. The mini-circles refer to information units of the external-structure and the mini-squares refer to information units of the virtual-structure (Kanizsa, 1985).

8.1   Occluding layers

Global and local completion

Adjacent pairs of surfaces may give rise to occlusion interpretations and some of these interpretations seem to falsify the simplicity principle. An illustration, designed by Kanizsa (1979), is presented in Figure 8.1A. For this figure, two interpretations are presented in Figures 8.1B and C. In Figure 8.1B, the background pattern is a regular polygon, I-int = 3, and in Figure 8.1C, the background pattern is a less regular polygon, I-int = 6. According to Kanizsa (1979), the regular polygon interpretation might be preferred at the conscious level of reasoning but at the level of perception the irregular polygon interpretation is preferred. Indeed, locally, at points of good continuation the irregular polygon code is simpler than the regular polygon code but, globally, it is more complex. Because Kanizsa (1979) assumed that the simplicity principle should apply to the global shape, he considered the irregular polygon interpretation as a

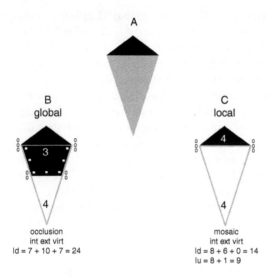

Figure 8.2 Pattern A either can be taken as a regular pentagon occluded by a triangle (B) or as a mosaic of two triangles (C). The latter mosaic interpretation is preferred although the code of the black pentagon in B is simpler than the code of the black triangle in C (Boselie, 1994). However, the whole dissociated code of B is more complex than the whole dissociated and the whole unified code of C. The mini-circles refer to units of external load and the white mini-squares refer to units of virtual load (Boselie, 1988).

falsification of the simplicity principle. In other words, local simplicity seems to overrule global simplicity. However, as shown in Figure 8.1, according to the dissociated codes, the irregular polygon interpretation is simpler than the regular polygon interpretation.

Figure 8.2A, which was designed by Boselie (1988), evokes a similar effect. Its global interpretation in Figure 8.2B organizes the stimulus as a black regular pentagon, I = 3, occluded by a grey triangle. Its local interpretation in Figure 8.2C reflects a mosaic of a black triangle, I = 4, and a grey triangle. Notwithstanding these loads, the latter local mosaic interpretation is preferred. So, also for this figure the simplicity principle seems to fail. However, this is not true according to structural information theory (SIT). As shown in Figure 8.2, both the dissociated representation and the unified representation of this mosaic interpretation are simpler than the dissociated occlusion representation.

Integrating local and global simplicity In the above two illustrations, the internal structure load I-int alone would not predict the judged preferences. This seems to falsify the global simplicity principle and seems to emphasize the visual relevance of local effects. However, the external and virtual loads I-ext and I-virt of the dissociated representations account for these local effects and restore the adequacy of the global simplicity principle. Whereas the internal structure belongs to the view-independent component of a dissociated representation, both the external and virtual structures belong to its view-dependent component, and it is to the merit of van Lier's integration model that it expresses the loads of all these structures in common terms, namely in terms of structural information and not partly in terms of structural information and partly in terms of probability (see Chapter 7). This way, the view-dependent factor is just as decisive as the view-independent factor. This is analogous to the components of the Bayes rule. Applied to perceptual organization, the conditional component of the Bayes rule deals with the view-dependent structure and is just as decisive as the prior component which deals with the view-independent structure.

Van Lier *et al.* (1994; see also van Lier, 1996) analysed 144 line drawings stemming from various earlier studies, namely twenty-five patterns from Buffart *et al.* (1981), twenty-seven patterns from Boselie (1988), and ninety-two patterns from Boselie and Wouterlood (1989). About 50 per cent of the patterns of the latter two sets evoke local effects. In all three studies, the preferred pattern interpretations were established by letting the subjects draw the occluded pattern parts. For 96 per cent of these figures, van Lier's predictions appeared to agree with the preferred visual interpretations. The correct predictions, purely on the basis of I-int, I-ext, and I-virt separately, amounted to 52 per cent, 65 per cent, and 49 per cent, respectively. Correct predictions based on the sum of a pair of these loads were higher, about 80 per cent, but lower than the predictions based on the sum of all three loads together. A few wrong predictions can be attributed to the measure of virtual load. This load counts each individual hidden turn and line segment irrespective of their regularity. Probably, this may lead to a visually implausible over-estimation of I-virt in case the virtual structure reveals a highly redundant regularity.

Various follow-up studies were published elsewhere by de Wit (2004), de Wit and van Lier (2002), van Lier (1999, 2000, 2001, 2003), van Lier *et al.* (1995, 1997), van Lier and Wagemans (1999). The assumption that perception prefers to deal with an overall criterion like simplicity has already been defended by other authors such as Buffart and Leeuwenberg (1983), Koffka (1935), Restle (1982), and Sekuler and Palmer (1992). This assumption contrasts to the view that visual phenomena, and especially the illustrated local effects in pattern completion, are mainly determined by local junctions. Some proponents of the latter are Barrow and Tenenbaum (1981), Boselie (1988, 1994), Boselie and Wouterlood (1989, 1992), Biederman (1987), Chapanis and McCleary (1953), Dinnerstein and Wertheimer (1957), Kellman and Shipley (1991), and Rock (1983). Next, we illustrate such an attempt to explain local completion effects by local cues.

A local approach Boselie (1988) showed that loads, based on internal structures only, are not sufficient to predict perceptual pattern interpretations, especially those revealing local effects (see Figures 8.1 and 8.2). To account for local effects, van Lier *et al.* (1994) introduced the above discussed integration model involving dissociated representations. At the time, Boselie (1994) proposed another solution for the same problem. He accepted the global simplicity principle based on internal structures only, but he assumed local cues that were supposed to overrule this simplicity principle. In fact, he distinguished between T-junctions and t-junctions. As is shown at the top of Figure 8.3, the vertical and the horizontal shaft of a T-junction delineate each one region whereas the vertical shaft of a t-junction delineates two regions. His claim was that, irrespective of the global simplicity principle, T-junctions evoke occlusion interpretations and t-junctions evoke mosaic interpretations.

Boselie (1994) tested various sets of four black-and-white patterns on grey backgrounds. In Figure 8.3, one set is illustrated. Figures 8.3A and B show T-junctions and Figures 8.3C and D show t-junctions. The task was to rate the patterns on a scale from mosaic to occlusion, and to draw the occluded parts. Indeed, Figures 8.3A and B were judged as occlusion patterns and Figures 8.3C and D as mosaic patterns. So, the outcomes agreed with Boselie's predictions.

Indeed, the effects of the local junctions overrule a simplicity principle based on internal structures only. For instance, the simplest internal structure of Figure 8.3D predicts the occlusion interpretation whereas the mosaic interpretation is preferred and predicted by the t-cue. However, notice that, for Figure 8.3, all visual interpretations are also predicted by a simplicity principle based on internal, external and virtual structures, as SIT uses nowadays. Furthermore, such simplest SIT codes are also compatible with the visual interpretations of Figures 8.4A and B, which contrasts with Boselie's approach. The first figure merely deals with T-junctions, so, Boselie would incorrectly predict the occlusion interpretation. The second pattern merely deals with t-junctions so, Boselie would incorrectly predict the mosaic interpretation.

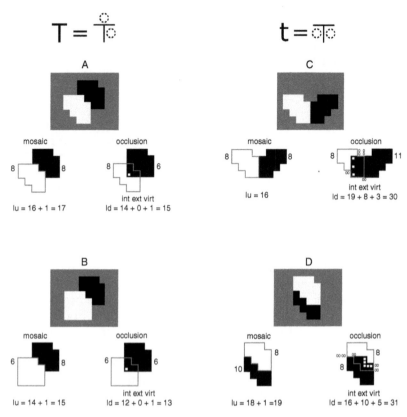

Figure 8.3 According to Boselie (1994), the T-junctions A and B evoke occlusion interpretations, and the t-junctions C and D evoke mosaic interpretations, irrespective of the simplicity of the shapes involved. The model proposed by van Lier *et al.* (1994), however, predicts these interpretations from the simplest unified or dissociated representations. The mini-circles refer to units of external-structure information and the white mini-squares refer to units of virtual-structure information (Boselie, 1994).

Subjective contours

An illusion, discovered by Schumann (1900), is evoked by a black pattern with a hole at its centre. The illusory effect is a white shape in between the black parts. This white shape appears slightly brighter than the white of the paper and is characterized by so-called 'subjective' contours. Figure 8.5A_1 is an example designed by Erhenstein (1941). It reveals a visually extra white disk at its centre. Figure 8.5A_2 illustrates a pattern without this illusory effect.

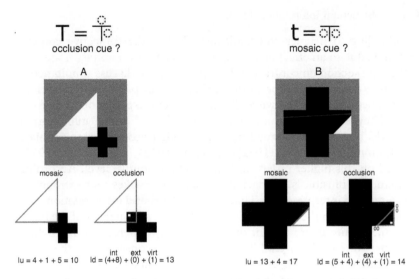

Figure 8.4 The T-junctions in A should evoke an occlusion interpretation and the t-junctions in B should evoke a mosaic interpretation (Boselie, 1994) although their visual interpretations are opposed. Their visual interpretations are predicted from their SIT loads. The mini-circles refer to external-structure load units and the white mini-squares refer to virtual-structure load units.

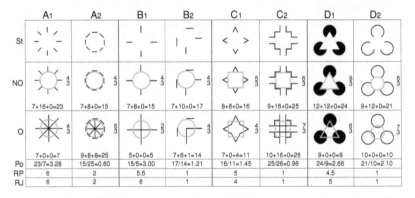

	A1	A2	B1	B2	C1	C2	D1	D2
NO	7+16+0=23	7+8+0=15	7+8+0=15	7+10+0=17	8+8+0=16	9+16+0=25	12+12+0=24	9+12+0=21
O	7+0+0=7	9+8+8=25	5+0+0=5	7+6+1=14	7+0+4=11	10+16+0=26	9+0+0=9	10+0+0=10
Po	23/7=3.28	15/25=0.60	15/5=3.00	17/14=1.21	16/11=1.45	25/26=0.96	24/9=2.66	21/10=2.10
RP	6	2	5.5	1	5	1	4.5	1
RJ	6	2	6	1	4	1	5	1

Figure 8.5 Row 1 presents eight experimental stimuli, that is, two from each set A, B, C, and D. Row 2 presents the contours (grey) of white shapes being in front of the empty central areas of the black stimuli. Row 2 also presents the dissociated loads of these non-occlusion interpretations (NO). Row 3 presents the contours of the same white shapes being in front of completed versions of the black stimuli. Row 3 also presents the dissociated loads of these occlusion interpretations (O). Row 4 presents the theoretical preference strengths (Po) of the occlusion interpretations. Row 5 presents their ranks (RP) per set. The average ranks (RJ) of the judged subjective contours per set are indicated in row 6.

According to Brigner and Gallagher (1974), the subjective contour illusion is due to an effect of simultaneous brightness contrast. Later on, in the next section on contrast and assimilation, we discuss simultaneous brightness contrast as a superposition effect of transparent colours. Frisby and Clatworthy (1975) gave a slightly different explanation at sensory level. They attributed the illusion to an effect of lateral inhibition at line ends, but they also argued that some higher order mechanism plays an additional role. Coren (1972), Gregory (1972), and Kanizsa (1979) focused on this higher order mechanism at a cognitive level. According to them, the illusion is stronger if the stimulus evokes more strongly a figure-ground interpretation. That is, a figure-ground interpretation with a black pattern on the overall white background, and in front of the black pattern, a white figure which, due to contrast, is perceived as brighter than the white of the overall background. As a consequence, the white foreground shape reveals contours. These contours are called subjective contours because, in the stimulus, this white foreground shape is not really brighter than the white of the overall background.

Van Tuijl and Leeuwenberg (1982) tested the latter idea by investigating whether the strength of the subjective contour illusion correlates with the theoretical preference strength for completing the black pattern behind the illusory foreground. The target of the preference measure is the simplest interpretation involving a completed black pattern, and this target is contrasted to the simplest interpretation without a completion of the black pattern. To specify this further, Van Tuijl and Leeuwenberg (1982) noticed that this subjective contour phenomenon is not an authentic illusion. After all, without having been explained what the illusory phenomenon is, and without knowing what to look for, subjects hardly experience an illusory effect. Therefore, they decided that the two interpretations to be contrasted should comprise the same potentially illusory foreground, which partly occludes a completed black pattern in case of the target interpretation (O) but not in case of the alternative interpretation (NO). The preference strength measure Po for the target (load of NO divided by load of O) then indicates the relative strength of the occlusion interpretation, which by the idea above, is assumed to predict whether and, if so, how strongly the potentially illusory foreground is indeed perceived as part of the stimulus. Hence, both interpretations involve two layers and are to be described by dissociated codes. Next, we go into more detail on these codes for the two experimental patterns shown in row 1 of Figures 8.5A$_1$ and A$_2$.

The non-occlusion code (NO) of Figure 8.5A$_1$ represents the stimulus (I = 4, see Figure 7.2B′) and a disk (I = 3), here indicated by its contour, in front of the empty central area of the stimulus. So, I-int = 7.

Furthermore, I-ext = 16 (see Figure 7.3C). Obviously, I-virt = 0, as the foreground does not occlude any stimulus part. In fact, this holds for each NO code. The occlusion (O) represents the simplest completed version of the stimulus. It describes crossing lines starting from an external invisible octagon (I = 4). Furthermore, it deals with a white disk (I = 3) that occludes the central part of the completed stimulus version. So, I-int = 7. Besides, I-ext = 0. Also, I-virt = 0, because the occluded part merely deals with linearly continuing lines without turns (see Chapter 7).

The NO code of Figure 8.5A_2 describes a regular octagon with gaps (I = 4) and a disk (I = 3) in front of its central empty area. So, I-int = 7. Due to the eight contour-segments of the regular octagon being tangent to the illusory disk, I-ext = 8 (see Figure 7.3B). The occlusion code (O) represents the simplest completed version of the stimulus and is shown in Figure 8.5, column 2, row 3. Its internal structure comprises an octagon with gaps being extended with radial lines towards the centre of the pattern (I = 6) plus a disk (I = 3). So, I-int = 9. Again, I-ext = 8 like it is for the NO interpretation. Besides, I-virt = 8 due to the virtual turns between the radial lines and the octagon segments. The turns in the centre of the pattern do not contribute to I-virt as they are not described by the simplest code of the background. As Po < 1, the prediction is absence of subjective contours.

In fact, the latter case reflects a paradoxical feature of subjective contour illusions, namely, the illusion of a brighter foreground is weaker the more the shape of this foreground is more explicitly present in the stimulus. The stimulus in Figure 8.5A_2 almost coincides with the contour of the disk. Likewise, in Figure 8.5C_2, the stimulus already exposes a large part of the contour of the square that is supposed to present the illusory foreground. Also this stimulus hardly evokes a subjective contour illusion.

In the study by Van Tuijl and Leeuwenberg (1982), four sets (ABCD) were involved, each comprising six patterns (row 1 in Figure 8.5 gives two examples from each set). The patterns within each set were similar in various respects and therefore well comparable. The first three sets were made up by variants of Ehrenstein patterns. The patterns in the last set were designed by Kanizsa (1976, 1979). In Figure 8.5, row 2 presents the NO interpretations and their dissociated loads, row 3 presents the O interpretations and their dissociated loads, row 4 presents the theoretical preference strengths Po, and row 5 presents their ranks RP per set.

The procedure was as follows. Sixty-four participants were tested individually. In each trial, two patterns were presented and the task was to indicate the pattern with the strongest subjective contour illusion. By testing all pair-wise combinations (fifteen) per set, the judged illusory strengths of the patterns were established. Their ranks RJ are indicated in row 6 of Figure 8.5.

The results were as follows. The Spearman rank-correlations between RP and RJ within the sets A, B, C, and D are r = .91, r = .98, r = .84, and r = .84, respectively. The three theoretically higher illusory patterns per set were judged significantly higher than the three theoretically lower illusory patterns (p < .01; sign-test and chi-square). So, the results were roughly in line with the predictions.

The earlier predictions by Van Tuijl and Leeuwenberg (1982) were of about the same level, but their measure was different. Their overall Po was a weighted sum of Po on a central code level and Po on a primitive code level. The first Po accounts for structural pattern aspects and the second Po accounts for metrical pattern aspects such as the number of line segments in patterns. Indeed, this number contributes to the illusory effect (Dumais and Bradley, 1976; Frisby and Clatworthy, 1975; Kennedy, 1978). In contrast, we use a single Po measure. It deals with dissociated codes that describe internal, external, and virtual structures. Generally, their internal structures account for structural pattern aspects and the external and virtual structures account for metrical pattern aspects such as the number of line segments in patterns.

8.2   Translucent layers

Above, we considered stimuli that can be interpreted as opaque layers with a foreground partly occluding the background. Then, perception tends to complete the background pattern behind the occluding part. Hence, the dissociated representation involves a virtual structure. In this section, we attend to stimuli that can be interpreted as partly overlapping translucent layers. Then, the background is still visible. Hence, there is no need to complete the background pattern and the dissociated representation does not deal with a virtual structure.

Line patterns

Van Tuijl and Leeuwenberg (1980) tested the visual segmentation of twenty patterns. A subset of seven patterns is illustrated in row 1 of Figure 8.6. Two subdivisions are contrasted to each other. Row 2 presents the segments of subdivision 1 and its load I_1. Row 3 presents the segments of subdivision 2 and its load I_2. The theoretical preference strength P for subdivision 2, being $P = I_1/I_2$, is indicated in row 4. For eighteen patterns in the experiment holds $P > 1$ and for two patterns holds $P = 1$. The

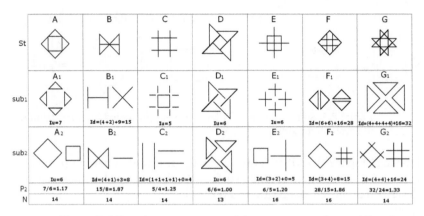

Figure 8.6 Row 1 presents seven of the twenty experimental line drawings. Row 2 shows the segments of subdivision 1 and its load I_1. Row 3 shows the segments of subdivision 2 and its load I_2. The theoretical preference for subdivision 2 is indicated in row 4. The numbers of subjects (N) who preferred subdivision 2 are presented in row 5 (Nmax = 16).

numbers of subjects (N) that preferred subdivision 2 are presented in row 5.

The task was as follows. In each trial, a pattern was presented and the subject had to mentally establish the preferred segmentation. After five seconds, two subdivisions were presented side-by-side below the pattern. The task was to indicate, as fast as possible, the preferred segmentation. There were sixteen participants, and the presentation order was randomized.

Before we discuss the results of the experiment, we make a digression to clarify a few aspects of coding. The reason is that these aspects are, in our view, not directly obvious. This also holds for some concrete pattern descriptions that we will discuss.

Generally, the simplest mosaic description is a unified code and the simplest description of a foreground-background interpretation is a dissociated representation. Furthermore, in many cases, it is more efficient to take a stimulus as a wire and not as a surface because a wire is not constrained by scanning order (clockwise or anti-clockwise) and does not need to be described by all its turns. Of course, each given pattern component of the subdivision should be described by an isolated and well identifiable part of the code.

The codes we illustrate describe a few patterns of Figure 8.6. In Figure 8.7, these patterns are presented once more, using the same

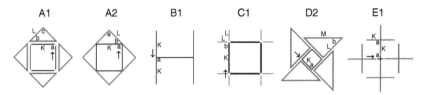

Figure 8.7 Some patterns of Figure 8.6 are presented in more detail to illustrate their coding.

labeling. Figure 8.7A1 is represented by a virtual square superstructure and a subordinate triangle surface. In the next code, the square is described at the left-hand side and the isosceles triangle at the right-hand side:

4 * (a K{S[(b)(L),(c)]K})

Figure 8.7A2 is represented by two square wires, one inside the other. In the next code, the inside square is described at the left-hand side and the outside square at the right-hand side, while the turn b determines the relation between the two squares:

4 * (aK)bS[S[((L)),((a))]]

Figure 8.7B1 comprises an H shape, described efficiently by making use of a 180° turn. The primitive code is as follows:

{K}180°{K}aLa{K}180°{K}

The description of Figure 8.7C1 also makes use of a 180° turn. Its partly simplified code is as follows:

4 * (K{L}b{L}180°)

Like Figure 8.7A1, Figure 8.7D2 deals with an invisible square superstructure. This time, the subordinate structure is an open isosceles triangle and therefore a wire object. As the superstructure fixates one of its turns, this figure can be described in a less complex way than Figure 8.7A1. Its partly simplified code is as follows:

4 * (a K{L bM b L})

Figure 8.7E1 can be described by a dissociated representation of four independent crosses, each represented by two independent lines, I = 2 + 2 + 2 + 2 = 8, but the unified representation of a nested hierarchy is more efficient, I = 6. It represents the pattern by a rotation around the centre. The primary component of the subordinate structure is an invisible line segment. At its end, a cross is attached. This time, this cross cannot be described by a dissociated pair of two independent lines, $I = 2$, but should be represented by a hierarchical rotation of four small lines, $I = 3$. Its code is:

$$4 * (a\ \underline{K}\{4 * (a\ \{K\})\})$$

Figure $8.6F_1$ can be described by a dissociated representation of two structures on two planes. Each structure, consisting of two symmetrical isosceles triangles, can be described by a unified representation ($I = 6$). The coincidental relations between the two structures contribute to I-ext $= 16$. Figure $8.6G_1$ consists of four isosceles triangles on four different planes. Also, their coincidental relations contribute to I-ext $= 16$.

Having clarified these coding aspects, we now turn to the results of the experiment. As said, for eighteen patterns holds $P > 1$ for subdivision 2. Indeed, for fifteen of them, N was significantly in favour of subdivision 2 according to the chi-square test ($N > 11$, $p < .05$). For two patterns holds $P = 1$. For one, $N = 10$, and for the other, $N = 13$. Hence, all in all, the predictions are supported well by the actually preferred pattern segmentations.

As said in the Introduction, this subsection deals with stimuli that can be interpreted as partly overlapping translucent layers. Indeed, most experimental stimuli are described as partly overlapping translucent layers, but not all. The exceptions are Figures 8.6A and D. In the studies discussed next, there are no such exceptions. Steadily, the double-layer interpretation will be the target of the preference measures.

Transparency

One of the first researchers who studied the transparency phenomenon was Metelli (1974). He mainly focused on the colour conditions under which transparency is apparent. The study of transparency by Leeuwenberg (1976), not only within the visual domain but also within the auditory domain, was on form aspects of stimuli, as follows.

Visual transparency Fourteen patterns were designed, each consisting of two differently coloured transparent subpatterns, one partly overlapping the other. Figure 8.8 shows two extreme exemplars of this set. Figure 8.8A clearly reveals a transparent subpattern in front of a black subpattern. Figure 8.8B rather is conceived of as a mosaic of differently coloured surface parts.

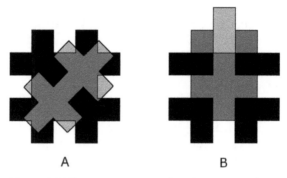

A   B

Figure 8.8 Two extreme exemplars from a set of experimental stimuli (Leeuwenberg, 1976). Pattern A clearly presents a transparent surface in front of a black background. In B, the transparent composition of the same two components is hardly visible, and the pattern is preferably seen as a mosaic of parts (Leeuwenberg, 1978).

The preference measure (PT) for transparency is specified by the ratio of the mosaic (M) load and the transparency (T) load: $P_T = I_M/I_T$. The simplest mosaic description is a unified representation of the mosaic parts together with their connections. The transparency interpretation is described by the dissociated pattern representation of two independent transparent patterns, one on top of the other. For Figures 8.8A and B, the theoretical preference strengths are as follows:

A	B
$P_T = I_M/(\text{I-int} + \text{I-ext})$	$P_T = I_M/(\text{I-int} + \text{I-ext})$
$P_T = 167/(14 + 0) = 11.90$	$P_T = 30/(14 + 40) = 0.56$

The task was to rank-order all fourteen patterns according to their perceived transparency. There were forty participants. The Spearman rank-order correlation between the preference strength values and the averaged transparency judgments was $r = .86$ and was significant.

Auditory cocktail-party phenomenon Above, we dealt with visual transparency, that is, with stimuli which can be interpreted as compositions of adjacent mosaic parts but which are preferably interpreted as two overlapping patterns. In the auditory domain, there are also stimuli that give rise to two such options. An instance is Bach's Violin Partita No. 2. It is a series of alternating high and low pitch tones which can be perceived as a single sequence of tones with large intervals but which is rather perceived as two separate simultaneous melodies, one at high pitch level and

T = high

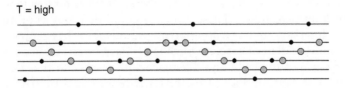

T = low

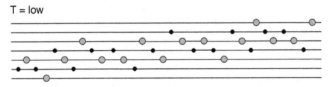

Figure 8.9 Two melodies consisting of small notes (A series) and alternating large notes (B series). In the experiment (Leeuwenberg, 1976), the A tones were presented to the left ear and the B tones to the right ear. Thereafter, either the A or the B melody was presented. The task was to judge whether this melody was a component of the previously presented combined melody. The recognition was better for the top melody than for the bottom melody, and this effect is predicted from the transparency measure.

the other at low pitch level. This phenomenon is known as 'streaming' (van Noorden, 1975). Leeuwenberg (1976) made an attempt to evoke such an auditory transparency effect on the basis of melodic structure instead of on the basis of pitch.

The experiment dealt with twelve series, each consisting of seventy-two tones. Two extreme exemplars are shown in Figure 8.9, each presenting a series of alternating notes. The submelody, indicated by small notes, was called an A series and another submelody, indicated by large notes, was called a B series. The whole combination of an A series and an alternating B series was called a C series.

The task was as follows. In each trial of the experiment, the tones of the A series were presented to the left ear, alternated with the tones of the B series presented to the right ear, that is, steadily one tone was presented to the left ear and thereafter one tone to the right ear. After this dichotic presentation of the C series, either the A or the B series was presented and the task was to judge whether this subseries was recognized as a component of the previously presented C series.

To clarify the predictions that were made about this streaming effect, the A, B, and C series are first represented by codes. To this end, the tones of each series are replaced by numbers, low ones for low tones and high ones for high tones. These numbers could be taken as primitives, but their intervals are more appropriate primitives as they represent the melody independent of absolute pitch level. Each interval is supposed to represent each number by the difference with respect to the preceding number. The first number of the series is represented by the interval between this number and a virtual number such that the interval leads to the simplest final description. We illustrate this as follows:

tones		numbers		intervals		code	load
C E G F	=>	1 3 5 4	=>	2 2 2 −1	=>	3*(2) −1	2

Tone C is represented by number 1 which, at interval level, is represented by 2 which leads to the simplest description of all intervals together.

The transparency strength of each melody was specified by: $P_T = I_C/(I_A + I_B)$. For the upper series in Figure 8.9 holds $P_T > 1$ and for the bottom series holds $P_T < 1$. Thus, the expectation was that the A and B melodies are better recognized as components of the C series in the upper series than in the bottom series.

The results of the experiment were as follows. In line with this expectation, the correlation was $r = .86$ between P_T and the recognition of A and B series, averaged over all nineteen participants, was significant. So, not only pitch but also melody may evoke streaming or auditory transparency.

Neon illusion

The so-called neon illusion was discovered by Varin (1971) and, later on, rediscovered independently by van Tuijl (1975, 1979). This illusion can be evoked by patterns with two colours, for instance, black and blue. The effect is an illusory spreading of the blue colour within a certain area on places beyond the blue lines. Figure 8.10A presents an illustration. All lines are black, except those within the central square. These are blue. Seen from some distance, a blue glow is perceived everywhere within the subjective contours of the central square, that is, an illusory spreading of the blue colour beyond the blue lines.

As shown by van Tuijl and de Weert (1979), the illusion merely takes place under the sensory condition that the brightness of the neon colour (blue) is in between the brightness of the lines (black) and the brightness of the background (white). This is satisfied by the colours in Figure 8.10. According to van Tuijl and Leeuwenberg (1979), there is also a form determinant of the illusion. The neon code should be simpler

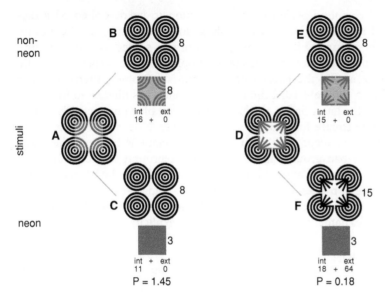

Figure 8.10 Two interpretations of A are presented in B and C. The non-neon interpretation (B) presents a pattern of black disks and a white square foreground surface with blue lines. This white surface is here presented by a grey surface. The neon interpretation (C) presents a pattern of black disks illuminated by a blue square. The neon code is simpler than the non-neon code. In contrast, the neon code (E) of D is more complex than the non-neon code (F). The numbers refer to loads. The coloured version of this figure is presented in the separate colour section of this book.

than the non-neon code. The neon code represents a black pattern and a blue foreground to be described by a dissociated representation. This foreground also can be taken as a blue light projected on the black pattern. For the stimulus in Figure 8.10A, this neon concept is illustrated in Figure 8.10C (the numbers refer to loads). In various respects, the concept of this illusion agrees with that of the subjective contour illusion (see preceding section). A minor difference is that in the neon illusion, the foreground is transparent whereas in the subjective contour illusion the foreground is opaque.

With respect to the alternative interpretation, the same argument is used as the one for subjective contours. Namely, the neon phenomenon is not an authentic illusion. Without explaining the illusory phenomenon or pointing out what to look for, subjects hardly experience an illusory effect. Therefore, also the non-neon interpretation is supposed to deal with a foreground-background composition to be described by a dissociated representation and possibly giving rise to subjective contours of the foreground. Like the foreground in non-subjective contours, the foreground in the non-neon code is an opaque white surface. The only difference is that the latter surface comprises a blue pattern. For the stimulus in Figure 8.10A, the non-neon concept is illustrated in Figure 8.10B. In the latter figure, the grey square with blue lines actually stands for a white square foreground with blue lines. Notice that the external load of this concept deals with the spatial relations between the black lines of the background and the square foreground surface. The blue lines on this surface are not relevant. So, not only for the neon code but also for the non-neon code of Figure 8.10A holds: I-ext = 0.

Like the subjective contour illusion, the neon illusion reveals a paradoxical feature, namely, the more the stimulus explicitly reveals the illusory shape the weaker the illusion is. Figure 8.10D presents an illustration. The contours of the candidate illusory square are almost completely presented by the stimulus. Indeed, for this stimulus, the non-neon code is simpler than the neon code. For the non-neon code, illustrated in Figure 8.10E, the I-ext = 0 whereas for the neon code, illustrated in Figure 8.10F, the I-ext = 64 (the thick lines are taken as single lines). Also, the I-int of the neon code is higher than that of the non-neon code. So, the prediction is a non-neon interpretation. This interpretation misses the illusory spreading of the blue on places beyond the blue lines, and this implies a relatively high concentration of blue within the lines. Hence, the prediction is a higher hue of blue in the case of the non-neon illusion than in case of the neon illusion. Indeed, this prediction seems correct, as can be seen by comparing Figure 8.10A and Figure 8.10D.

In the experiment by van Tuijl and Leeuwenberg (1979), thirty-two patterns were involved. Six of them are presented in row 1 of Figure 8.11. Row 2 presents the non-neon (Nn) interpretations with their loads, and row 3 presents the neon (N) interpretations with their loads. Row 4 presents the preference strength P_N of the neon interpretation, where $P_N = I_{NN}/I_N$. The thirty-two patterns were subdivided into sixteen pairs of similar patterns, designed such that the P_N of one pattern (A) is always larger than the P_N of the other pattern (B). Figure 8.11 illustrates three of such A–B pairs. The theoretical dominance of P_A over P_B is specified by P_A/P_B and is indicated in row 5. The ranks of these ratios within the experimental set of stimuli are indicated by $R(P_A/P_B)$ in row 6.

We briefly comment on Figures $8.11A_1B_1$. Their non-neon interpretations deal with a foreground surface with black lines. This foreground has a square shaped hole. The background is a grid of blue lines. These blue lines miss any coincidental relation with the contours of the square

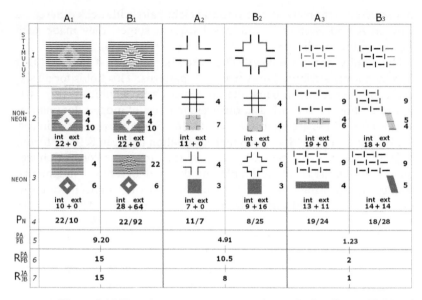

Figure 8.11 Row 1 presents some experimental stimuli (van Tuijl and Leeuwenberg, 1979). Row 2 presents the non-neon components with their internal loads and row 3 presents the neon components with their internal loads. Row 4 presents the theoretical preference strengths P_N of the neon interpretation. Row 5 presents P_A/P_B quotients. Their ranks are indicated in row 6. The average ranks of judged neon dominances of A over B are indicated in row 7. The coloured version of this figure is presented in the separate colour section of this book.

hole in the foreground surface. The neon interpretations deal with black line patterns and blue transparent squares on the foreground. The neon code of Figure 8.11A_1 does not comprise black lines that involve coincidental relations with this square. The neon background of Figure 8.11B_1 has the same components as those of its non-neon code. The only difference is that all the components in the neon background are black. This time, all black background lines involve coincidental relations with this square.

There were two tasks. The first task was performed by thirty-six participants. In each trial, an A–B pair was presented to each subject, and the task was to indicate the pattern that revealed the strongest neon illusion. In the second task, performed by fourteen other participants, all sixteen pattern-pairs were presented on a table. The subject had to focus on the neon dominance of A over B patterns and to order the dominance strengths. In fact, subjects performed the task from global to local. First, they selected eight pairs with strong and eight pairs with weak differences between A and B stimuli, and in subsequent stages, they made such choices within subdivisions.

The results were as follows. The outcome of the first task was that more neon was attributed to A than to B patterns. This holds for all sixteen pairs. For fourteen pairs, the differences were significant ($p < .01$; sign-test). For the second task, the average ranks of judged dominances are relevant. These are indicated by R(JA/JB). Some are presented in row 7 of Figure 8.11. The Spearman rank correlation between R (PA/PB) and R (JA/JB) was: $r = .94$; $p < .01$. Precisely the same rank correlation was found between the theoretical ranks and the median ranks of judgments. Besides, all Spearman rank correlations of individual subjects were significant, $p < .01$, and ranged from $r = .72$ to $r = .98$. The Kendall's coefficient of concordance among subjects amounted to $W = .75$.

Finally, we attend to a general coding effect. The exclusion of I-ext hardly appears to change the rank orders of the loads and hardly affects the rank orders of the load proportions. The Spearman rank correlation between R (PA/PB) and R (JA/JB), merely based on I-int, is $r = .91$, whereas it is $r = .94$ if based on I-int + I-ext. In fact, the exclusion of I-ext also minimally affects the load rankings involved in the earlier discussed translucent phenomena, such as subjective contours, transparency, and line drawings. In other words, generally, I-ext appears to correlate with I-int. As the external structure, which accounts for metrical pattern aspects, depends on the hypothetical internal structure, which accounts for structural pattern aspects, we tend to conclude that, in all these visual phenomena, metrical pattern aspects play a subordinate role with respect to structural aspects.

Contrast and assimilation

A grey surface within a white–black background may evoke either contrast or assimilation effects. Contrast effects occur if the grey is judged as being opposed to the surrounding colour, and assimilation effects occur if the grey is judged to tend towards the surrounding colour (von Bezold, 1874). In fact, the assimilation effect is an offshoot of the transparency phenomenon.

Helson (1963) performed experiments of grey lines on a black-and-white background. He showed that contrast prevails if the width of the grey lines is relatively small (see Figure 8.12A) and assimilation prevails if the width of the grey lines is relatively large (see Figure 8.12B).

Leeuwenberg (1982b) showed that also the form of the grey area evokes assimilation or contrast effects. For all tested stimuli, the size of the grey

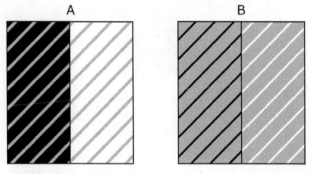

Figure 8.12 A and B present grey lines on black-and-white back-grounds. If the width of the grey lines is relatively small (see A) a contrast effect prevails: the grey within the black area seems brighter than the grey within the white area. If the width of the grey lines is relatively large (see B) an assimilation effect prevails: the grey within the black area seems darker than the grey within the white area (Helson, 1963).

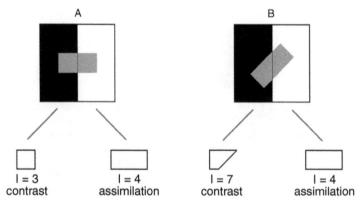

Figure 8.13 A and B present each a grey rectangle on a black–white background. The vertical lines divide the rectangles in equal parts. Argued is that contrast effect prevails if each of these parts are simpler than the rectangle (see A), and that assimilation effect prevails if they are more complex than the rectangle (see B) (Leeuwenberg, 1982b).

area was kept constant. Moreover, the line that divides the background into equal white and black areas also divides the gray area into two equal parts. Figure 8.13 illustrates two stimuli.

Two codes of the grey areas are relevant. One code describes one of the two equal local parts. For Figure 8.13A, this part is a square, and for Figure 8.13B, it is a trapezoid. The other code describes the whole grey

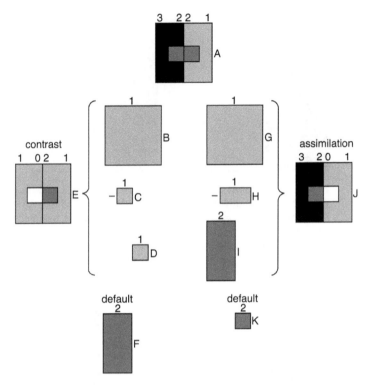

Figure 8.14 For stimulus A, two compositions are illustrated. Each composition deals with transparent layers. The numbers refer to degrees of darkness. B, C, D, and F contribute to the contrast composition E, and G, H, I, and K contribute to the assimilation composition J. The distinctive components are C and H. It means that, if C is simpler than H, the contrast interpretation is favoured, whereas if H is simpler than C, the assimilation interpretation is favoured (Leeuwenberg, 1982b).

rectangle. Notice that these two codes are complementary in the sense that the code of the whole shape fixates the form of the rectangle while the code of the part fixates the orientation of the rectangle (see Chapter 6). The square is part of a horizontal rectangle and the trapezoid is part of a tilted rectangle. Presumably, because the two codes are complementary, they are involved in opposite visual effects. Our claim is that the contrast interpretation is favoured if the local part is simpler than the global form, and that the assimilation interpretation is favoured if it is more complex than the global form. This claim is supported by the effects which emerge in Figure 8.13, and it may be explicated as follows.

Figure 8.14A presents degrees of darkness by numbers. The left black background part is represented by 3, the central grey by 2, and the right

light-grey background part by 1. In line with the vectorial colour analysis
of Beck (1966) and Metelli (1974), the colour number of superimposed
transparent layers equals the sum of their separate colour numbers. By
using this rule Figure 8.14A can be obtained by two compositions of
transparent layers.

One composition is presented at the left of Figure 8.14. It comprises
a global light-grey (1) frame (Figure 8.14B). Superimposed are a darkness decreasing (-1) small square at the left of the centre (Figure 8.14C)
and a darkness increasing (1) small square at the right side of the centre
(Figure 8.14D). So far, the composition (Figure 8.14E) reflects the contrast interpretation, namely, the small left square is brighter (0) than
the small right square (2). To obtain the stimulus in Figure 8.14A,
this outcome has to be completed by a global shadow (2) projected
on the left half (Figure 8.14F). The other composition is presented at
the right of Figure 8.14. It again comprises a global light-grey (1) frame
(Figure 8.14G). Superimposed are a darkness decreasing (-1) rectangle
in the centre (Figure 8.14H) and a global shadow (2) at the left (Figure
8.14I). The composition (Figure 8.14J) reflects the assimilation interpretation, namely, the small left square is darker (2) than the small right
square (0). To obtain the stimulus in Figure 8.14A, this outcome has to
be completed by a small dark square (2) on the right half of the centre
(Figure 8.14K).

To establish the distinctive form component of each composition,
their common form components are canceled, namely, the large squares
(Figures 8.14B and G), the large vertical rectangles (Figures 8.14F
and I), and the small squares (Figures 8.14D and K). The distinctive component of the contrast composition is one part of the central
area, here a square (Figure 8.14C), and the distinctive component of
the assimilation composition is the whole central area, here a rectangle
(Figure 8.14H).

The distinctive characteristics of assimilation and contrast effects can
be paraphrased by starting from the assumption that, in both cases, the
whole left-hand area (including the local part) is taken to be illuminated
less than the whole right-hand area (also including the local part). Then,
for the assimilation effect, the crucial condition is that the two local
parts (which have the same proximal colours, i.e., the same amounts
of light received by the retina) are preferably taken as belonging to one
relatively simple object, and that they are therefore assumed to have the
same proper colours (these are inherent distal object properties disre-
garding illumination). Hence, the assumption of same proper colours
gives rise to the inference that the only difference between the two local
parts is the difference in illumination. For the contrast effect, about the
reverse applies. Then, the crucial condition is that the two local parts are

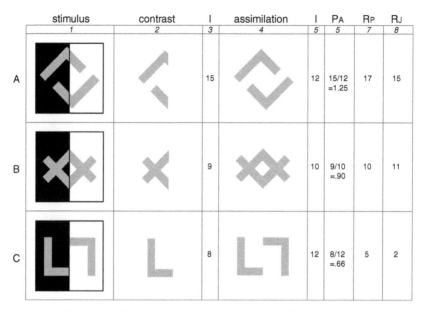

stimulus	contrast	I	assimilation	I	PA	RP	RJ
1	2	3	4	5	5	7	8
A		15		12	15/12 =1.25	17	15
B		9		10	9/10 =.90	10	11
C		8		12	8/12 =.66	5	2

Figure 8.15 Column 1 presents experimental stimuli (Leeuwenberg, 1982b). Columns 2 and 3 present contrast components and their loads. Columns 4 and 5 present assimilation components and their loads. Column 6 presents the theoretical preference strengths PA of the assimilation interpretation. Column 7 presents their rank-order RP. Column 8 presents the average judged assimilation ranks RJ (Leeuwenberg, 1982b).

preferably taken as relatively simple separate objects which might have different proper colours. Because they have the same proximal colours despite the different illuminations, the inference is made that they indeed have different proper colours (which compensate for the different illuminations).

The stimuli in the experiment by Leeuwenberg (1982b) were twenty grey patterns, each with a black-and-white background, and displayed on separate sheets. Three exemplars are shown in column 1 of Figure 8.15. Columns 2 and 3 present the crucial contrast components and their I-loads. Columns 4 and 5 present the crucial assimilation components and their I-loads. Column 6 presents the theoretical preference strength of assimilation PA, that is, the ratio of the contrast load and the assimilation load. Column 7 presents its rank-order RP within the experimental set of stimuli. Column 8 presents the average ranks of judged assimilation by RJ.

There were thirty participants and the task was to rank-order the twenty stimuli according to their visual assimilation strength. There was no time limit and the participants were free to correct their responses.

The Spearman rank correlation between the theoretical preference ranks R_P and the average judged assimilation ranks R_J, amounted to: $r = .81$ and was significant. The Pearson correlation between the theoretical measures P_A and the average judged assimilation ranks R_J also amounted to $r = 81$. The concordance (W) among subjects' judgments was significant too: $W = .82$, $p < .001$. In our view, the outcomes support the given hypothesis about the form determinant of brightness contrast and assimilation.

According to Helson (1963), pattern compactness, defined by surface divided by contour length, contributes to pattern unity, so that a higher compactness may lead to more assimilation responses. In our experiment, the correlation between the compactness of the experimental patterns and their assimilation judgments was $r = .24$. Because this correlation is very low, we conclude that the main determinant of assimilation judgments in our experiment was not pattern compactness but the form determinant illustrated in Figure 8.14.

In all studies discussed so far in this chapter, the preference strength measure was used as predictor. This measure contrasts two pattern codes, namely, usually the simplest code and a less simple code. The simpler code is supposed to be preferred, but the assumption is that both codes are actually generated. Indeed, it is obvious that the preferred code is generated. However, it is less obvious that a non-preferred code is generated too. Then, a further question is whether one or more non-preferred codes are generated. In the next section, we discuss such issues.

8.3   Rivalry

The local approaches of pattern completion, discussed at the end of section 8.1, assume that the visual interpretation of a pattern is the single visual solution determined straightaway by one or more stimulus cues. Competition processes are supposed to be relevant but merely at local stimulus levels and merely during the process towards the solution. Attneave (1982) characterized this as follows: perception minimizes processing costs by instantiating locally cooperative hill-climbing procedures. Furthermore, according to Perkins (1983), this minimal search suggests that the human perceiver proceeds along paths of highly reliable recognitions and inferences in order to avoid detours for checking parallel alternatives.

Our preference strength measure, however, is not compatible with these local approaches. Our measure rather presupposes a choice among all rivaling pattern interpretations. This idea was suggested by Herbart (1816) for the broad cognitive domain of sensations and drives. For the domain of perception, the idea of parallel activation of pattern interpretations has been defended by Gregory and Gombrich (1973) and Kurbat (1994), and experimentally investigated by Gottschaldt (1929), Palmer (1977), Reed and Johnsen (1975), and van Tuijl and Leeuwenberg (1980) by using part-probe or embedded-figure detection tasks. The idea of simultaneously present rivaling interpretations is also at the heart of connectionist modeling (Churchland, 1986, 2002; Churchland and Sejnowsky, 1990, 1992; Smolensky, 1988).

Earlier, in Chapter 3, we argued that linear process-stage models insufficiently explain shape interpretations, mainly because of the detour characteristics of perception. The phenomenon of pattern completion, in particular, reveals detours that do not stem from pure local cues. Of course, then, the main question is whether pattern completion is a visual phenomenon. In our view, it is a visual phenomenon for the following reason. There is no doubt that subjective contours but also transparency, neon effect, and assimilation versus contrast are visual phenomena. However, all of them are explained as versions of pattern completion (Rock, 1983). Hence, it is implausible that precisely pattern completion itself is not a visual phenomenon. There is also direct experimental evidence for the visual level of pattern completion. Some studies were reported in Chapter 1 (Gerbino and Salmaso, 1987; Kanizsa, 1985). Some other studies are reported next.

Concurrent completions

Here, we review four experiments performed in the 1990s. These experiments were set up to demonstrate the concurrent visual presence of preferred and non-preferred completion interpretations.

Experiment 1 We first briefly review a study by Sekuler and Palmer (1992). They used Beller's (1971) primed-matching paradigm to assess the subject's perception and the process course of pattern completion. Each trial comprised a prime followed, after a short interval, by two test patterns. The task was to judge whether these test patterns were equal or not, and the reaction time was measured. Figures 8.16A, B, and C show typical prime patterns and Figures 8.16D and E show typical test pairs. In the analysis of the data, only correct 'yes' responses were considered.

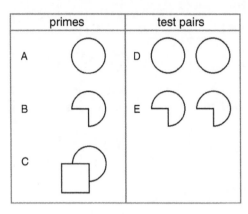

Figure 8.16 The primed-matching paradigm was used by Sekuler and Palmer (1992) to study visual pattern completion. Each trial dealt with a prime (A, B, or C), an interval, and two test patterns (D or E). The task was to judge, as fast as possible, whether the test patterns were equal. Primes A and C had about the same facilitating RT effects on testing D and the same negative reaction time (RT) effects on testing E. The visual completion in C appeared to occur within about 200 ms (van Lier *et al.*, 1995).

The results were as follows. Prime A facilitated the test of D but not of E. Equally, prime B facilitated the test of E but not of D. Crucial was the observation that, already within a processing time (prime plus interval) of about 200 milliseconds (ms), primes A and C have about the same positive facilitating effects on the test of D and the same negative effects on the test of E. So, apparently, prime C is interpreted as an occlusion pattern within a period that is commonly taken as the visual processing time. This suggests that pattern completion is a visual phenomenon.

Experiment 2 In the occlusion patterns of Sekuler and Palmer (1992), the global completion coincided with the local completion based purely on good continuation. In another study, Sekuler *et al.* (1994) used the primed-matching paradigm to investigate patterns whose global completions differed from local completions. Figure 8.17A shows an instance of an occlusion prime. Its globally completed background shape, shown in the test pair in Figure 8.17F, reveals three axes of symmetry, whereas its locally completed background shape, shown in the test pair in Figure 8.17G, reveals one axis of symmetry. For prime durations of 150 ms up to 1,000 ms, the effects of the occlusion prime were compared with the effects of the non-occlusion primes with

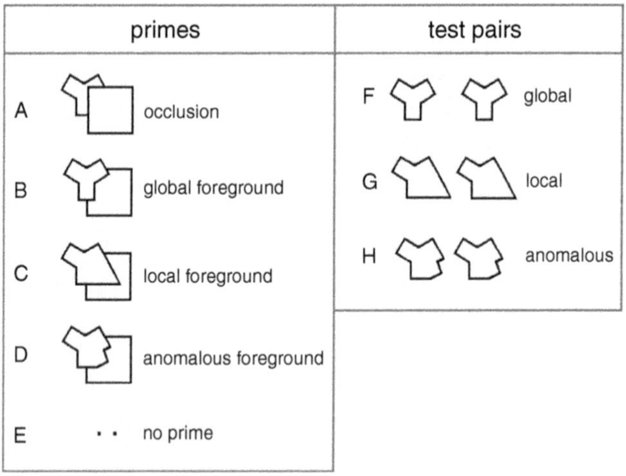

Figure 8.17 Prime A and test pairs F and G were used by Sekuler *et al.* (1994). Their study was set up to show that global completion is not dominated by local completion. Van Lier *et al.* (1995) applied the same primed-matching paradigm to the primes A to E and to the test pairs F to H. His question was: does the dominance of one type of completion (global or local) exclude the other type of completion (local or global), or might the non-dominant completion be generated as well? (van Lier *et al.*, 1995).

the non-occluded globally or locally completed shape. The effects of occlusion primes appeared to be similar to those of non-occluded globally completed primes. Sekuler *et al.* (1994) concluded that, for their set of stimuli, pattern completions were not dominated by a local process. That is, at an early stage of completion, the occlusion shapes revealed a maximum of symmetry.

Experiment 3 The just mentioned studies set the stage for the research of van Lier *et al.* (1995). They again used the primed-matching paradigm of Sekuler *et al.* (1994) but with a different goal. The question was whether or not the prevailing type of completion (global or local) excludes the generation of the other type of completion. The study dealt with six pattern sets. In Figure 8.17, one set is shown. The experimental design differed from the previous designs in the following respects. First, anomalous completions of the occlusion prime were added (Figure 8.17H) to contrast them to local and global completions. Second, to prevent any bias effect of the square in the occlusion primes (Figures 8.17A), also the non-occlusion primes (Figures 8.17B, C, and

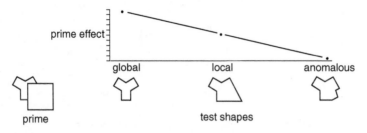

Figure 8.18 Some results of van Lier *et al.* (1995). The graph presents effects of the occlusion prime on the test pairs FGH shown in Figure 8.17. These prime effects gradually decrease from global to local to anomalous test pairs and suggest the presence of non-dominant completions.

D) were combined with a square. Third, a no prime condition was introduced (see Figure 8.17E) to serve as baseline condition. The prime effect (PE) was expressed by reaction time (RT) in the baseline condition minus the RT in the target conditions.

The procedure agreed with that of the experiments of Sekuler and Palmer (1992). Each trial began with a fixation point presented for 500 ms, followed by an empty screen for 50 ms. Subsequently, the prime appeared for 750 ms, and 17 ms thereafter, the two test patterns were shown, one at the left and one at the right. In addition, a rectangle appeared at the centre of the top of the screen to avoid misleading apparent motion effects. The test pair remained on the screen until a response was given. Subjects responded by pushing one of two buttons to answer whether or not both test shapes were equal. Subjects received visual feedback on their response time and correctness. The analysis merely applied to the 'yes' response times on identical test shapes.

The results showed priming effects of the occlusion prime (Figure 8.17A), being maximal on global test pairs (Figure 8.17F), intermediate on local test pairs (Figure 8.17G), and minimal on anomalous test pairs (Figure 8.17H). This pattern of results, shown in the graph in Figure 8.18, also was found for the other five sets of patterns. The gradual decrease in priming effect supports the idea that both global and local completions are generated by the perceptual system.

Experiment 4 There still is a reserve about the preceding study. It is possible that only the global completion is generated and that the priming effect on the local test pairs is due to a spreading of completions that are more or less similar to the global completion. This

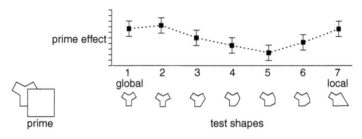

Figure 8.19 Some results of van Lier *et al.* (1995). The graph presents effects of the occlusion prime on seven test pairs varying from global to local features. The dip in between the global and local test pairs favours the notion that the visual system generates multiple completions (van Lier *et al.*, 1995).

spreading effect may affect the local test pair more than the anomalous test pair. In order to control for such a spreading effect, many more anomalous completions were added (van Lier *et al.*, 1995). These completions ranged, with small changes, from global to local completions. In Figure 8.19, seven test patterns are shown. The rationale is that if the priming on the local completion is due to a spreading effect based on the similarity with the global completion, the priming effect would gradually decrease from global to local test pairs. In fact, there were nine different primes: the occlusion prime, seven foreground primes, and the no prime. In each trial, one of these primes was followed by one of fourteen test pairs, seven identical and seven non-identical test shapes. The experimental procedure was the same as in the previous experiment. Again, only test pairs with identical test shapes were analysed.

The prime effects of the occlusion prime on the seven test pairs varying from global to local features did not reveal a gradually decreasing function, but revealed two peaks, one around the global test pairs and one around the local test pairs. The drop around the central test pairs differed significantly from the two peaks. This pattern of the amounts of priming opposes the idea that the priming effect on the local completion is simply due to a spreading of the priming effect caused by the presence of the global completion. The priming effects therefore once more indicate the special status of global and local completions. In fact, the data support the notion that multiple completions are generated by the visual system. That is, within the present prime duration time of 750 ms, one occlusion pattern might evoke global, local, and perhaps even other completions. In fact, a similar conclusion can be drawn from various other studies

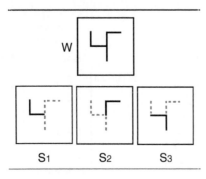

Figure 8.20 Stimuli in an experiment by Mens and Leeuwenberg (1988) designed to test whether suppressed pattern interpretations are yet generated. Each trial comprised a whole pattern W (10 ms) and a subpattern S (10 ms) presented in W-S or S-W order. The task was to identify the S pattern among alternatives. S_1 is a component of the best, S_2 of the second-best, and S_3 of a bad interpretation of W. The dotted lines do not belong to the presented stimuli, and just help to indicate where the parts are located in W (Mens and Leeuwenberg, 1988).

(de Wit and van Lier, 2002; Gerbino and Salmaso, 1987; Shimaya, 1994; van Lier, 1999; van Lier and Wagemans, 1999).

Concurrent segmentations

Like the two experiments discussed above by van Lier *et al.* (1995), the experiment by Mens and Leeuwenberg (1988; see also Mens, 1988) was designed explicitly to show the concurrent presence of alternative interpretations. This time, however, the subjects' task was to identify stimulus parts. In each trial, a whole pattern (W) and a subpattern (S) were presented one after the other on the same spot with maximal overlap. There were three kinds of S patterns: S_1 is a component of the preferred interpretation; S_2 is a component of a second-best interpretation; and S_3 is a component of an anomalous interpretation of W. This preference order was established in a separate experiment and agreed with the information loads. Figure 8.20 illustrates a single W with S patterns.

The S and W patterns were presented each for 10 ms in S-W or W-S order. The stimulus onset asynchronies (SOAs) were 20, 40, 60, and 100 ms. The task was to identify the S pattern and to respond, after each trial, by a forced choice among possible S patterns. In the experiment, fifty participants were involved. After a training of 20 trials, 248 trials

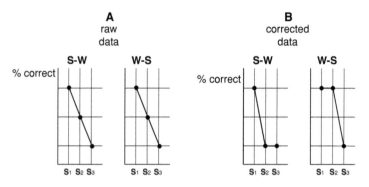

Figure 8.21 Results for the stimuli in Figure 8.20 (Mens and Leeuwenberg, 1988). A depicts the raw percentage correct detections without bias correction. Both S-W and W-S orders reflect the preference strength of S_1, S_2, and S_3 in W interpretations. B depicts the percentage correct detections after bias correction. This bias is supposed to merely stem from the processing of W. The S-W order reflects the preference strength of S_1 and S_2 in W interpretations whereas the W-S order reveals the concurrent presence of these interpretations irrespective of their preference (Mens and Leeuwenberg, 1988).

were given in random order: 2 (S-W, W-S) * 4 (SOA) * 3 (S) * 8 (W) = 192 plus 24 (S only, masked by a grid) plus 32 (W only). The dependent variable was the percentage correct detection.

The graphs for the various SOAs are similar. To attend to the common effects we present the results by the simplified and stylized graphs in Figure 8.21A. Notice that the graphs of both the S-W and the W-S conditions reflect the preference order of the preferred, second-best, and anomalous interpretations of W. That is, the percentage correct is high for S_1, mediocre for S_2, and low for S_3. Indeed, if W would have been presented alone (i.e., without a preceding or succeeding S), then one would expect this preference effect. The goal of the experiment, however, was not to assess this preference effect, but to assess the concurrent presence of alternative interpretations of W.

Therefore, a bias correction was applied, derived from the hits and false alarms per stimulus set (for details, see Mens and Leeuwenberg, 1988). The idea of this bias correction was that it cancels the difference in preference between interpretations of W so that, after bias correction, concurrently present interpretations can be identified by an equal detectability of their parts. Also in a simplified and stylized fashion, Figure 8.21B shows the percentage correct detection after bias correction. An analysis of variance of the bias-corrected data revealed a significant interaction between order (S-W versus W-S) and S (mainly due to S_1 versus S_2). That is, the corrected S-W graph shows a relatively low percentage correct S_2 detection with respect to the percentage correct S_1 detection, and the corrected W-S graph shows the same percentage correct for S_2 detection and S_1 detection.

A plausible explanation is as follows. The corrected scores in the S-W condition, on the one hand, are considered to be merely effects of the preferred W interpretation boosting or masking preceding S parts. S_1 coincides with a segment in the preferred W interpretation which, therefore, boosts S_1. Both S_2 and S_3 conflict with the preferred W interpretation which, therefore, suppresses S_2 and S_3. The corrected scores in the more interesting W-S condition, on the other hand, are supposed to be effects of the generated W interpretations irrespective of their preference. By the reasoning above, the lack of a difference between the succeeding S_1 and S_2 parts suggests the concurrent presence of both the best and the second-best interpretations of W. Mens and Leeuwenberg (1988) concluded therefore that, in general, the preferred interpretation of a stimulus is selected from among concurrently present alternative interpretations.

Summary

Van Lier et al. (1994) explained alleged falsifications of the global minimum principle, namely, so-called local effects of occlusion interpretations, by the globally simplest dissociated codes of these interpretations. These codes not only represent the view-independent internal structures but also the view-dependent external and virtual structures of the hypothetical components of a stimulus. Van Lier et al. (1994) showed that each of these structures plays their own role in perception. Furthermore, T and t junctions do not appear to be tenable as always-safe local cues for occlusion interpretations and mosaic interpretations, respectively.

The subjective contour illusion is categorized as an occlusion phenomenon. The transparency and the neon illusion deal with translucent layers. Their dissociated representation loads do not comprise any virtual load. The preference strength of the mentioned illusions is determined by the simplest 2-D mosaic load divided by the simplest 3-D double layer load. The preference strength of assimilation equals the quotient of the contrast load and the assimilation load. Contrast is determined by a local part and assimilation by the global form. All these illusions have been topics of earlier research but mostly with respect to metrical aspects. Here, the attention is merely focused on form aspects and we have shown that their visual effects are predicted well by SIT codes.

Finally, there is empirical evidence for the assumption that the visual interpretation results from a rivalry among various interpretations and not from local stimulus cues heading to a single unique visual solution. It is shown that not only the preferred but also the non-preferred representations are generated and remain accessible for some period.

9   Time effects

Introduction

As in Chapter 8, this chapter tests the preference of simplest pattern inter-pretations, this time using pairs of patterns whose codes are related asymmetrically: one pattern is a prototype and the other is a non-prototype. This means that the code of one pattern affects the code of the other pattern, but not vice versa. This chapter shows that this asymmetry may give rise to temporal order effects. Section 9.1 shows that simultaneously presented patterns may evoke a specific temporal order. This suggests a perceptual criterion for judged time direction. Section 9.2 deals with subsequently presented patterns which may induce a percept of simultan-eously presented patterns. The data suggest an estimation of the temporal integration span of perception.

9.1   Induced temporal order

Everyone is aware of the time course from early to late. However, if one is shown two photographs, for instance, then it is not obvious which cues are indicative of the order in which the two photos had been taken. In other words, what are the criteria people might use to judge the original temporal order? In this section, we elaborate on a genuinely perceptual criterion, and to set the stage, we begin by discussing two other criteria that have been proposed.

Entropy and knowledge

Inanimate nature exhibits a tendency from order to disorder. For instance, a building might fall apart but, spontaneously, a chaos of stones never turns into a building. This natural tendency, which often is referred to as 'entropy' in the broad sense, seems to be a plausible criterion for time direction. Notice that, like any criterion, it is not foolproof. That

181

A   B

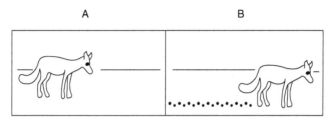

Figure 9.1 A and B present two snapshots. If the dots are taken as footprints and the animal as a fox, the most plausible temporal order is A-B. However, if the dots are taken as pieces of food and the animal is known to be walking backwards while eating, the plausible order is B-A. So, knowledge affects the judged order of events (Leeuwenberg, 2003a).

is, in inanimate nature, it does not capture processes from disorder to order, like in crystal formation. In fact, processes from disorder to order are common in animate nature. For instance, perception processes turn disorder (patches of light on the retina) into order (structured stimulus interpretations). Hence, entropy might be a plausible criterion for time direction, but meanwhile it is also a criterion for inanimate nature as opposed to animate nature (Monod, 1970; Prigogine and Stengers, 1984). This double function is illustrated next.

Consider a movie of the assembly of a car from various parts. The task is to judge whether the movie is played in forward mode or in backward mode. Taken as a criterion for time direction, entropy would suggest that it is played in backward mode; after all, the movie shows a process from disorder to order. Taken as a criterion for the involvement of an inanimate versus an animate actor, however, entropy suggests that it might yet be played in forward mode; after all, an animate actor may aim at disassembly but just as well at assembly. In other words, because of its double function, the criterion of entropy does not give an unequivocal indication of time direction (be it right or wrong).

Another criterion for judged temporal order is the mark criterion proposed by Reichenbach (1956) and suggested earlier by Descartes (1644/1953). This criterion holds that temporal order is judged on the basis of the assumption that a later event receives a mark of a preceding event. This is illustrated by the two snapshots, in Figure 9.1, of a fox (snapshot A) and of the same fox at another position together with footprints (snapshot B). The footprints are the traces of the fox in snapshot A and they belong to snapshot B, so, the mark criterion suggests that snapshot A must have preceded snapshot B. Notice that also this criterion is neither foolproof nor unequivocal, however. That is, suppose that the dots in snapshot B are actually pieces of food and that the animal is one that always walks backwards while eating food (presumably, he first cleans the food with its tail before he eats it). If this is known, then it is plausible that snapshot B is judged to have preceded snapshot A. Hence, the mark criterion is not unequivocal because it is subject to variable knowledge about the world.

Notice that, for the entropy and mark criteria, it does not matter whether two snapshots are presented simultaneously or successively. In the case of successive presentation, the judged original temporal order will not trigger an illusory reversal of the perceived presentation order, but at most, the conclusion that the snapshots were presented in the reversed original order (Ruyer, 1956). In other words, in the case of successive presentation, the snapshot will be experienced and scanned in the given presentation order. In the case of simultaneous presentation, the only difference is that viewers are free to scan the snapshots in one order or the other. The scanning order is not relevant to the entropy and mark criteria but, as we discuss next, it does affect the perceptual representation of snapshot pairs in a way that gives rise to a genuinely perceptual and unequivocal criterion for the judged original temporal order of simultaneously presented snapshots.

Visual recoding

In our view, the scanning order of snapshots triggers a forward context effect which is a genuine perception principle and which affects the perceptual representation of the snapshots. To illustrate this, we consider Figure 9.2. Figure 9.2A is unambiguous and Figure 9.2B is semi-ambiguous. That is, pattern A evokes a unique code which is much simpler than any rivaling code. Pattern B is less stable. It may evoke a unique simplest description, but its rivaling code is almost equally simple and, in fact, agrees with the simplest code of pattern A. Figure 9.2A is interpreted as a 3-D cube (**C**) and not otherwise. Figure 9.2B is preferably interpreted as a 2-D flower (**F**) and slightly less preferably as a 3-D cube (**C**).

Now, if Figure 9.2A is presented first, it evokes its preferred **C** interpretation which, due to the forward context effect, is expected to also evoke this **C** interpretation for the subsequently presented Figure 9.2B. If Figure 9.2B is presented first, however, it evokes its preferred **F** interpretation which is of no use for coding the subsequently presented

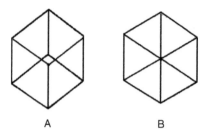

A   B

Figure 9.2 A is unambiguous and is perceived merely as a 3-D cube. B is semi-ambiguous. It is preferably seen as a 2-D 'flower' and slightly less preferably as a 3-D cube. If the patterns are presented successively, a forward context effect is expected. In the A-B order, both A and B are represented as cubes whereas, in the B-A order, B is represented as a flower and A as a cube. If the patterns are presented simultaneously but scanned in one order or the other, an additional backward context effect is expected. In the A-B order, both A and B are represented again as cubes whereas, in the B-A order, B is initially represented as a flower and A as a cube but, thereafter, B is re-interpreted as a cube and represented that way.

Figure 9.2A, and the latter is, therefore, again interpreted as **C**. Hence, in short, the A-B presentation and scanning order yields the **CC** codes, and the B-A order yields the **FC** codes. Notice that only the A-B order provides a flavour of Reichenbach's mark criterion in that, only in that order, the forward context effect implies that B is interpreted using the preceding A. This illustrates that the scanning order of snapshots affects their perceptual representation in the case of successive presentation. As we discuss next, we expect an additional effect of scanning order in the case of simultaneous presentation.

If, under simultaneous presentation, Figure 9.2A is scanned before Figure 9.2B then, as before, both figures evoke **C** interpretations. Furthermore, if Figure 9.2B is scanned first then, initially, it again evokes its preferred **F** interpretation whereafter Figure 9.2A again is interpreted as **C**. However, because the two patterns are simultaneously present and therefore both accessible, we expect that, thereafter, Figure 9.2B adopts the **C** interpretation of Figure 9.2A because, this way, the two figures together are represented by the simplest description. In other words, we expect that Figure 9.2B is interpreted initially as **F** but later on as **C**.

Notice that the latter recoding of B is expected to occur only if B is scanned first. If so, this interpretation change is an identifiable feature of the B-A order whereas the A-B order lacks such a feature. Hence, if the simultaneously presented patterns are scanned in the A-B order then there is no reason to have specific expectations about the judged original temporal order, but if they are scanned in the B-A order then this interpretation change (which has a positive effect in that it yields a simpler global description than obtained initially) might bias judgments towards the B-A order. As we discuss next, this was investigated in an experiment performed by Leeuwenberg (1974) and re-analysed by Collard and Leeuwenberg (1981).

The experiment by Leeuwenberg (1974) involved forty participants and comprised an inspection stage and a test stage. In the inspection stage, two catch patterns were presented one after the other, each for 5 milliseconds (ms) and without interval. These catch patterns were random line configurations and the brevity of the presentation prevented any access to their content. In the test stage, pairs of AB patterns were presented side-by-side during 2 seconds. Their distance exceeded 7 degrees visual angle, implying that the two patterns cannot be focused on simultaneously. In the presentations, their left-right positions were randomized to control for a bias thereof. The subjects were told that these patterns had already been presented, one after the other, in the inspection stage. The task was to indicate which pattern had been presented first during the inspection stage. The experiment involved three stimulus sets, and we expected that the proportions of A-first and B-first responses would differ per set. Next, we introduce these sets together with an analysis to justify the expected response proportions.

Set 1 comprised six experimental pattern pairs. Each pair consisted of an unambiguous A pattern and a semi-ambiguous B pattern. In Figure 9.3, this set is illustrated by the pattern pair in column 1 of row 1. Column 2 then illustrates the initial interpretations of the patterns when scanned in different orders, plus their loads. As we argued earlier, in case of the A→B scanning order, both patterns are interpreted as cubes (**C**). In case of the A←B scanning order, three interpretations are involved. The first refers to a flower (**F**) for B, the second to a cube (**C**) for A, and the third refers to a cube (**C**) again for B. The latter interpretation of B is not shown in the figure as it does not belong to the initial interpretations. The summated loads are indicated in column 3, showing that the summated load of the codings in the A→B order is lower than the summated load of the initial codings in the A←B order. As we argued above, precisely this load difference gives rise to the interpretation change in B, which is expected to provide a B-first cue. In fact, as we argue next, the expected response proportions can be specified in detail.

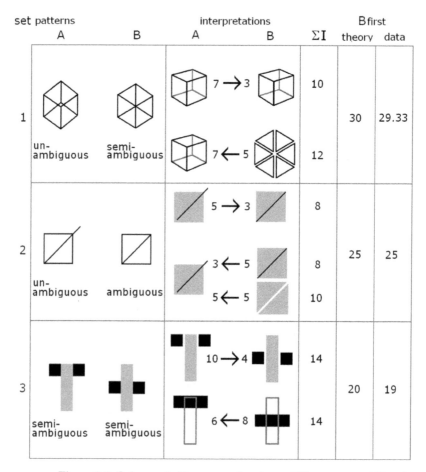

Figure 9.3 Column 1 illustrates, for three different sets, AB pairs involved in a judged temporal order study (Collard and Leeuwenberg, 1981). In set 1, A is unambiguous and B is semi-ambiguous; in set 2, A is unambiguous and B is ambiguous; in set 3, both A and B are semi-ambiguous. Column 2 illustrates the initial pattern interpretations for different scanning orders. The numbers refer to the initial pattern loads. Column 3 presents the summated initial loads (notice that, from set 1 to set 3, the load asymmetry decreases). Column 4 presents the expected, and column 5 the actual, numbers of B-first responses.

We assume that, to perform the task, participants scan the two pictures either in the A→B order or in the A←B order, with a 50 per cent chance each. Furthermore, we assume that participants try to infer a temporal order (to be attributed to the inspection stage) without being aware that the scanning order of the test patterns might affect their judgment. The following scheme can then be set up to estimate the percentages A-first and B-first responses for the two scanning orders:

orders:	50% A $\rightarrow$ B	50% A $\leftarrow$ B
interpretations:	50% CA $\rightarrow$ CB	50% CB $\leftarrow$ CA $\leftarrow$ FB
judgments:	A-first 25%	B-first 50%
	B-first 25%	

That is, the A→B scanning order, on the one hand, activates first the **CA** code and then the **CB** code. This is in line with the simplest interpretation of the entire display, so that it does not trigger an interpretation change and, therefore, does not yield any cue whatsoever. Hence, participants will guess that either A or B was first. The B→A scanning order, on the other hand, activates first the **FB** code, then the **CA** code, and finally the **CB** code. That is, then, there is a re-interpretation of pattern B to comply with the simplest interpretation of the entire display. Hence, this interpretation change is an identifiable cue which occurs only for the B→A order, and we assume that it therefore cues B-first responses. So, the overall expectation here is 25 per cent A-first responses and 75 per cent B-first responses. More specifically, for this set 1, the expected number of subjects giving B-first responses is thirty of the, in total, forty subjects.

Set 2 comprised two experimental pattern pairs. Each pair consisted of an unambiguous A pattern and an ambiguous B pattern with the restriction that one of the two simplest interpretations of B agrees with the simplest interpretation of A. In Figure 9.3, this set is illustrated by the pattern pair in column 1 of row 2. Column 2 then illustrates the initial interpretations of the patterns when scanned in different orders, plus their loads. In case of the A→B scanning order, both patterns are interpreted as a square plus line (**S**). This is in line with the simplest interpretation of the entire display, so, by the reasoning above, it yields no identifiable order cue. The A←B scanning order deals with two simplest interpretations of B. Under its **S** interpretation, again both patterns are interpreted as a square plus line (**S**), so, again, no identifiable order cue. The other simplest interpretation of B deals with triangles (**T**) but disagrees with any interpretation of A. So, only under this interpretation of B, the A←B coding order gives rise to an identifiable order cue in the form of an interpretation change. Hence, the following scheme can be set up to estimate the percentages A-first and B-first responses for the two scanning orders:

orders:	50% A → B	50% A ← B	
interpretations:	50% SA → SB	25% SA ← SB	25% SB ← SA ← TB
judgments:	A-first 25%	A first 12.5%	B first 25%
	B first 25%	B first 12.5%	

So, the overall expectation here is 37.5 per cent A-first responses and 62.5 per cent B-first responses. More specifically, for this set 2, the expected number of subjects giving B-first responses is twenty-five of the, in total, forty subjects.

Set 3 comprised four experimental pattern pairs. Each pair consisted of a semi-ambiguous A pattern and a semi-ambiguous B pattern, with the restriction that the one but simplest interpretation of A agrees with the simplest interpretation of B, while the one but simplest interpretation of B agrees with the simplest interpretation of A. In Figure 9.3, this set is illustrated by the pattern pair in column 1 of row 3. Column 2 then illustrates the initial interpretations of the patterns when scanned in different orders, plus their loads. In case of the A→B scanning order, both patterns are interpreted as mosaics (M), and in case of the A←B scanning order, both patterns are interpreted as occlusion patterns (O). In fact, both coding orders yield a simplest interpretation of the entire display, so, by the reasoning above, neither scanning order yields an identifiable order cue. Hence, the overall expectation here is 50 per cent A-first responses and 50 per cent B-first responses. More specifically, for this set 3, the expected number of subjects giving B-first responses is twenty of the, in total, forty subjects.

The results of the experiment were as follows. For all eight pairs of set 1 and set 2, more than twenty participants who delivered B-first responses (sign-test, $p < .01$). The four pairs of set 3 did not reveal preference biases. So, at ordinal level, the results are in line with the predictions. Even at ratio level, the results are remarkable. The numbers of subjects giving B-first responses to the six pairs of set 1 were 27, 27, 29, 30, 31, and 32. The average, 29.33, is close to the predicted number 30 of B-first responses. The numbers of subjects giving B-first responses to the two pairs of set 2 were 25 and 25. Both numbers are equal to the predicted number of B-first responses. The numbers of subjects giving B-first responses to the four pairs of set 3 were 17, 19, 20, and 20. The average, 19, is close to the predicted number 20 of B-first responses too. The correlation between these experimental numbers and theoretical numbers amounts to $r = 0.93$, and is significant.

To discuss these results, we start with a salient contrast. In sets 1 and 2, the unambiguous pattern A agrees with a prototype and the (semi)ambiguous pattern B agrees with a non-prototype (see Figures 2.3A and B). So, in this sense, the preferred order would be A→B. In fact, in column 3 of Figure 9.3, the arguments are presented, namely, the summated initial loads of the patterns are lower in the A→B order than in the reverse order. It is clear that the data in the experiment above disagree with this order based on (non-)prototypes. This is not surprising, however, considering that the experimental task was not to indicate the preferred order but to indicate the order that was supposed to have occurred in the inspection stage. Furthermore, the preferred order is independent of the scanning order, whereas in the experiment above, it is plausible that participants tested only one specific order. As we argued, this may or may not provide a temporal B-first order cue which participants can attribute to the inspection stage.

Furthermore, we already noted that, though only for the A-B order, visual recoding has a flavour of the mark criterion in that the forward context effect implies that B is interpreted using the preceding A. Visual recoding, however, is a genuinely perceptual factor which, unlike the mark criterion, is not affected by knowledge. On the other hand, the entropy criterion could, in principle, have had an effect in this experiment. After all, entropy reflects the tendency from order to disorder, that is, from simple to complex, so that it might affect the judged original temporal order of the simultaneously presented patterns. However, this factor was controlled for by keeping the number of pairs with B simpler than A equal to the number of pairs with A simpler than B. In fact, it is true that the data for six pairs agreed with the entropy criterion, but the data of all twelve pairs agreed with the visual-recoding criterion.

Finally, just as the entropy and mark criteria, also the visual-recoding criterion will not be foolproof in predicting the judged original temporal order of arbitrary pairs of simultaneously presented snapshots. The stimuli in the experiment, however, were such that (in)animacy and knowledge can hardly play a role. For such stimuli, the results show that the visual-recoding criterion, which is a genuinely perceptual criterion based on the simplicity principle, yields an unequivocal and remarkably accurate prediction of the response proportions. This suggests that it is indeed a factor in judged temporal order.

9.2   Induced simultaneity

In the previous section, we considered simultaneously presented patterns inducing a perceived temporal order. Here, we consider the opposite, namely, subsequently presented patterns inducing a percept as if they were presented simultaneously. This effect is shown in two studies. One is an experiment by Leeuwenberg *et al.* (1985). They used code-asymmetrical patterns like the ones of set 1 in Figure 9.3 (see also Mens, 1988). The other study is by van der Vloed *et al.* (2007), who used partly symmetrical and partly random configurations.

In the first study (Leeuwenberg *et al.*, 1985) the procedure was as follows. In each trial, a whole pattern (W) and a subpattern (S) were presented one after the other with a maximal spatial overlap. Both the W and the S patterns were presented each for 10 ms in different orders (W→S and W←S). The stimulus onset asynchrony (SOA) varied from 10 ms to 70 ms in steps of 10 ms. The task was to identify the S pattern and the subject had to select this pattern from twelve possible S patterns (forced choice). The dependent variable was the percentage correct detection. There were thirty participants. To each subject, 168 double stimuli were presented (twenty-four pairs, seven SOAs). Next, we first discuss the expected and the actual results, and then we argue that the results lead to an estimate of the temporal integration span.

Recency and masking

The actual stimuli are shown in Figure 9.4. In each of the four rows, one W pattern was combined with three S patterns in two different orders (W→S and W←S). S_1 and S_2 are code-asymmetrically related to W (see later). This does not hold for S_3. According to Michels and Turvey (1979), the detection of the last pattern of two serially presented patterns is positively affected by two factors. One is the recency of the last pattern. The other factor is the masking of the first pattern by the last pattern if the codes of the two patterns are incompatible. This leads to the following for the patterns in the first row of Figure 9.4.

The S1→W order is compatible and is indicated by a bold arrow. The zigzag code of S_1 is supposed to affect the interpretation of W. As a consequence, W is interpreted as a zigzag pattern too, though with a line. The W→S_1 order is incompatible and is indicated by a dotted arrow. W is interpreted as three triangles and S_1 as a zigzag. We expect that the detection of S_1 in this W→S_1 order is better than in the S_1→W order, for the above two reasons. That is, in the W→S_1 order, S_1 is not only recent but also masks W due to the incompatible coding relation (the latter means that S_1 becomes more isolated from W). The total effect

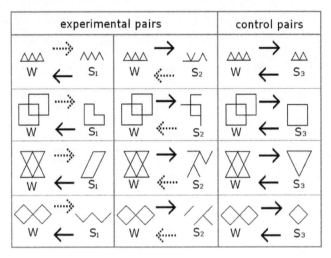

Figure 9.4 Stimuli of a study by Leeuwenberg *et al.* (1985). Columns 1 and 2 present pattern pairs whose orders give rise to code-asymmetry. Dotted arrows indicate incompatible orders (the code of the first pattern is of no use for the code of the second pattern) and normal arrows indicate compatible orders (the code of the first pattern is of use for the code of the second pattern). Column 3 presents pattern pairs whose two orders are both compatible. S patterns are parts of W patterns. In each trial W and S are presented each for 10 ms and with a maximal overlap. The SOA varies from 10 to 70 ms. The task was to identify the S pattern (forced choice) (Leeuwenberg *et al.*, 1985).

is that S_1 is better detected than in the $S_1 \rightarrow W$ order in which nothing special happens.

For the pairs $W \rightarrow S_2$ and $S_2 \rightarrow W$, the expectation is partly equal and partly different for similar reasons. On itself, S_2 is interpreted as a line with two V shapes. This interpretation is of no use for coding W. Hence, this time, the $S_2 \rightarrow W$ order is incompatible. In contrast, the interpretation of W is of use for coding S_2, namely, as three triangles minus three line segments. Thus, the $W \rightarrow S_2$ order is compatible. This time, we expect that S_2 is better detected in the $W \rightarrow S_2$ order than in the $S_2 \rightarrow W$ order, again for the two reasons above. That is, one reason is the recency of S_2 in the $W \rightarrow S_2$ order and the other reason is that, in the incompatible $S_2 \rightarrow W$ order, S_2 is masked by W. All in all, due to recency and masking, both S_1 and S_2 detection is better in the $W \rightarrow S$ than in the $S \rightarrow W$ order.

Furthermore, the S_3 detection is expected to be better in the $W \rightarrow S_3$ order than in the $S_3 \rightarrow W$ order but merely because of its recency in

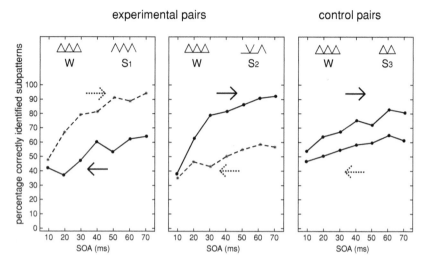

Figure 9.5 Results of the study by Leeuwenberg *et al.* (1985). The graphs correspond to the columns of Figure 9.4. Only the patterns in the first two graphs reveal code-asymmetry. Their orders are either incompatible, indicated by dotted arrows, or compatible, indicated by normal arrows. For all pairs it holds that the percentage correct S detection is higher in the W→S than in the W←S order. Presumably, this is due to the recency of S. An additional effect is supposed to stem from the masking of the first pattern by the second pattern in case of two incompatible patterns. Therefore, the detection gap between W→S and W←S is expected to be greater for S_1 and S_2 than for S_3. The results support this expectation for SOA larger than 20 ms. This brief period is taken as the visual integration time (Leeuwenberg *et al.*, 1985).

the W→S_3 order. We do not expect a masking effect because both orders, W→S_3 and S_3→W, are equally compatible. They miss any code-asymmetry. So, in total, there are predictions on the basis of recency and masking. The predicted effect of recency is that the S detection, in all conditions, is better in the W→S order than in the S→W order. The predicted effect of masking is that this detection gap between W→S and S→W is greater for S_1 and S_2 than for S_3.

The graphs in Figure 9.5 reveal whether these predictions were supported by the data. These graphs present the percentages correctly identified S patterns, averaged over all double stimuli, as a function of SOA. The upper curves deal with W→S and the bottom curves deal with S→W stimuli. Analysis of variance showed that the gaps between the upper and bottom curves for S_1 and S_2 patterns were significantly larger than the gaps for S_3 patterns (p < .001). These overall results agreed with the expectations. An additional analysis revealed that primitive pattern features, such as closure, contrast points, and number of angles, do not explain the outcomes.

Temporal integration span

A more refined analysis of the data in Figure 9.5 showed significant gap differences between S_1 and S_3 stimuli only for SOA $\geq$ 20 ms, and between S_2 and S_3 stimuli only for SOA $\geq$ 30 ms. This result gave, inversely, rise to the tentative conclusion that only within a period as small as about 20 ms two subsequent stimuli are processed as one integrated stimulus. Within this brief period the perceptual coding is supposed to be affected by subsequent stimuli and sensitive to backward context. In other words, this period reveals no effect that can be attributed to the difference between incompatible and compatible pattern relations.

In principle, this integration period restricts the forward context effect of a prime on a subsequent target pattern. A prime should have a code that is fixated and insensitive for recoding, implying that the SOA between prime and target should anyhow exceed this integration period. It is not clear whether forward context effect beyond this integration period is the result of perception (see Chapter 1.2). It might be due to a post-perceptual process of expectation (Mens and Leeuwenberg, 1994). Similar restrictions on contextual interactions have been shown in micro-genetic experiments by Bachmann and Allik (1976) and by Calis et al. (1984).

The foregoing findings and arguments can also be given a neurophysiological interpretation. This interpretation was triggered by van der Vloed et al.'s (2007) experiment which suggests a variable temporal integration span and which is next discussed briefly as leg up to this neurophysiological interpretation.

Van der Vloed et al. (2007) considered pattern pairs consisting of one part surrounding another, each part being either symmetrical (S) or random (R) (see Figure 9.6). Both parts were presented for 200 ms, but the two parts could be presented synchronously (SOA = 0) or asynchronously with an SOA of 20, 40, 60, 80, or 100 ms. The task of the participants was to discriminate partly symmetrical stimuli (for SOA > 0, presented in the orders RS and SR; see Figure 9.6, rows 1 and 2), from either completely random stimuli (RR; see Figure 9.6, row 3) or completely symmetrical stimuli (SS; see Figure 9.6, row 4).

One result was that, for all SOAs, both RS and SR were discriminated better from SS (error proportion around .2) than from RR (error proportion around .5) if the centre part is random and the surrounding

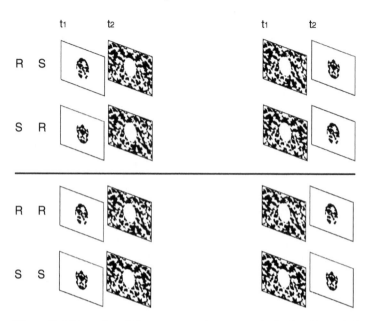

Figure 9.6 Rows 1 and 2 present partly symmetrical stimuli consisting of a random part and a symmetrical part; the random part could be the centre part or the surrounding part, and it could be presented first (RS) or last (SR). Row 3 presents stimuli consisting of two random parts (RR) and row 4 presents stimuli consisting of two symmetrical parts (SS) (van der Vloed *et al.*, 2007).

part symmetrical, and discriminated better from RR (error proportion around .15) than from SS (error proportions around .35) if the centre part is symmetrical and the surrounding part random. This result is not surprising, because it reflects the well-known fact that, in symmetry perception, the centre part is more important than the surrounding part (Barlow and Reeves, 1979). The novel result, however, was that SR showed no difference between SOA = 0 and SOA > 0, whereas RS did. That is, in SR, participants seemed to perceive just as much symmetry or randomness for SOA > 0 as for SOA = 0 (i.e., discrimination from RR and SS remained the same when SOA increased), but in RS, they seemed to perceive more symmetry or less randomness for SOA > 0 than for SOA = 0 (i.e., discrimination from RR was better and discrimination from SS was worse for SOA > 0 than for SOA = 0).

The latter result suggests that, in SR, the temporal integration span is up to 100 ms, whereas in RS, backward masking occurs in that the symmetrical part masks the preceding random part. This backward masking is perhaps understandable, but then, why does SR not also show an effect of (backward or forward) masking? In other words, the difference between SR and RS cannot be attributed to masking alone and must also be due to something specific to the perceptual difference between symmetry and random information. We think that the difference between SR and RS can be understood neurophysiologically by taking into account spatio-temporal factors in the visual hierarchy in the brain. We are aware that this neurophysiological picture (which we give next) may be too simplistic on details, but it seems to reflect a basic principle of when and how backward masking might occur, and thereby, it goes further than just establishing that it occurs.

The visual hierarchy can be said to start in the primary visual area V1 in the occipital lobe, which is followed by higher (or later) visual areas and, eventually, by a smooth transition to non-visual cognitive levels. The idea now is that the representation of an incoming stimulus is built up hierarchically under the motto that (less-structured) parts are represented in lower areas than their organization into (more-structured) wholes. This idea is analogous to Hubel and Wiesel's (1968) distinction between (low-level) simple cells and (high-level) complex cells, but it is more general in that we assume that 'parts' and 'wholes' refer to constituents of representations rather than just to areas in a stimulus. We further assume that top-down attentional processes access a resulting representation in the reversed order (Ahissar and Hochstein, 2004; Hochstein and Ahissar, 2002), that is, from wholes to parts, so that higher-level constituents of representations have primacy over lower-level constituents – this agrees with the superstructure-dominance hypothesis (see Chapters 6.2, 10.1, and 10.2).

Applied to van der Vloed et al.'s (2007) cases of SR and RS with SOA = 0, the foregoing idea implies that the (hardly structured) random part is represented relatively low and that the (highly structured) symmetrical part is represented relatively high. The same occurs in SR with SOA > 0, because then, the representation of the symmetry settles relatively high and the representation of the subsequently presented random part remains relatively low – just as when the parts are presented simultaneously. In RS with SOA > 0, however, the symmetry information (on its way to being represented relatively high) passes through the relatively low areas where the representation of the preceding random part resides – thereby, it affects (i.e., perturbs or masks) this representation of the random part, resulting in a percept that contains less randomness than there really is.

This explains van der Vloed et al.'s (2007) data, and it also seems to agree with the data in Leeuwenberg et al.'s (1985) study (see Figure 9.5).

That is, by the idea above, backward masking occurs when (a part of) a representation at some level in the visual hierarchy is perturbed by new visual information that is to be represented at the same or at higher levels. Such a perturbation does not occur in the compatible orders (old and new information leave the same trace at that level) but does occur in the incompatible orders. For instance, in the incompatible order $W \rightarrow S_1$, both W and S_1 are fairly structured but in different ways (triangles versus zigzag) so that the representation of S_1 will affect the representation of the preceding W up to its highest level. Furthermore, in the incompatible order $S_2 \rightarrow W$, the higher-structured W will be represented higher than the lower-structured S_2, and on its way to this higher level, it will leave a different trace at the lower level where the preceding S_2 is represented, so that the representation of S_2 will be affected.

In sum, the temporal integration span in vision seems to be about 20 ms in general, but it may also be longer depending on the structural relationships within and between subsequently presented stimuli. This is, first, a factor to be reckoned with in experiments involving priming or masking (see also Hermens and Herzog, 2007), and second, it asserts that structural factors are at least as relevant as spatio-temporal factors (probably also in, e.g., apparent motion; see Moore *et al.*, 2007).

Summary

This chapter deals with pairs of patterns with code asymmetries. Of each pair, one pattern is unambiguous and the other pattern is semi-ambiguous, that is, the rivaling code is almost as simple as the simplest code. Furthermore, the simplest code of the unambiguous pattern is compatible with the rivaling, one but simplest, code of the semi-ambiguous pattern, whereas the simplest code of the semi-ambiguous pattern is of no use to represent the unambiguous pattern. As a consequence, the code of the unambiguous pattern affects the code of the ambiguous pattern, but not the other way around. Section 9.1 shows that two simultaneously presented patterns of this kind can suggest that they must have occurred earlier in a specific order, namely, from the semi-ambiguous to the unambiguous pattern. The reason is that only this order deals with an identifiable recoding cue. Section 9.2 shows a reversed effect and provides an estimation of the time span within which two subsequently presented patterns are perceived as simultaneously presented patterns. This time span is supposed to stand for the temporal integration span within which backward context effects may still take place. One study showed that this temporal integration span is about 20 ms in case of code-asymmetrical patterns. Another study, presenting patterns consisting of a symmetrical part and a random part, showed that the temporal integration span may be up to 100 ms if the symmetrical part precedes the random part, but that it is also about 20 ms if the symmetrical part succeeds the random part. A neurophysiological interpretation of the effects in both studies suggests that structural factors are at least as relevant as spatio-temporal factors.

10   Hierarchy effects

Introduction

This chapter is on visual effects of hierarchy. The first two sections
deal with the hierarchy between the superstructure and the subordinate
structure in the simplest code of a pattern. The hypothesis is that the
superstructure plays a more dominant role in perception than the subordinate structure. Section 10.1 tests this hypothesis directly by way of
unity and duality judgments and by way of primed object matching, and
section 10.2 tests this hypothesis by way of mental rotation to match
mirrored objects. The latter study is reported more extensively as it deals
with rather indirect effects of superstructure dominance. Section 10.3
attends to view-dependent effects of frames on pattern concepts. These
frames are not superstructure components of the target pattern itself, but
rather agree with the coordinates determined by the context of the target
pattern.

10.1   Superstructure dominance

Unity and duality

Van Bakel (1989) studied pictures each presenting two objects. His question was whether a picture was perceived as a unitary configuration of
subcomponents or rather as two separate objects. In other words, he
tested whether a picture was judged as a unity or as a duality. His goal
was to test the superstructure dominance hypothesis. To this end, he
used the kinds of stimuli depicted in Figure 10.1. This figure presents
a set of four object pairs together with their visualized structural information theory (SIT) codes. The top component of each code presents
the superstructure and the bottom component presents the subordinate
structure. In Figures 10.1A and C, the superstructure consists of two
parts, whereas in Figures 10.1B and D, the subordinate structure consists of two parts. The set is furthermore balanced as follows. The code

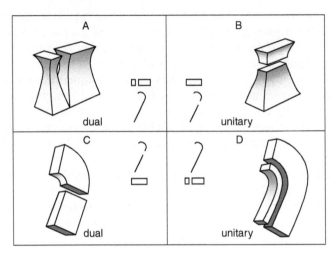

Figure 10.1 Four double objects with their visualized SIT codes (van Bakel, 1989). In each code, the superstructure is presented above the subordinate structure. Of A and C, only the superstructure is divided in two parts, and of B and D, only the subordinate structure is divided in two parts. A and C are judged more as dual objects than B and D. The conclusion is that the superstructure is visually more dominant than the subordinate structure (Leeuwenberg and van der Helm, 1991).

hierarchy in Figure 10.1A is opposed to the code hierarchy in Figures 10.1C, and the code hierarchy in Figure 10.1B is opposed to the code hierarchy in Figure 10.1D. The superstructures in Figures 10.1A and B are smaller than the subordinate structures, and the superstructures in Figures 10.1C and D are larger than the subordinate structures. Now, the superstructure dominance hypothesis implies that the superstructure is decisive and gives rise to expect that, notwithstanding these variables, a configuration with a divided superstructure is perceived as more dual and less unitary than a configuration with a divided subordinate structure. It means that Figures 10.1A and C are perceived more as dual than Figures 10.1B and D are.

The actual experimental procedure was as follows. In each trial of the experiment, two object pairs were presented. Of one pair, the superstructure was subdivided, and of the other, the subordinate structure was subdivided. The task was to indicate which stimulus was preferably perceived as a 'dual object' as opposed to a 'unitary object'. Obviously, the codes were not shown to the subject.

In fact, various sets of four double objects were tested. Each double object was randomly presented four times due to the variation of left-right order and of orientation. The study dealt with two experimental versions each for fifteen participants. In one version, the perceived 3-D space between the two objects was kept constant. Six sets were involved and only the judgments of double objects with the same code hierarchy were compared, so only A-B and C-D pairs. As a consequence, each subject got forty-eight pairs of double objects. In another version, the projective 2-D distance between the object parts was kept constant. Nine sets were involved and the judgments of all double objects were compared with each other in all combinations. So, each subject got 144 pairs of double objects.

The average judgments over subjects of both versions significantly ($p < .01$) supported the superstructure dominance hypothesis. It means that double objects with a divided superstructure were rather judged as dual objects than double objects with a divided subordinate structure. Also within subjects there was significant support.

Object matching

To provide a more direct test of superstructure dominance, van Lier *et al.* (1997) designed an experiment using the primed-matching paradigm of Sekuler and Palmer (1992). In each trial, a prime pattern was presented for 500 milliseconds (ms). After 17 ms, two equal or unequal drawings of test objects were shown until the response of the subject was given. For each of thirty-one participants, the task was to judge, as fast as possible, whether the two test objects were equal. The unequal test objects belonged to the catch trials and were not involved in the analysis (see Chapter 8.3). The expectation was that a prime pattern which agrees with the superstructure in the code of the test object facilitates the identification of the test objects more than a prime pattern which agrees with the subordinate structure. The facilitation is indicated by prime effect (PE), and is expressed as a negative function of reaction time (RT) as follows:

$$PE = RT \text{ (no-prime)} - RT \text{ (prime)}$$

The RT (no-prime) is taken as a base line to control for effects of irrelevant factors, such as the complexity of test patterns.

The test objects of the experiment are shown in Figures 10.2A to H. Obviously, the codes were not shown to the subjects. The prime patterns are presented in Figures 10.2K to N. They merely deal with circle and square components. The unclosed code components were not used as primes because in the projections of the test objects they are present in too many variations. The primes were presented in two ways.

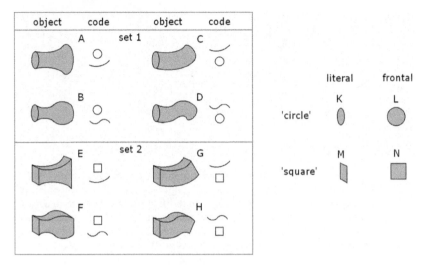

Figure 10.2 A to H present test objects in a primed-matching study (van Lier *et al.*, 1997). In each visualized code, the superstructure is presented above the subordinate structure. K to N are prime patterns, L and N are frontal patterns, and K and M are their actual projections. Each trial dealt with a prime (500 ms), an interval (17 ms) and two equal or different test objects. The task was to judge, as fast as possible, whether the test objects are equal. The data support superstructure dominance (van Lier *et al.*, 1997).

Figures 10.2L and N present the primes in a 'frontal' fashion, that is, as they would appear in the frontal-parallel plane. These primes are supposed to agree with the view-independent representations of the test object components. Figures 10.2K and M present the primes in a 'literal' fashion. They agree with the actual projections of the test object components. The assumption is that these primes not only reveal representational similarity but also physical similarity with the components of the test objects. In the experiment, each prime was combined with each test object. Furthermore, each prime-test pair was presented in two orientations, one in an upright orientation and the other in a 90° turned orientation.

An analysis of variance (ANOVA), applied to PE data, showed that, for literal primes, the superstructure and the subordinate structure primes, each on themselves, provide significant prime effects. This holds partly for frontal primes, namely only for the superstructure primes.

The results are shown in Figure 10.3A. The PE of the superstructure primes was significantly higher than the PE of the subordinate structure

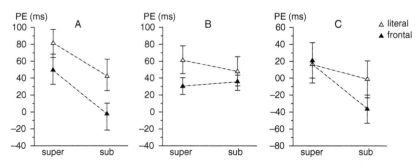

Figure 10.3 Results for the stimuli in Figure 10.2 (van Lier *et al.*, 1997). PE stands for prime effect. A reveals superstructure dominance: PE of the superstructure primes is higher than PE of the subordinate structure primes. This holds for both literal and frontal primes. B presents the data of a control study. This time, the objects A to H in Figure 10.2 are primes and K to N are test patterns. As expected, these data do not reveal any superstructure dominance. C presents PE of the first experiment minus PE of the control study. These differences support superstructure dominance merely for frontal primes.

primes (p < .05). This holds for both literal and frontal primes. Thus, the main expectation about the superstructure dominance is supported by the data.

The PE of the literal primes were significantly higher than those of the frontal primes (p < .01). This outcome may be related to the assumption that the literal primes both reveal representational and physical similarity with the test object components, whereas the frontal primes merely reveal representational similarity. All other interaction effects were not significant.

The foregoing shows that matching (then to be encoded) hierarchical stimuli is better when the superstructure component is primed than when the subordinate-structure component is primed. Inversely, however, we do not expect a differential effect on matching such components if they are primed by a (then already encoded) hierarchical stimulus. To test this, van Lier *et al.* (1997) conducted a control experiment in which the roles of the components and the objects were reversed. So, the objects in Figures 10.2A to H were used as primes and Figures 10.2K to N were used as test patterns. To the same thirty-one subjects the primes were again presented for 500 ms. However, the interval between the prime and the test patterns was not 17 ms but 50 ms. In all other respects, this control experiment was the same as the previous main experiment.

The assumption is that, after the priming stage, the simplest code of the object in the prime is available. That is, we assume that, then, the hierarchy between the superstructure and the subordinate structure in the prime has been established and that, subsequently, the superstructure component and the subordinate-structure component are equally accessible. The latter implies that the separate components (i.e., not so much their hierarchical relationship in the prime) can exert equally a priming effect on matching such components. In other words, the prediction is that matching superstructure and subordinate structure components is affected equally by these object primes.

An ANOVA analysis showed that the PE on superstructure and on subordinate-structure test patterns, each on their own, are significant. This holds both for literal and frontal test patterns. The results are shown in Figure 10.3B. The PE on the superstructure test patterns is not higher than the PE on the subordinate-structure test patterns. This holds for both literal and frontal primes. Thus, this outcome supports our expectation about the equivalence of the superstructure and the subordinate-structure effects of the prime objects once their simplest hierarchical codes have been established. Furthermore, the PE on the literal test patterns was not significantly higher than those on the frontal test patterns. The other interaction effects were also insignificant.

In fact, this control experiment, from objects to components, provides information about the accessibility of superstructures and subordinate structures in object codes irrespective of their hierarchical relationships. These hierarchical relationships are only involved in the previous experiment from components to objects. This implies that the hierarchical dominance of the superstructure over the subordinate structure will be prominently revealed by the difference between the PE of experiment 1 minus the PE of this control experiment 2. In Figure 10.3C, this surplus effect is presented. It shows, though only for frontal primes, that the PE of the superstructure was significantly higher than the PE of the subordinate structure ($p < .05$).

In our view, this outcome supports that the superstructure dominance is actually restricted to effects of representational component primes on whole objects whereas the effects of whole object primes on representational components rather reflect the concurrent presence of these components in the representation of whole objects. The same conclusion was drawn by other researchers, for instance, by Beller (1971) and by Sekuler and Palmer (1992) with respect to the role of representational similarity of prime and test shapes in a matching task, but also by Mens and Leeuwenberg (1988). As was reported in Chapter 8.3 and illustrated by Figure 8.21, the latter authors showed that component priming of whole

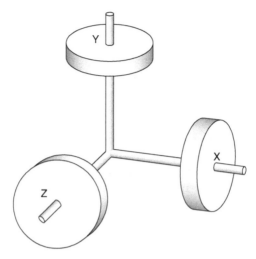

Figure 10.4 The disks indicate rotations about X, Y, and Z axes. These rotations are supposed to be mentally performed during the experiment.

patterns affects their segmentation preference, whereas whole pattern priming of components reflects the concurrent presence of preferred and not-preferred segmentations.

10.2   Mental rotation

The experiment performed by Leeuwenberg and van Lier (2005) tested the superstructure dominance hypothesis in an indirect way. Therefore, here, it is discussed more extensively. It involved again a matching task, but in contrast to the previous study, this study focused not on the super-structures and subordinate structures themselves, but on cues supplied by these structures. A second difference deals with the matching task. Each trial presented a mirror-symmetrical display of two objects, and the task was to assess whether a 180° rotation about the X, Y, or Z axis would turn one object into the other.

Figure 10.4 shows how rotations about the X, Y, and Z axes were indicated by disks. Figure 10.5 illustrates a mirror-symmetrical display of two objects. Note that this symmetry applies to the presented objects and not to their projections. The 180° X-rotation of one of the two objects, say of the object in Figure 10.5A, does not lead to the mirror version in Figure 10.5B. Thus, the 180° X rotation does not lead to a match. In contrast, both the 180° Y and Z rotations do lead to the mirror version. The outcome of the three tests is indicated by: X−, Y+, Z+.

A   A'

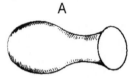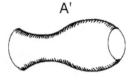

Figure 10.5 The combination of A and B presents a mirror-symmetrical display. The 180° X, Y, and Z rotations of A lead to, respectively, a mismatch, a match, and a match with B. The outcome, in shorthand, is X−, Y+, Z+ (Leeuwenberg and van Lier, 2005).

The display in Figure 10.5 is mirror symmetrical about the Y-Z plane. The orthogonal of this plane is the X-axis and is called the 'alignment axis'. In fact, in all illustrations we merely use the X-alignment axis as the standard axis of the display. Y and Z alignment axes were also used in the experiment.

The further discussion of this study comprises two parts. One part deals with the explanation of data by object cues and the other part deals with the way these cues can be replaced by code cues. In the first part, it is argued that each 180° rotation about the X, Y, or Z axis goes together with an object property that guarantees that the rotation turns an object into its mirror version. So, such an object property can be taken as cue for a matching rotation (Quinlan, 1995). Furthermore, it is established how well the object cues explain the matching data of the experiment by Leeuwenberg and van Lier (2005). In the second part, it is examined which object cues can be represented by recognition by components (RBC) codes (Biederman, 1987) and by SIT codes. Properties of some code components appear to be code cues for matching rotations. Furthermore, it is established how well these code cues explain the matching data of the experiment.

Object cues

As said, for each 180° matching rotation about the X, Y, or Z axis, there is an object property that can be used as cue for matching objects. To establish each of these object cues, use is made of Figure 10.6 that presents objects by transparent cubes. The cube in Figure 10.6A is supposed to stand for the first object of two sequentially presented objects. Its corners are marked by numbers. Two transformations are applied to this cube. One is mirroring (M). Its outcome is presented in Figure 10.6B. The other transformation is one of the three 180° rotations. Their outcomes are presented in Figures 10.6C, C′, and C″. Each of these outcomes

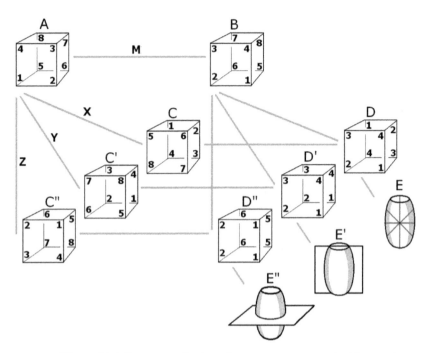

Figure 10.6 By means of cubes whose corners are marked by numbers, the cue for each 180° rotation is derived that turns an object into its mirror version. A is the standard cube that stands for the first of two objects. Two transformations are applied to this cube to obtain the mirror version. One is the mirroring (M) presented by B. The other is one of the three 180° rotations. These rotations are presented by C, C′, and C″. The combination of B with C, C′, and C″ is, respectively, presented by D, D′, and D″. The numbers in the latter cubes reveal the object cues. For a 180° X rotation, the cue is point-symmetry (D); for a 180° Y rotation, the cue is mirror-symmetry about the Y-X plane (D′), and for a 180° Z rotation, the cue is mirror-symmetry about the Z-X plane (D″). By E, E′, and E″ the cue features are illustrated by vase shapes (Leeuwenberg and van Lier, 2005).

is combined with the outcome of mirroring. This implies that different numbers in the same corner of the two cubes are replaced by one of these numbers, say, the lowest number. The combined results are presented by Figures 10.6D, D′, and D″. Their numbers reveal the object cues of each rotation. Figures 10.6E, E′, and E″ illustrate these cues by vase shapes. Next, we describe each cue.

A 180° X rotation of Figure 10.6A causes a top–bottom and a front–rear exchange of the numbers in the figure. These exchanges, shown in Figure 10.6C, in combination with the left–right exchanges of M, lead to the cube in Figure 10.6D. This cube reveals equal numbers on its diagonals. In other words, it is characterized by point-symmetry. Accordingly, this kind of symmetry is the object cue for a 180° matching X rotation. Figure 10.6E illustrates this cue for a vase shape.

A 180° Y rotation of Figure 10.6A causes a front–rear and a left–right exchange of the numbers in the figure. These exchanges, shown in Figure 10.6C′, in combination with the left–right exchanges of M, lead to the cube in Figure 10.6D′. This cube reveals equal fore–back numbers. In other words, it is characterized by mirror-symmetry about the Y-X plane. Accordingly, this kind of symmetry is the object cue for a 180° matching Y rotation. Figure 10.6E′ illustrates this cue for a vase shape.

A 180° Z rotation of Figure 10.6A causes a left–right and a top–bottom exchange of the numbers in Figure 10.6A. These exchanges, shown in Figure 10.6C″, in combination with the left–right exchanges of M, lead to the cube in Figure 10.6D″. This cube reveals equal top–bottom numbers. In other words, it is characterized by mirror-symmetry about the Z-X plane. Accordingly, this kind of symmetry is the object cue for a 180° matching Z rotation. Figure 10.6 E″ illustrates this cue for a vase shape.

Figure 10.6 merely deals with object cues for mirror symmetrical displays along the X alignment axis. The general cue rule for any alignment axis is as follows. A mirror rotation about the alignment axis is cued by the object's point-symmetry (P), and a mirror rotation about another axis is cued by the object's mirror-symmetry (M) about the plane determined by the rotation axis and the alignment axis. Before we show how the object cues can be predicted from code cues, we first discuss the experiment to explore how well the P and M cues might have affected the matching performance.

In Figure 10.7, the experimental objects are shown in standard orientations. In the experiment, these objects were combined with their mirror versions under varying orientations. One set of items, shown in row 2, consists of solid objects. Rows 3 and 4, respectively, present their visualized RBC and SIT codes (see next subsection). Another set, shown in row 5, consists of surface objects. Rows 6 and 7, respectively, present their visualized RBC and SIT codes (see next subsection). The top row indicates whether a rotation of an object around the X, Y, or Z axis matches (+) or mismatches (−) with its X-aligned mirror version. Care was taken that there are as many matches as mismatches per rotation. To construct a critical set of objects, we excluded objects for which all rotations lead to a match (X+, Y+, Z+) or to a mismatch (X−, Y−, Z−).

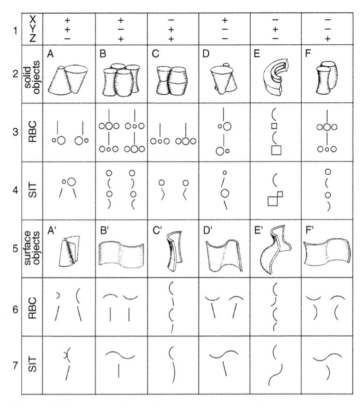

Figure 10.7 An overview of the experimental objects and their properties. Row 1 presents the matches (+) and mismatches (−) for 180° rotations about X, Y, and Z axes (for the standard display with an X alignment axis). Row 2 presents solid objects (A to F). Rows 3 and 4, respectively, present their visualized RBC and SIT codes discussed in the next subsection. Row 5 presents surface objects (A' to F'). Rows 6 and 7, respectively, present their visualized RBC and SIT codes discussed in the next subsection (Leeuwenberg and van Lier, 2005).

To exclude orientation sensitive bias effects, for instance, of vertical symmetry (Goldmeier, 1937/1972; Mach, 1886), objects and displays were tested under varying orientations. In Figure 10.8, these varying orientations are illustrated for object C in Figure 10.7. The rows deal with the X, Y, and Z orientations of the objects on themselves. The columns deal with the X, Y, and Z alignment axes of the displays. In each cell, the three 180° X, Y, and Z rotations are indicated together with information about their match (+) and mismatch (−) effects. Also

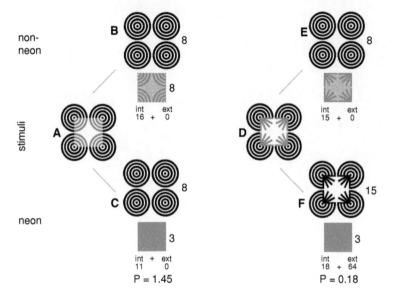

Figure 8.10 Two interpretations of A are presented in B and C. The non-neon interpretation (B) presents a pattern of black disks and a white square foreground surface with blue lines. This white surface is here presented by a grey surface. The neon interpretation (C) presents a pattern of black disks illuminated by a blue square. The neon code is simpler than the non-neon code. In contrast, the neon code (E) of D is more complex than the non-neon code (F). The numbers refer to loads.

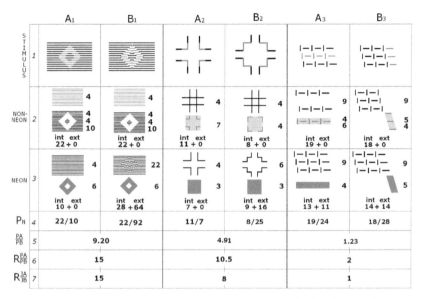

		A₁	B₁	A₂	B₂	A₃	B₃
STIMULUS	1						
NON-NEON	2	4 / 4 / 4 / 10 / int ext 22 + 0	4 / 4 / 4 / 10 / int ext 22 + 0	4 / 7 / int ext 11 + 0	4 / 4 / int ext 8 + 0	9 / 4 / 6 / int ext 19 + 0	9 / 5 / 4 / int ext 18 + 0
NEON	3	4 / 6 / int ext 10 + 0	22 / 6 / int ext 28 + 64	4 / 3 / int ext 7 + 0	6 / 3 / int ext 9 + 16	9 / 4 / int ext 13 + 11	9 / 5 / int ext 14 + 14
P_N	4	22/10	22/92	11/7	8/25	19/24	18/28
$\frac{PA}{PB}$	5	9.20		4.91		1.23	
$R\frac{PA}{PB}$	6	15		10.5		2	
$R\frac{JA}{JB}$	7	15		8		1	

Figure 8.11 Row 1 presents some experimental stimuli (van Tuijl and Leeuwenberg, 1979). Row 2 presents the non-neon components with their internal loads and row 3 presents the neon components with their internal loads. Row 4 presents the theoretical preference strengths P_N of the neon interpretation. Row 5 presents P_A/P_B quotients. Their ranks are indicated in row 6. The average ranks of judged neon dominances of A over B are indicated in row 7.

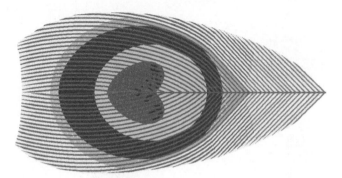

Figure 12.7 The beauty of a peacock's feather is explainable under the assumption that the separately coloured feather strips belong to the means and that the envelopes of the colours belong to the effect. The fact that the feather shape is quite unrelated to the circular colour patterns explains the beauty of a peacock's feather.

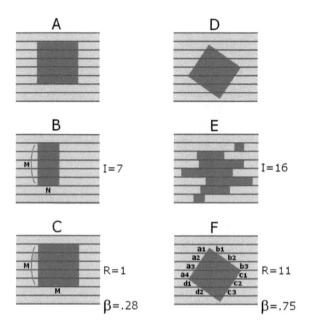

Figure 12.8 Patterns A and D present simplified feathers. In A, the blue square is related and in D the blue square is unrelated to the grid structure. The configurations below these patterns, namely BC and EF, illustrate the assessments of the loads I and the additional regularity R. The β of D appears to be higher than the β of A. The argument for the beauty of D explains the beauty of the peacock's feather (see Figure 12.7).

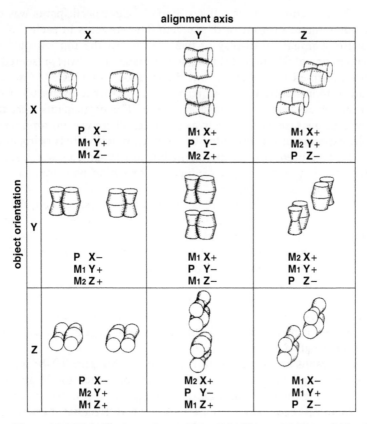

Figure 10.8 This illustrates how object C in Figure 10.7 is combined in the experiment with its mirror version. The rows present the X, Y, and Z orientations of the objects themselves. The columns present the varying X, Y, and Z alignment axes. In each cell, the three 180° X, Y, and Z rotations are indicated together with their correct positive or negative matches and together with their object cues P, M1, and M2, where P stands for point-symmetry, M1 stands for the mirror-symmetry cued by a high hierarchical code component, and M2 stands for the mirror-symmetry cued by a low hierarchical code component (see next subsection) (Leeuwenberg and van Lier, 2005).

indicated is whether these effects can be cued by the object's mirror-symmetry (M) or point-symmetry (P). The M1 and M2 indices are clarified in the next subsection. Notice that, due to the balance between matches and mismatches for each rotation (see row 1 in Figure 10.7), each M and P cue deals with the same number of + and – matches across all experimental trials.

The procedure was as follows. Each of eight participants was seated about 1 metre in front of the screen. The stimulus in each trial was a mirror-symmetrical display of two objects. At the top left part of the screen, one of the three disks, shown in Figure 10.4, was presented. This disk informed the subject about the rotation to be tested. The subject had to indicate, by yes or no responses, whether a given 180° rotation of one object leads to the mirror version. The participants were told to perform the task as accurately as possible. There was no time pressure. The experiment was preceded by eighteen practice trials being different from those used in the experiment but of the same object types. Only during this practice stage, feedback information was given about the correctness of the response.

The presented stimuli were composed as follows. In total, there were two object sets (solid and surface), six objects per set, three individual object orientations (X, Y, and Z), three alignments axes of displays (X, Y, and Z), and three kinds of 180° test rotations (X, Y, and Z). This leads to 324 different object pairs. To each participant, these stimuli were presented twice, in two different blocks, each block in a different random order. The experiment was done in two runs, each lasting about an hour. Half of the participants first received two blocks of solid objects in the first run and two blocks of surface objects in the second run, and the other half vice versa.

The results are presented in Figure 10.9. In Figure 10.9A and B, the average proportions correct responses are presented for M and P cued tasks. In Figure 10.9C and D, the average reaction times are presented for M and P cued tasks. Figure 10.9A and C differentiate between blocks 1 and 2, and Figure 10.9B and D differentiate between solid and surface objects. Significant differences (LSD, $p < 0.05$) between connected data points are indicated with an asterisk.

The data reveal three effects. First, Figures 10.9A and C show that the performance in block 2 is more accurate than in block 1. So, experience with the task improves the overall performance. Second, Figures 10.9B and D show that the task for solid objects is performed more accurately and faster than for surface objects. Third, the accuracy data in Figure 10.9A show an M > P effect within blocks. The RT data in Figure 10.9C do not reveal this effect within blocks. Figures 10.9B and D reveal differential effects: neither the accuracy nor the RT data on solid objects support any difference between M and P, but both accuracy and RT data on surface objects reveal an M > P effect.

We evaluate these results as follows. The first effect, that experience with the task improves the overall performance, hardly applies to

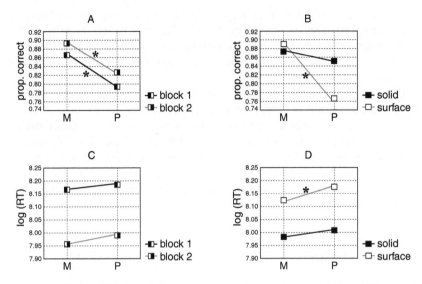

Figure 10.9 A and B present proportions correct and C and D present reaction times as functions of M (mirror-symmetry) and P (point-symmetry) cues. A and C differentiate between the first and second halves of each experiment. B and D differentiate between solid and surface objects. The asterisks indicate significant differences (LSD, p < 0.05) between connected data points (Leeuwenberg and van Lier, 2005).

mental rotation. In our view, it rather applies to the object cues and is an indication that these cues have played a role during mental rotation. For the remaining two effects, however, the object cues do not supply an explanation. After all, these cues equally stem from solid objects as from surface objects. Our main concern is that these cues explain neither the M > P effect nor why this effect merely deals with surface objects. Next, we examine whether codes might represent the object cues and, thereby, explain the M-P effects.

Code cues

To find out whether codes explain the M-P effects, we attend to the RBC and SIT codes presented in Figure 10.7 in a visualized form. This form is subject to the following five conventions: (1) foreground subshapes are represented below background subshapes; (2) the axis of each subshape is indicated above the cross-section and the superstructure is indicated above the subordinate structure; (3) only the object's top axis or super-structure is indicated in the code; (4) only the object's left cross-section or subordinate structure is indicated in the code; and (5) an RBC cross-section that expands from top to bottom is represented from left to right by small and large cross-sections.

The codes in Figure 10.7 reveal the following general features. The RBC representations of both solid and surface objects are multiple codes. They describe each stimulus by two or four separate geons. Also SIT uses multiple codes but only for solid objects. They describe each solid object by two or more superstructures, each with their own subordinate structure (see Figure 7.15G). The SIT codes of open surface objects consist of single codes, that is, each object is described by just one superstructure and one subordinate structure (see Figure 7.15E).

The implications are as follows. A subcode of a multiple code does not convey sufficient information about the M and P of the whole object. Even all its subcodes together do not supply this information as they do not explicitly describe the relationship between the subobjects. So, the RBC representations of both solid and surface objects and the SIT codes of solid objects do not capture M and P properties. So, in all these cases the expectation is indifference (i.e., the expectation is M = P). This does not hold for SIT codes of surface objects. It is true that the components of these codes do not convey P cues but they do convey M cues. The arguments for the latter claim are as follows.

The fact that components of single SIT codes do not capture P cues will just be shown by a few falsifications. Both the circle superstructure and the S-shape subordinate structure of each object in Figure 10.5 are point-symmetrical but the object is not point-symmetrical. Furthermore, Figures 10.7A′ and F′ are point-symmetrical objects but the components of their codes are not point-symmetrical. So, codes of surface objects do not convey P cues.

On the other hand, the superstructure of a single code captures an M cue for the following reason. All subordinate structures are equal and have the same orientation with respect to the superstructure. Therefore, mirror-symmetry of the superstructure around a plane perpendicular to the superstructure applies to any two subordinate structures anchored at symmetrical points of the superstructure. This implies that the mirror-symmetry of the superstructure applies to the whole object. So, as the mirror-symmetry of the whole object is a cue for a 180° matching rota-tion, the mirror-symmetry of the superstructure alone is a cue for a 180° matching rotation. Figure 10.7E′ presents an illustration. Its super-structure reveals mirror-symmetry around the Y-X plane. Therefore, this symmetry is a cue for a 180° matching rotation about the Y axis.

Also the subordinate structure of a single code captures an M cue. The reason is like that for the superstructure. In a SIT code, all subordinate structures are equal and have the same orientation with respect to the superstructure. Therefore, the mirror-symmetry of one subordinate structure around a plane parallel to the superstructure applies to all subordinate structures, that is, to the whole object. For instance, the subordinate C-curve of Figure 10.7F$'$ is mirror-symmetrical around the Z-X plane which is parallel to the superstructure. As a consequence, the whole object is mirror-symmetrical around this plane. So, the overall expectations are as follows:

RBC	SIT	
Solid objects	$M = P$	$M = P$
Surface objects	$M = P$	$M > P$

The two indifferent $M = P$ expectations from the multiple RBC and multiple SIT codes about solid objects agree with the data shown in Figures 10.9B and D. For surface objects the RBC expectation $M = P$ disagrees with the experimental data whereas the SIT expectation $M > P$ agrees with the data.

Single SIT codes give rise to an extra prediction, namely, from the assumption that the superstructure plays a more dominant role than the subordinate structure (Leeuwenberg and van der Helm, 1991). If M1 is the mirror-symmetry captured by the superstructure and M2 is the mirror-symmetry captured by the subordinate structure (see Figure 10.8), the expectation is $M1 > M2$. Notice that this difference cannot be derived from a multiple code. In that case the expectation is $M1 = M2$. So, the specific expectations are as follows:

RBC	SIT	
Solid objects	$M1 = M2$	$M1 = M2$
Surface objects	$M1 = M2$	$M1 > M2$

To verify these expectations, the data in Figure 10.9 are presented again in Figure 10.10, but this time, the data for the M cued task are split into those for the M1 and M2 cued tasks.

For solid objects, Figures 10.10B and D do not reveal any significant effect. This observed indifference, indicated by $M1 = M2 = P$, agrees

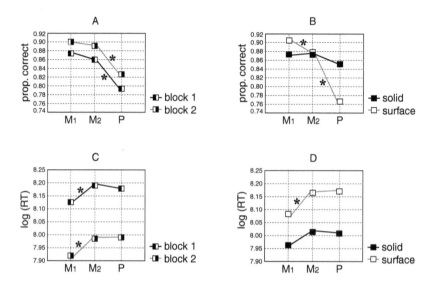

Figure 10.10 A and B present proportions correct and C and D present reaction times as functions of M1 cues (mirror-symmetry of high-level code components), M2 cues (mirror-symmetry of low-level code components), and P (point-symmetry) cues. A and C differentiate between the first and second halves of each experiment. B and D differentiate between solid and surface objects. The asterisks indicate significant differences (LSD, $p < 0.05$) between connected data points (Leeuwenberg and van Lier, 2005).

with the expectations of both RBC and SIT codes. For surface objects, an M1 > M2 effect is revealed both by the accuracy data in Figure 10.10B and by the RT data in Figure 10.10D. In combination with the earlier M > P effect (Figure 10.9) the data tend to point to an overall M1 > M2 > P effect. Only the accuracy data for surface objects explicitly support the M2 > P relation. The RT data neither support this relation nor reveal a decreasing trade-off effect that would be expected from the relatively low accuracy for P.

Generally, the data support our expectations. However, there are alternative explanations that we discuss here. Our explanation of the M > P effect based on rotation is as follows. In line with the suggestion of the instruction, both P and M cued matching tasks are performed by rotating one object and by comparing the rotated object with the mirror object. However, for M cued tasks there is another option, namely, by rotating the whole display and by comparing the rotated display with the given display. This rotation merely applies in the case of an M cue. There-fore, it may favour the M response. This explanation, however, is not quite satisfactory. First, the explicit instruction of the task is to rotate one object instead of the whole display. Second, the two options cannot be performed simultaneously but only the first option, being in line with our instruction, is useful for both P and M cued matching tasks. Third, this rotation bias explains neither the M = P effect for solid objects nor the M1 > M2 effect for surface objects.

A topic of discussion is the tool used by participants of the experiment to perform the task. Is it mental rotation or a code cue? Notice that these two tools are quite different. The mental rotation process deals with view-dependent features of images such as their orientations (Cooper, 1976; Finke, 1980; Kosslyn, 1981) whereas code cues are properties of view-independent object representations. In favour of mental rotation is the fact that most participants reported to perform the task that way. In contrast, cues explain the differential outcomes of symmetries. At least, SIT codes of surface objects explain their M > P and M1 > M2 effects. In our view, the combination of mental rotation and cueing is most plausible (Leeuwenberg and van der Helm, 2000; Takano, 1989; Tarr, 1995). Regarding their interaction, there are two options. One is suggested by Corballis (1988): the cue provides an index for the matching task and this strategy is complemented by mental rotation as a double check. The other option stems from Hochberg and Gellman (1977): the mental rotation process is guided by cues. They observed a facilitation of mental rotation due to unique and unambiguous landmark features of patterns. This option is also supported by our observations reported in Chapter 11.2. In our view, the latter option is the most plausible one.

Finally, in our study the mirror-symmetry is a relatively frequent fea-ture of objects involved in the experiment. Besides, it is a characteristic of whole displays. So, there is, anyhow, an imbalance between global displays and local item cues in favour of mirror-symmetry. To avoid this unbalance, an option would be to extend the experiment with point-symmetrical displays. However, all such displays give rise to symmetrical cues and not to point-symmetrical cues. This conclusion can be derived from the strategy shown in Figure 10.6. So, such an extension would not undo the unbalance. Notwithstanding this circumstance, the mirror-symmetry of displays does not explain all data. It does not explain the M = P effect for solid objects. In fact, there is even reason to expect a larger M > P effect for solid objects than for surface objects because, accidentally, there are two solid objects (Figures 10.7D and F) which are symmetrical around the same planes as their global displays whereas there are no surface objects with such properties.

10.3   Orientation frames

In Chapter 3.2 we argued that structural complexity determines the hierarchy between the superstructure and the subordinate structure, and that metrical size determines the perceived hierarchy between the global shape and the substructure if structural complexity is indifferent with respect to structural hierarchy. Here, we focus on the orientations of superstructures and global shapes and we show how they determine perceived properties of subpatterns. We first present a code technical account of the way a subpattern is affected by its superstructure, and then, of the way a subpattern is affected by its global shape.

Superstructures

Palmer and Bucher (1982) made a study of the visually preferred pointing directions of equilateral triangles. In principle, a single equilateral triangle is ambiguous in this respect. It means that its three angles equally point in directions along their symmetry axes. Yet, there is a favoured pointing direction if one of the sides of the triangle is vertical or horizontal. Then, the favoured pointing direction is perpendicular to this vertical or horizontal. Without doubt, this is because the vertical or horizontal are dominant natural orientations (Rock, 1973).

Of more interest are the effects, shown by Palmer and Bucher (1982), of configurations consisting of a few equilateral triangles, for instance, of those presented in Figures 10.11A, D, E, and H. They demonstrated that certain alignments of the triangles induce reference axes that favour pointing directions that might disagree with the local pointing direction of a single triangle as induced by its vertical or horizontal side. For instance, the visual pointing direction of the three triangles in Figure 10.11D appears to be top-right whereas each triangle on itself favours the leftward direction. Furthermore, the visual pointing direction of the triangles in Figure 10.11H tends to point bottom-right whereas each triangle on itself favours the upward direction.

We will attempt to explain these favoured pointing directions from codes. First we attend to global configuration effects. The simplest SIT code of each configuration describes a linear superstructure of three subordinate equilateral triangles. The subcode representing the equilateral triangle, however, reveals rotation invariance but not a unique bilateral symmetry with a pointing direction. So, if the task is to judge the pointing direction, the simplest code does not give an unequivocal cue about which direction might be chosen. Therefore, we assume that resort is

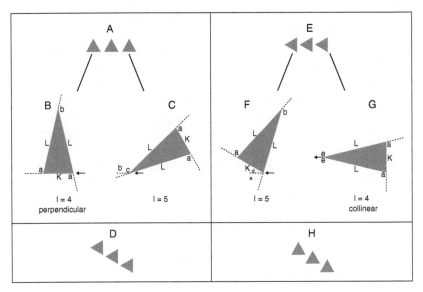

Figure 10.11 A, D, E, and H present configurations of equilateral triangles. The orientations of their superstructures seem to evoke specific pointing directions of the triangles. In A and D the orientation of the superstructure agrees with the orientation of their baselines, and the triangles appear to point perpendicular to these baselines. In E and H the orientation of the superstructure agrees with the orientation of the symmetry axes, and their pointing directions appear to be in line with these axes. The favoured pointing direction of a single triangle is perpendicular to the side that either is horizontal or vertical. All the effects are derived from the one but simplest stimulus codes.

taken to a second-best rivaling code (which is assumed to be concurrently present; see Chapter 8.3). According to this code, the equilateral triangle is taken as a member of a broader class, namely, of isosceles triangles characterized by unique pointing directions. The orientation of the superstructure is used as the initial scanning orientation of each triangle. For explaining a local effect of a single triangle the natural vertical or horizontal is used as the initial scanning orientation.

Now we steadily will describe two differently oriented isosceles triangles in the context of the horizontal orientation of the superstructure. So, the initial scanning orientation is horizontal and is indicated by an arrow. The predicted pointing direction is supposed to belong to the isosceles triangle with the simplest load. Figures 10.11B and C, respectively, present an upright and an oblique pointing triangle. With respect to the horizontal orientation of the superstructure in Figure 10.11A they are represented as follows:

KaLbLa → K S[(a)(L), (b)]	c LaKaL b → c S[(L)(a), (K)]b

The first code, I = 4, is simpler than the second code, I = 5. Hence, the upward pointing direction, being perpendicular to the superstructure, is predicted to be favoured. Notice that this pointing direction also is predicted from the natural horizontal orientation of one side of the triangle. Thus, global and local effects coincide. The same two codes also represent the two options of Figure 10.11D whose superstructure is tilted. So, also of this figure the predicted pointing direction of the triangles is perpendicular to the superstructure. However, this time the global and local effects do not coincide. After all, the orthogonal of the superstructure is oriented top-right whereas the local pointing direction, predicted from the natural vertical orientation of one side of the triangle, is leftward (see code of Figure 10.11B).

In Figure 10.11E, the horizontal superstructure agrees with the symmetry axis of the whole configuration and its orientation is horizontal too. With respect to the scanning orientation, that agrees with this horizontal, Figures 10.11F and G are represented as follows:

dKaLbLa → d K S[(a)(L), (b)]	e LaKaLe → S[(e)(L)(a), (K)]

This time the first code, I = 5, is more complex than the second code, I = 4. Thus, the leftward pointing direction of Figure 10.11G is predicted to be preferred. This orientation also is induced by the natural vertical orientation of one side of the triangle (see code of Figure 10.11B). Thus, the global and local effects coincide. Furthermore, Figure 10.11H has a bottom-right oriented superstructure and the predicted pointing direction agrees with this orientation. However, this time the global and local effects do not coincide. After all, the just mentioned global pointing direction differs from the local upward pointing direction derived from the natural horizontal orientation of one side of the triangle (see code of Figure 10.11B).

Global shapes

Figures 10.12A, D, E, H are square subpatterns within rectangular frames and Kopfermann (1930) has shown that the subpatterns in the first two figures are preferably interpreted as squares. Furthermore, he has shown that the subpatterns in the last two figures can be interpreted

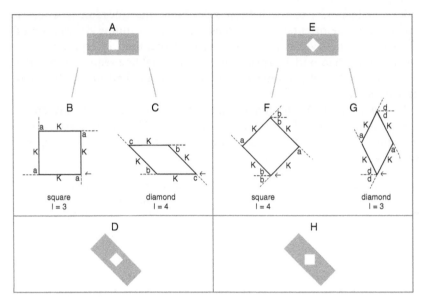

Figure 10.12 A, D, E, and H present square shaped subpatterns within rectangular frames. The interpretations of these subpatterns appear to be affected by these frames. If the subpatterns are parallel to these frames (AD) they are seen as squares (B) and not as diamonds (C), and if the subpatterns are oblique with respect to these frames (EH) they are seen as diamonds (G) and not as squares (F). The favoured interpretation of a subpattern, on itself without frame, is a square if one side is horizontal or vertical. All the effects are derived from the one but simplest stimulus codes.

as squares but also as diamonds. At least, they are more preferably perceived as diamonds than the subpatterns in the first two figures. In the first two figures, the sides of the subpatterns are parallel to the sides of their frames, and in the latter two figures none of the subpatterns' sides is parallel to the sides of their frames. So, orientation relations between subpatterns and frames seem to evoke the mentioned interpretation bias.

Here we will examine whether these interpretations can be derived from SIT representations. Notice, however, that the simplest SIT code, being a dissociated representation, describes a subpattern just as a square. So, it does not reveal the interpretation bias observed by Kopfermann (1930). Therefore, we explore whether the concurrently present rivaling code explains this bias (Chapter 8.3). This is a unified representation of a 2-D pattern, namely, of a rectangle with a hole. According to this representation, the subpattern is represented in relation to the rectangular frame, that is, as a deviation from the orientation of one of the rectangular sides, for instance, of the longest side. Now, the question is whether the longest side orientation, taken as the initial scanning orientation of the subpattern, gives rise to a square or a diamond interpretation. A square and a diamond are quadrangles with equal line segments, but the difference is that of the square all angles are equal and of the diamond only opposed angles are equal.

In Figure 10.12A, the longest side of the rectangle is a horizontal. The square and the diamond interpretation are illustrated, respectively, in Figures 10.12B and C. With respect to this horizontal they are represented as follows:

Square	Diamond
KaKaKaKa $\rightarrow$ 4*(Ka)	KbKcKbKc $\rightarrow$ 2*(S[(K),(b)] c)

The code of the square, $I = 3$, is simpler than the code of the diamond, $I = 4$. So, the square code is predicted for Figure 10.12A. This prediction equally applies to Figure 10.12D though for another global orientation.

In Figure 10.12E, the orientation of the rectangle is horizontal again but the orientation of the subpattern is oblique. The square and diamond interpretation are illustrated, respectively, in Figures 10.12F and G. With respect to this horizontal these interpretations are described as follows:

Square	Diamond
b KaKaKaKa $\rightarrow$ b 4*(Ka)	d KeK d d KeK d $\rightarrow$ S[S[((d))((K)),((e))]]

This time, the code of the square, $I = 4$, is more complex than the code of the diamond, $I = 3$. So, the diamond code is predicted for Figure 10.12E. The same prediction holds for Figure 10.12H though for another global orientation.

Finally, we make a comment on the relation between the global frames and the enclosed subpatterns in Figure 10.12. These global frames appear to determine the orientations of the local subpatterns and not the other way around. Exchange of the global and local shapes does not evoke the presented effects. For instance, if Figure 10.12H would be replaced by a tilted rectangle within a not-tilted square, the square is not affected by the rectangle and remains a square. In fact, also the code of a surface with a hole excludes this reversal. According to this code, the surface is an anchor for the hole but the hole is not an anchor for the surface. After all, a hole without a surface makes no sense.

In summary, the mentioned effects can be explained from codes, but not from the simplest codes. They can be explained by codes that are hidden but not quite hidden. They belong to the one but simplest descriptions and are therefore still supposed to be accessible in the context of the mentioned tasks.

Summary

The first two sections in this chapter deal with the hierarchy within the simplest pattern code, namely, between superstructure and subordinate structure. The hypothesis is that the superstructure plays a more dominant role in perception than the subordinate structure. Section 10.1 tests the hypothesis directly. One study shows that the judged unity and duality of objects is more affected by the unity and duality of their superstructures than that of their subordinate structures (van Bakel, 1989). Another study demonstrates that object matching is more facilitated by superstructure primes than by subordinate-structure primes (van Lier et al., 1997). Section 10.2 verifies the hypothesis indirectly, namely, by testing effects of code cues for the rotations that match objects in mirror displays (Leeuwenberg and van Lier, 2005). Cues stemming from superstructures appear to be more effective than cues stemming from subordinate structures. Section 10.3 shows that the superstructure of a series of equilateral triangles appears to affect the visual pointing direction of each separate triangle (Palmer and Bucher, 1982). These effects are explainable from SIT codes. Equally, a square, enclosed by a global frame, might be perceived either as a square or as a diamond. The orientation of the subpattern with respect to its frame appears to be decisive. These visual interpretations are explainable from SIT codes.

Part III

Extensions

In Parts I and II, the focus was on structural information theory (SIT) and perception. This Part III deals with topics at the margins of these two domains. One chapter is on perception beyond SIT and another is on SIT beyond perception.

Chapter 11 is concerned with visual perception, in a way that is beyond but still related to SIT. Two topics are discussed. One deals with a measure of metrical information load. This load reflects quantitative aspects of visual form. The relation between metrical and structural information is also considered. The other topic deals with the question of whether visual representations differentiate between an object and its mirrored version, and with the role visual representations might play in handedness discrimination.

Chapter 12 makes use of SIT but its application is beyond the prototypical domain of perception. Two topics are discussed. One deals with series of alphabetic letters and their inferred extrapolations. Experiments reveal a preference for extrapolations yielding simplest global representations. The other topic deals with evaluative pattern qualities such as salience, interestingness, and beauty. Attempts are made to specify measures of these qualities and to illustrate their relevance.

11 Perception beyond SIT

Introduction

Obviously, there are many topics of perception beyond structural information theory (SIT). Examples are colour perception, binocular rivalry, and the physiology of visual processing. Here, we discuss two topics which lie outside the scope of SIT but which, like SIT, deal with form perception.

Section 11.1 deals with a measure of metrical information load and its relevance for perception. This load does not refer to structural aspects, being the topic of SIT, but to quantitative or metrical aspects of visual form, especially of line lengths and turns. It is expressed by the amount of 'change' and its visual relevance is shown by complexity judgments.

Section 11.2 deals with the issue of whether objects and their mirrored versions are represented by handedness sensitive or handedness insensitive codes. A relevant question is whether, for handedness discrimination, mental rotation is needed or merely used to verify a response. Another question is whether either kind of codes provides a cue for the kind of rotation to be applied during the mental rotation test.

11.1 Metrical information

Cherry (1961), Gabor (1946), Mackay (1950), and van Soest (1952) made the distinction between structural and metrical information. The amount of structural information is called logon-content and the amount of metrical information is called metron-content. Structural information refers to pattern dimensions, descriptive parameters, or degrees of freedom, whereas metrical information refers to quantitative variations within structural dimensions. For instance, the lengths and widths of rectangles vary within a wide range. In effect, quantities are predicates of dimensions and not the other way around. So, conceptually, metrical information is subordinate to structural information (see also Chapter 3.2). Indeed, a quantitative change on some dimension only accidentally causes a structural change. For instance, if the length of a rectangle becomes equal to the width, the pattern changes into a square, and if the lengths and widths of a square become different, the pattern changes into a rectangle. After all, structural information deals with categorically identical and categorically different pattern elements and not with their actual sizes. The topic of this section, however, is about these sizes.

Earlier (in Chapter 7.1) we said that pattern elements that are not noticeably different are considered as identical and are, therefore, represented by equal symbols in SIT codes. The range of stimuli that are confused is a topic that concerns metrical aspects of patterns and has been the topic of stimulus discrimination research by Erikson and Hake (1955). They observed that, if a line of 7 centimetres (cm) is shown during an inspection stage, any line presented in a test stage with a length in between 6.5 and 7.5 cm is judged to be similar to the line in the inspection stage. Expressed in selective information terms (Shannon and Weaver, 1949), this means that the information transfer of length is slightly less than 3 bit. Generally, the visual selective information transfer pro dimension (e.g., length, width, or angle) appears to be about 2.5 bit (Anderson and Fitts, 1958; Pollack and Klemmer, 1954; Quastler, 1955). For patterns varying in N respects or dimensions, a maximum transfer has been established that is somewhat less than N * 2.5 bit. In addition, Erikson and Hake (1955) have shown that the visual dimensions are not affected by learning. They tested an over-learned set of rectangular patterns whose length and width dimensions correlate and thus actually vary one-dimensionally. Therefore, they expected 2.5 bit information transfer but established 4.2 bit transfer. So, the two visual dimensions of a rectangle appear not to be affected by the knowledge of the actual stimulus set (Garner, 1962, 1974).

This section is about a measure of metrical information and, indeed, the selective information theory (Shannon and Weaver, 1949) provides such a measure. To evaluate its perceptual role we briefly sketch a few of its characteristics. The selective information of a message deals with the number of alternative options. A message that misses any alternative, for instance, 'grass is green' is not informative, whereas a message that excludes alternatives, for instance, 'the flower is blue', is informative. In effect, the selective information deals with the amount of uncertainty reduction in a guessing game. It equals the number of yes or no answers (being the number of 'bits') to find the solution. Indeed, the selective information measure can be used in perception research to establish, for instance, the mentioned visual resolution of pattern elements. However, the measure assumes knowledge about the alternative options of a message. Therefore, it is hardly compatible with perception (see Chapter 1.2). Moreover, the measure it is not about the content of a message. It merely deals with a formal aspect of the message's information. We illustrate this as follows: a closed testament that hides two equally probable options, namely, the heritage of a castle or nothing, supplies, at the moment of its opening, just one bit of selective information, whatever the outcome might be. However, for the heir this information is not that indifferent.

Load as amount of change

In our view, there is a metrical pattern representation that, analogous to a structural code, describes the content of a pattern, namely, as a construction recipe. Of course, its role comes across in case structural information is not distinctive (see Chapter 3.2). By way of introduction, we consider two Gestalt cues that merely deal with metrical information. One is the so-called proximity cue and the other is the good continuation cue. The grouping effect by proximity is triggered by short distances between pattern elements. Therefore, the assumption is that metrical load is a positive function of distance. In our view, this metrical load has a broader domain. The shortest connection between two points is a straight line. So, the distance between two points equals the length of this mediating line. Therefore, we assume that metrical load equally is a positive function of the length of a line. According to Dember (1965), the underlying reason is that more effort is involved in the construction or imagination of a long line than of a short line. The good continuation cue deals with turns and its grouping effect is hampered by angular changes, especially, of acute angles (Dember, 1965). For this reason we assume that metrical load is a positive function of angular change, that is, the outside angle between a preceding and a subsequent contour segment.

The next figures illustrate visual effects of metrical line and turn loads. Figure 11.1A, designed by Kanizsa (1979), illustrates a visual effect of line length (this effect is also known as Petter's law; Petter, 1956). For this figure, we consider two occlusion concepts. The interpretation of a thin rectangle in front of a fat rectangle, illustrated in Figure 11.1B, implies the virtual filling-in of two long contours (dotted lines) whereas the interpretation of a fat rectangle in front of a thin rectangle, illustrated in Figure 11.1C, implies the virtual filling in of two short contours (dotted lines). So, the visual preference for the latter foreground-background interpretation can be attributed to the low metrical load of the virtual contours.

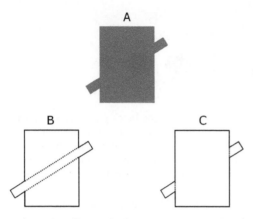

Figure 11.1 B and C illustrate two occlusion interpretations of A. The dotted lines accentuate the virtual foreground contours. These are larger in B than in C. So, the metrical load of B is larger than that of C. This explains the preference for C (Kanizsa, 1979).

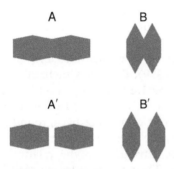

Figure 11.2 Both A and B can be interpreted as single surfaces or as the compositions of surfaces, shown in A′ and B′ respectively. The composition concept is attributed to B rather than to A because the transition from B to B′ implies a lower increase of metrical turn load than the transition from A to A′.

Figures 11.2A and B illustrate turn effects of pattern segmentations shown by Wouterlood and Boselie (1993). Probably, these figures are preferably conceived as single surfaces. Yet, there is some tendency to take the patterns as compositions of two separate symmetrical segments. These compositions are illustrated by Figures 11.2A′ and B′, respectively. The tendency is stronger for Figure 11.2B than for Figure 11.2A. The metrical load based on angular change explains these preferences as follows. Each concave turn c contributes $2*(c)$ angular change to

A   B

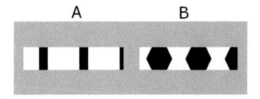

Figure 11.3 In A, the lengths of the black parts are shorter than those of the white parts. In B, the turns of the black parts are more obtuse than those of the white parts. So, in both patterns, the metrical load of the black parts is less than that of the white parts. This explains why the black parts are perceived as foreground patterns (Hanssen *et al.*, 1993).

the summated angular changes of 360° along the contour of a convex shape. Hence, the angular changes involved in both compositions are equal and more than in the single figures, but the amount of angular change involved in the single Figure 11.2B is more than in the single Figure 11.2A. Precisely therefore, the increase of angular change involved in the transition from Figure 11.2B to Figure 11.2B′ is less than the increase of angular change involved in the transition from Figure 11.2A to Figure 11.2A′. The line lengths involved in both transitions are equal.

The previous figures illustrate effects of virtual lines and turns. The next figure, designed by Kanizsa (1979), illustrates metrical effects of actually presented lines and turns involved in foreground-background interpretations. Figure 11.3A is preferably conceived of as a series of small vertical black rectangles in front of a white background instead of as a series of large horizontal white rectangles in front of a black background. This outcome can be attributed to the relatively small line lengths of the black rectangles. Their metrical length load is relatively low. Figure 11.3B is preferably conceived of as a series of convex black polygons in front of a white background instead of as a series of concave white polygons in front of a black background. This outcome can be attributed to the relatively small angular changes in the convex black polygons. Their metrical turn load is relatively low. Next, we consider the question how to express length and turn loads in common terms.

In explaining the previous illustrations, for simplicity, metrical load is taken as a linear function of line length and angular deviation. However, according to a concept underlying both line length and turn loads, this function is not linear. The argument is as follows. A structural description describes subsequent operations or moves that are involved in the construction of the stimulus (see Chapter 6). Similarly, metrical information content refers to virtual moves involved in the construction of the pattern. Its load reflects the amount of 'change' needed to evoke these motions. As is said, this idea stems from Dember (1965). The concept of change, that applies both to line lengths and turns, can be illustrated by a ball in a soccer game. To kick the ball over a long distance, more effort is needed than to kick it over a short distance. Furthermore, to let the ball make an acute turn a stronger kick is required than to let it make an obtuse turn. From a physical point of view, the amount of change is not expressed by force or energy but by impulse **p**. Hence, we assume that the $\sum \mathbf{p}$ needed to move a ball along the trajectory of a pattern is the **M**-load of the pattern. In our view, this assumption is justified by the perceptual observations by Runeson and Frikholm (1981). They showed that subjects are well able to estimate stimulus properties in line with the laws of physics. Notice that during the perception of static patterns, we neither assume a motion of actual scanning nor an analogous physical motion in the brain.

To obtain a well calculable and useful **M**-load measure we introduce some simplifications. First, we assume a space without resistance. However, if the speed of the motion would be constant, the **p** involved in a short distance would be equal to the **p** involved in a long distance. To avoid this insensitivity for line length, the rule can be considered to keep the scanning time constant per pattern. Indeed, in that condition, the impulse needed to produce a large pattern will be larger than the impulse needed to produce a small pattern. Yet, there is still the problem that the **M**-load measure does not differentiate between length proportions. To avoid this insensitivity, we make a second assumption, namely, of a constantly accelerated motion that, like a rocket, starts with zero speed. As a consequence, we merely have to account for the **p** at turns for changing directions and at the end of the pattern for stopping the motion. This **M**-load measure, which differentiates between line lengths, length proportions, and turns, is specified as follows.

We first consider the load of a single line with length **L** (Figure 11.4A). The termination of the motion of a continuously accelerating object along this line is supposed to be achieved by a frontal collision. According to the laws of dynamics, the impulse needed to stop this object equals $\mathbf{p} = \mathbf{mv}$, where **m** stands for the mass and **v** for the velocity of the object. Furthermore: $\mathbf{v} = \mathbf{at}$, and $\mathbf{L} = \mathbf{at}^2/2$ so that $\mathbf{t} = \sqrt{(2\mathbf{L}/\mathbf{a})}$, where **a** stands for acceleration and **t** for duration. Hence: $\mathbf{p} = \mathbf{m}\sqrt{(2\mathbf{aL})}$. Different values of **m** and **a** do not affect the predictions, so, without loss of generality, we can attribute to them the following convenient values: $\mathbf{m} = 1$ and $\mathbf{a} = \frac{1}{2}$. So, $\mathbf{p} = \sqrt{\mathbf{L}}$ for stopping the object. In other words, the metrical load of a single line is: $\mathbf{M} = \sqrt{\mathbf{L}}$.

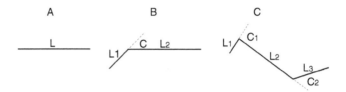

Figure 11.4 A, B, and C show serial line patterns. **L**, **L1**, **L2**, and **L3** stand for line lengths and **C**, **C1**, and **C2** for turns. The longest line in each pattern is supposed to have a normalized length of 1.

The load of an angular turn **c**, shown in Figure 11.4B, at the end of line **L1** and at the beginning of line **L2** is specified as follows. A maximal turn **c** = 180° deals with a maximal frontal collision. This collision involves the impulse to stop ($\mathbf{p} = \sqrt{\mathbf{L1}}$) and an equal impulse ($\mathbf{p} = \sqrt{\mathbf{L1}}$) to return the object. So, $\mathbf{p} = 2\sqrt{\mathbf{L1}}$. For a less acute turn **c** < 180° the impulse exerted on the moving object is part of the maximal impulse at **c** = 180°. This part agrees with the impulse component sin (**c**/2) exerted at the actual turn **c**. This sinus function of the turn ranges from 0 to 1. So, $\mathbf{p} = \sin(\mathbf{c}/2) * 2\sqrt{\mathbf{L1}}$ at the first turn of a pattern.

For Figure 11.4B, one still has to specify the impulse load for stopping the motion at the end of **L2**. Here, it is important to notice that the speed of the object is not hampered at turn **c**. In other words, the object cumulatively accelerates along the whole trajectory **L1** + **L2**. Thus, the impulse load for stopping the motion at the end of **L2** equals $\mathbf{p} = \sqrt{(\mathbf{L1} + \mathbf{L2})}$. So, the total metrical load **M** involved in the trajectory of Figure 11.4B is:

$$\mathbf{M} = \sin(\mathbf{c}/2)^{*}2\sqrt{(\mathbf{L1})} + \sqrt{(\mathbf{L1} + \mathbf{L2})}$$

To quantify this expression, we normalize the longest line to have length 1. So, **L2** = 1. As **L1** = 1/2 **L2** and **c** = 60°, the total metrical load is:

$$\mathbf{M} = \sin(60°/2)^{*}2\sqrt{(0.5)} + \sqrt{(0.5 + 1)}$$

For Figure 11.4C, being the kind of pattern used in the next experiment, the total metrical load is specified by extending the same procedures, as follows:

$$\mathbf{M} = \sin(\mathbf{C1}/2)^{*}2\sqrt{(\mathbf{L1})} + \sin(\mathbf{C2}/2)^{*}2\sqrt{(\mathbf{L1} + \mathbf{L2})}$$
$$+ \sqrt{(\mathbf{L1} + \mathbf{L2} + \mathbf{L3})}$$

Notice that the M load obtained by scanning an asymmetrical pattern in one order is not necessarily equal to the M load obtained by scanning

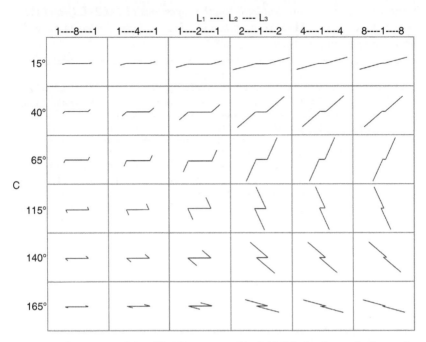

Figure 11.5 Stimuli in Hanssen *et al.*'s (1993) judged complexity study. The columns discern length proportions (**L1-L2-L3**) and the rows refer to turns (**C**) (Hanssen *et al.*, 1993).

the pattern in the reversed order. The model's final M load is taken to be the lowest of the two.

The **M**-load measure was tested by Leeuwenberg (1982a) who analysed the Müller-Lyer illusion effects observed by Restle and Decker (1977). A better test, however, was performed by Hanssen *et al.* (1993), using nearly the same stimuli in a judged complexity task. Therefore, next, we only discuss the latter study.

Judged complexity

In Hanssen *et al.* (1993), the test patterns were point-symmetrical line drawings each consisting of three line segments: a horizontal central line and two equal wings. The experimental set comprised thirty-six patterns with six different line-length proportions and six different angles. In Figure 11.5 such a set is presented. There were four versions of this set. One dealt with patterns with a constant sum of line lengths and

Table 11.1 *The columns deal with length proportions* (**L1-L2-L3**) *and the rows with turns* (**C**). **M** *refers to ranked metrical load and* **J** *refers to ranked judged complexity (Hanssen et al., 1993).*

	L1–L2–L3												
	1–8–1		1–4–1		1–2–1		2–1–2		4–1–4		8–1–8		total	total
	M	J	M	J	M	J	M	J	M	J	M	J	M	J
15°	1	1	2	2	3	4	7	7	5	3	4	6	22	23
40°	6	5	8	8	10	10	14	9	12	11	11	12	61	55
65°	9	13	13	15	15	19	22	21	$18\frac{1}{2}$	16	17	14	$94\frac{1}{2}$	98
C 115°	16	18	21	20	25	29	31	26	28	27	26	25	147	145
140°	$18\frac{1}{2}$	17	23	30	27	23	35	34	32	32	30	28	$165\frac{1}{2}$	164
165°	20	24	24	22	29	31	36	36	34	35	33	33	176	181
total	$70\frac{1}{2}$	78	91	97	109	116	145	143	$129\frac{1}{2}$	124	121	118	666	666

a second with their mirror-images. A third dealt with patterns whose longest distance between pattern points was kept constant and a fourth dealt with their mirror-images.

In the experiment, 176 participants were involved. To each subject, thirty-six stimuli of one set were presented. The task was to order the patterns from simple to complex. There was no time limit and corrections were allowed. No definition of complexity was given. Subjects were told to avoid associations with known objects and to avoid grouping on the basis of pattern similarity.

Table 11.1 presents the data for the thirty-six stimuli averaged over the four experimental sets. The columns refer to length proportions and the rows to turns. Within the cells, the ranks of the **M**-loads are presented at the left side and the averaged judged complexity ranks are presented at the right side. In the last row and in the last column, the summated ranks are indicated.

The results were as follows. The Kendall rank correlation between the **M**-load ranks and judged complexity ranks was r = .95. The Spearman rank correlation was r = .97. The Kendall measure of concordance (between the rankings of patterns with a constant sum of line lengths and the rankings of patterns whose longest distance between pattern points were kept constant) was W = .94. The ranking of the **M**-load totals and the ranking of the judged complexity totals of length proportions at the bottom row correlate perfectly. From left to right, both rank orders are: 1, 2, 3, 6, 5, 4. The sinus term in the model is supported by the Pearson correlation between the **M**-load totals and the judged complexity totals of the last columns at the right side: $r = .99$. According to the sign-test the interaction between length and turn effects is significant at the level $p < .001$ between columns, and at the level $p < .01$ between rows.

To strengthen our model choices, we consider some alternative **M**-load options that, beforehand, might seem plausible but that appear to be unsatisfactory:

(1) One option is to use **M**-loads of the literal lengths of the lines within the experimental patterns with a constant sum of line lengths. Then, however, the ranking of the load totals of length proportions is 1, 2, 3, 5, 5, 5, whereas the ranking of their summated judged complexity is 1, 2, 3, 6, 5, 4. Besides, the correlation between the ranked loads and the ranked judged complexity of individual patterns is $r = .67$, which is clearly lower than the correlation, $r = .95$, for the load with standard length $L = 1$.

(2) Another option is to use **M**-loads of the literal lengths of the lines within the patterns whose longest distance between pattern points is kept constant. Then, however, the ranking of the load totals of length proportions is 6, 1, 5, 3, 4, 2, which disagrees completely with the ranking of judged complexity. Besides, the ranked loads and the ranked judged complexity of individual patterns hardly correlate, $r = .45$.

(3) If the shortest line is taken as standard, the summated **M**-load ranks of length proportions is 5, 3, 1, 2, 4, 6 which, however, correlates negatively with the observed summated judged complexity ranks.

(4) If the first line is taken as standard, the ranking of the **M**-load totals of length proportions is 6, 5, 1, 4, 3, 1 which, however, does not correlate with the ranking of judged complexity.

(5) If $p = L$ instead of $p = \sqrt{(L)}$, the Kendall rank correlation would be: $r = .90$ instead of $r = .95$, and the Spearman rank correlation would be: $r = .90$, instead of $r = .97$. Besides, this simplification is not justifiable from the point of view of physics.

(6) If in the load, the cumulative lengths are replaced by single preceding lengths, the difference between the load for a 1-Q-1 proportion and the load for a Q-1-Q proportion ($Q = 8, 4, 2$) would be equal for all turns. Hence, all summated turn loads are equal to each other. The data do not support this outcome. Besides, also this proposal is not justifiable from the point of view of physics.

Finally, we make some comments on the relation between metrical load and other measures. The first is about metrical load versus structural load. In fact, so far, all stimuli used for testing metrical load were equal in a structural respect. The argument was that the metrical load plays a

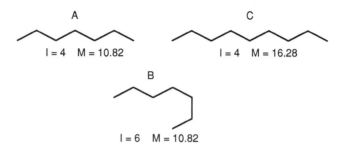

Figure 11.6 A is metrically as complex as B but structurally simpler. Visually, A is simpler than B. B is metrically simpler than C but structurally more complex. Visually, B is more complex than C. So, visual complexity seems to be determined mainly by structural load.

differentiating role between codes only in case their structural loads are the same. This implies that if, inversely, metrical load is kept constant, then structural load is supposed to be decisive. Figures 11.6A and B illustrate this case. Both figures have the same M-load but the first figure is structurally simpler than the second figure. Also, visually, the first figure is simpler than the second. Moreover, the structural load is decisive in case the structural and metrical loads are opposed. For instance, Figure 11.6B is structurally more complex but metrically simpler than Figure 11.6C. Indeed, Figure 11.6B is visually more complex than Figure 11.6C. This illustration supports the idea that the visual effect of metrical load is subordinate to that of structural load.

Also, the relation between metrical load and figural goodness is a topic. Commonly, metrical load correlates with weight of evidence or figural goodness (see Chapter 6.2). Figures 11.6A and C are illustrations. Of the first figure both the metrical load and the figural goodness are lower than those of the second figure, and this might seem somewhat contra-intuitive. However, notice that the roles of these two qualities are different. Figural goodness is a property of the selected code, and like structural load, metrical load determines code selection. So, figural goodness merely is a spin-off effect of this selection.

11.2   Image versus mirror-image

Children learn the name 'blue' for blue and 'red' for red. However, in an earlier stage, they are already sensitive to these colours. In other words, these colours belong to innate visual categories. Only their customary names have to be learned. The same holds for shapes like a straight line and a curve or for the directions upwards and downwards. The main

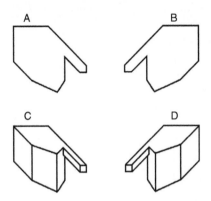

Figure 11.7 A is an image and B is its mirror image. In 2-D space these patterns are different. However, in 3-D space they are equal, namely, B is the back side of A. C is the projection of an object and D is the projection of its mirrored version. In 3-D space these objects are unequal (Leeuwenberg and van der Helm, 2000).

question of this study is whether the concepts left and right are also innate visual categories and whether there is an intrinsic visual sensitivity for these concepts. If this is not the case, then one has to conclude that not only their labels 'left' and 'right' but also the underlying concepts themselves have been learned.

Usually, the term handedness is used to refer to the hand preference of people, that is, some are right-handed and others are left-handed. Here, we use the term handedness as referring to the property that distinguishes an asymmetrical object from its mirror version. So, our initial question of whether there is an intrinsic visual sensitivity for the concepts left and right is reflected by the question whether there is an intrinsic visual sensitivity for the handedness of an object. To be clear, most people are well able to assess that a left-hand shoe and a right-hand shoe are different, but the focus here is on the handedness of each shoe separately. Later on, we compare a handedness-sensitive coding system and a handedness-insensitive coding system and we test their properties against experimental data on handedness discrimination to establish which system is tenable. Before that, we consider some properties of image and mirror-images and we discuss how this topic has been approached earlier in philosophy and perception research.

Figure 11.7B is the mirror image of Figure 11.7A. In 2-D space these images are differently handed, like the letters **d** and **b**. This means that these images cannot be mapped onto each other by a translation or rotation in the picture plane. This handedness difference appears only if

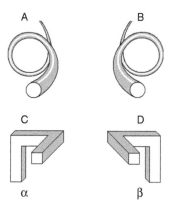

Figure 11.8 A is an uncommon left-turning corkscrew. B is a usual right-turning corkscrew. C and D are stylized versions of A and B, respectively. C is called an α screw and D is called a β screw (Leeuwenberg and van der Helm, 2000).

both images are asymmetrical. A 2-D image which is mirror-symmetric about some axis, for instance the letter E, is always identical to its mirror image. The same holds for 3-D objects. If mapping would be allowed through 3-D space, however, even asymmetrical 2-D images are identical to their mirror images, so, there would be no handedness difference. For instance, if both images are drawn on a transparent sheet, the Figure 11.7B is identical to Figure 11.7A seen from the rear. This also holds for Figures 11.7C and 11.7D taken as 2-D images. They also can be taken as 3-D objects but then these objects remain unequal. In 3-D space, an asymmetrical 3-D object and its mirrored version are differently handed. Corkscrews are the most elementary objects that are asymmetrical in 3-D. Figure 11.8A depicts an anti-clockwise or left-turning corkscrew. A differently handed version is shown in Figure 11.8B. It is the common clockwise or right-turning corkscrew, to be used for opening bottles. Stylized versions of these corkscrews are the α and β screws in Figures 11.8C and D, respectively. As we will show later on, these screws can be used as the building blocks of descriptions of complex 3-D objects.

To introduce our approach, we review debates on images and mirror-images among philosophers and perception researchers in the given order. Kant (1783) was one of the first philosophers with ideas on this topic. He drew attention to the following paradox. On the one hand, all distances within an image are equal to those within its mirror image. For instance, if 3, 4, and 5 cm are the lengths of the sides of a triangle, the sides of the mirrored triangle have the same lengths. This equality also applies to the angles of the two triangles (Deutsch, 1955). On the other hand, an image and its mirror image are different. Not their equality but their difference was essential to Kant (1783). Also for Newton (1687/1960), the difference was essential. According to him, the space within an object is not determined by its internal distance relations but by its coordinates in an absolute external space. For instance, the space within a left-hand glove does not match the space within a right-hand glove. Hence, according to these views, handedness differences follow from the unique descriptions of objects as opposed to their mirrored versions.

Leibniz (1714) had an opposite view. He considered the common structure of images and mirror images as essential. The difference is accidental and merely a matter of viewpoint. After all, the mirror-image of a 2-D image is equal to this image seen from the back. This backside is accessible by rotation in 3-D space. Analogously, the mirror image of a 3-D object, for instance of a left-hand glove, equals its back side being accessible by rotation in 4-D space. In fact, this 4-D back side of a left-hand glove is its inside out and equals the right-hand glove. The conclusion by Freudenthal (1962) was in line with Leibniz's view but deals with a complementary aspect. He formally proved that the leftness or rightness of a turn is not definable. This implies that the difference between an asymmetrical object and its mirrored version is not definable. Nowadays, the views of Freudenthal and Leibniz are generally accepted and the views of Kant and Newton are not (Gardner, 1964; Weyl, 1952).

In fact, the controversy among perception researchers is similar. Analogous to the view of Kant (1783) and Newton (1687/1960) that the handedness of an object is somehow specifiable, is the assumption by Corballis (1988) that the brain deals with an innate asymmetric reference frame. The interaction between this frame and a pattern is assumed to establish the unique form of the pattern (i.e., as opposed to its mirrored version), irrespective of its orientation. He took the mental rotation heuristic for discriminating images and mirror images (which he observed in his experiments) as merely a double check of the handedness difference which, in his view, is already revealed by the difference between the visual codes. His view is more or less shared by Cohen and Kubovy (1993) and Pylyshyn (1973). Analogous to the conclusion by Freudenthal (1962) and Leibniz (1714) that the handedness of an object cannot be defined, is the conviction by perception researchers such as Cooper (1976), Finke (1980), Hinton and Parsons (1981), and Shepard and Metzler (1971), that visual codes do not explicitly represent an object and its mirrored version differently. As a consequence, handedness discrimination requires mental rotation of images (see Chapter 1.1).

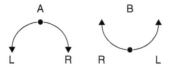

Figure 11.9 Both a hill shape and a valley shape are scanned from their centres in two directions. So, a hill-shape is described by **LR** and a valley shape by **RL**.

To obtain a clear position on handedness discrimination, Leeuwenberg and van der Helm (2000) considered two coding systems and their properties. One is called the H-system, referring to handedness. It explicitly represents left and right turns by different code labels, which implies that its codes already allow for handedness discrimination (so that, to this end, mental rotation is not required). The other system is called the M-system, referring to mirror symmetry. It explicitly represents bilateral symmetries, which implies that its codes do not allow for handedness discrimination (so that, to this end, mental rotation is required). In all other respects, the two systems were kept equal. Next, each system is introduced and evaluated against experimental results taken from the literature on handedness discrimination.

The handedness-sensitive system

The handedness-sensitive system, or the H-system, explicitly represents a left turn in a line pattern by another label than a right turn. That is, a left turn is represented by **L** and a right turn by **R**. To prevent coding ambiguity, we avoid global clockwise or anti-clockwise scanning of the pattern. Instead, we propose a local scanning of each hill shape and of each valley shape in the contour. This scanning starts, in both directions, from the centre of the hill shape or of the valley shape. Thus, the hill shape in Figure 11.9A is represented by **LR** and the valley shape in Figure 11.9B is represented by **RL**. As a consequence, the description of any 2-D pattern has an even number of symbols. Within this coding approach, we represent a line pattern merely as a series of hill and valley shapes. We disregard their angular degrees and line lengths. Furthermore, a code represents the positions of pattern elements merely stimulus analogously, that is, elements at the left-hand side of the pattern are represented at the left-hand side of the code and elements at the right-hand side of the pattern are represented at the right-hand side of the code. In other words, the stimulus-analogous order of code elements as such does not yet give rise to any conclusion.

H-cues for handedness As has been argued by Levelt (1996), any attribution of a left or right direction is bound to an agreement or rule, and here we show that there is a rule by which a unique handedness can be attributed to any asymmetrical pattern or object on the basis of its code in the H-system. As an introduction to this rule we consider a few peculiarities of the H-system.

One is that a completely symmetrical pattern is represented by a completely asymmetrical code (i.e., a code without any local symmetry of two equal symbols around the centre of the code). A simple illustration of this symmetry-inversion is presented in Figure 11.9A. This hill shape is completely symmetrical whereas its **LR** code is completely asymmetrical. A more complex illustration is a series of a hill, a valley, and hill shape. This pattern is completely symmetrical whereas its code **LRRLLR** is completely asymmetrical. Inversely, a completely asymmetrical code always describes a completely symmetrical pattern.

A completely symmetrical pattern is equal to its mirror version and is therefore not handed. Any deviation from complete symmetry renders the pattern asymmetrical and therefore handed. So, by the symmetry-inversion property of H-codes, an asymmetrical pattern is represented by a code having, at least, one local symmetry. Such a local symmetry is given by two equal symbols around the centre of the code. Inversely, such a code always describes an asymmetrical pattern. Now, by convention, we take the L or R symbol involved in the most central local code symmetry to specify the handedness of the pattern. Here, this rule is illustrated in Figure 11.10.

Figure 11.10A is taken as a standard pattern and Figures 11.10B, C, and D are obtained by 180° rotations of this pattern around the **z**, **x**, and **y** axes, respectively (see Figure 10.4). So, in the picture plane, Figure 11.10B is equal to Figure 11.10A and Figures 11.10C and D are their mirror-images. The codes straightaway supply the handedness cues of the patterns. The most central local code symmetries in the codes of Figures 11.10A and B reveal the same handedness cues **R**, that is, they reveal that these figures are equally handed. Similarly, the most central local code symmetries in the codes of Figures 11.10C and D reveal the handedness cues **L**. They imply that these figures are equally handed but differently handed than the previous two figures. This implies that by using codes of the H-system, handedness discrimination does not require mental image rotation.

H-system

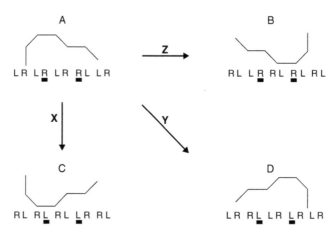

Figure 11.10 A, B, C, and D are 2-D patterns in the picture plane. The 180° rotations about the **z**, **x** and **y** axes turn A into B, C, and D, respectively. A and B are equal. Also, C and D are equal but 2-D mirror images of A and B. The H-system code supplies a handedness cue, namely, the most central pair of symmetrical symbols. These symbols are underlined. For A and B these are **R** symbols. For C and D these are **L** symbols (Leeuwenberg and van der Helm, 2000).

There are similar code cues for the handedness of 3-D objects but first we attend to the way screws are represented. As said, the basic handedness elements of objects are the stylized α and β screws introduced by Figures 11.8C and D. Their coding is, analogous to the coding of 2-D turns, centrifugal. Each screw has a central component, called the screw-axis, and two outer components (Takano, 1989). The screw-axis can be indicated by **x**, **y**, or **z**, depending on whether its orientation agrees with the x, y, or z-axis, respectively (see Figure 10.4). A screw whose central component agrees with, for instance, the x-axis is briefly called an x-screw. One outer component describes a 3-D aspect of the screw. If this outer component is oriented forward it is indicated by **f**, and if it is oriented backward it is indicated by **b**. The other outer component refers to a 2-D aspect. If this outer component with respect to the central screw axis is anti-clockwise it is indicated by **L** and if it is clockwise it is indicated by **R**.

Obviously, this coding is view dependent. In fact, there are twelve different points of view of an α screw and twelve different points of view of a β screw. All these screw versions are shown in Figure 11.11 with

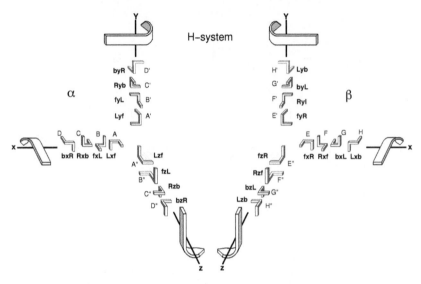

Figure 11.11 A to D″ present subsequent 90° backward **x**, **y**, and **z** rotated versions of the α screw. Equally, E to H″ present the subsequent 90° backward **x**, **y**, and **z** rotated versions of the β screw. The backward rotations are indicated by bended arrows. Each screw is represented by three code components. The central screw legs are indicated by **x**, **y**, and **z** axes. The **f** refers to a forward and the **b** to a backward screw leg. **L** stands for an anti-clockwise turn and **R** for a clockwise turn with respect to the screw's centre (Leeuwenberg and van der Helm, 2000).

their codes. To clarify the organization of this figure we first consider the α screws. Figures 11.11A to D depict four x-screws aligned along the x-axis. These screws are subsequent 90° backward rotated screw versions starting from Figure 11.11A. At the end of these screws the backward rotation around the x-axis is indicated by a bended arrow. The figure presents two more bended arrows, one for the y-screws in Figures 11.11A′ to D′ aligned along the y-axis and one for the z-screws in Figures 11.11A″ to D″ aligned along the z-axis. Notice that the spatial relation between each bended arrow and its four screws is precisely the same as that between the first bended arrow and the x-screws. This way, also the 90° backward y- and z-rotations are fixated (Pani *et al.*, 1996). Notice further that the organization of β screws, presented in Figures 11.11E to H″, is just the mirror image of the aforementioned whole organization of α screws.

Now, we attend to the codes. Inspection of Figure 11.11 reveals that all α screw codes comprise specific combinations of outer components.

H–system

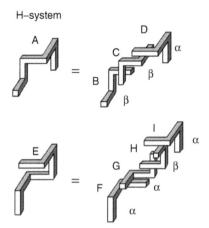

Figure 11.12 A is composed of the three partly overlapping screws β, β, and α, which are presented separately by B, C, and D, respectively. The right-turning nature of the central β screw is taken to characterize the handedness of the total object. E is composed of the four partly overlapping screws α, α, β, and α, which are presented separately by F, G, H, and I, respectively. The α screw is involved in the most central local symmetry of two identical screws around the centre of the chain. The left-turning nature of this screw is taken to characterize the handedness of the total object.

These combinations either are **f L** or **b R**. Of all β screw versions the outer components merely consist of **f R** or **b L** combinations. So, these combinations are valid handedness cues for single α and β screws. Notice that, whereas the screw codes are initially viewpoint dependent, they are meanwhile view-independent representations of screws.

The handedness cues mentioned above identify a screw as an anti-clockwise or left-turning α screw or as a clockwise or right-turning β screw. By this local identification, also the handedness of a chain of screws can be fixated. We illustrate this first for a chain of an uneven number of screws. The object in Figure 11.12A can be described by a chain of three overlapping screws, which are presented separately in Figures 11.12B, C, and D. They are identified as β, β, and α screws, respectively. Each pair of successive screws shares two legs. Now, notice that any chain of an uneven number of screws is anyhow asymmetrical. Therefore, we can take the central screw to characterize the handedness of the chain, and therewith, of the total object. So, the R stemming from the central β screw characterizes the handedness of the object in Figure 11.12A.

The handedness of a chain of an even number of screws can be assessed analogously to the way the handedness is assessed for a 2-D pattern (see Figure 11.10). We recall the procedure once more. According to the symmetry-inversion property of H-codes, an asymmetrical object is presented by a chain of screws having, at least, one local symmetry. Such a local symmetry is given by two equal screws around the centre of the chain. Inversely, such a chain always presents an asymmetrical object. By convention, we take the L or R of the screw involved in the most central local code symmetry to specify the handedness of the total object. This convention is illustrated for the object in Figure 11.12E which consists of the four screws α, α, β, and α, presented separately in Figures 11.12F, G, H, and I, respectively. The α screw is involved in the most central local symmetry, so that the L stemming from this α screw is taken to characterize the handedness of the total object.

H-cues for rotation As said, H-codes do not need mental rotation to assess whether two objects are equally or differently handed, but if it would still make use of mental rotation, for instance, as a double check, it would need a rotation cue. Such a cue is supposed to be supplied by the object codes and is supposed to indicate, beforehand, which is the minimal rotation that might lead to a match. Without such a cue, many rotations should be tested. The question is whether H-codes supply such cues, and if so, which ones. For the answer we check the cued rotations of four cases to which H-codes give rise. We leave out the 180° rotations unless they cannot be replaced by 90° rotations. The cued rotations will be illustrated by Figure 11.11.

Case 1 deals with two screws sharing all components. Then, their codes cue a 90° rotation around the common screw axis, for instance the backward x-rotation of Figure 11.11A to B. However, as these codes merely reveal different permutations of the same outer components they are indistinguishable. As a consequence, they do not differentiate between a backward and a forward rotation, for instance, between the backward x-rotation of Figure 11.11A to B and the forward x-rotation of Figure 11.11B to A. In fact, there is not even any distinction between different and same codes. So, also two 0° rotations belong to the options. All in all, two codes give rise to four options.

Case 2 deals with two screws that merely share the outer components. Then, their codes cue two 90° rotations around the third axis. For instance, they cue the forward z-rotation of Figure 11.11A towards B' and the backward z-rotation of Figure 11.11B towards B'. Neither Figure 11.11A nor Figure 11.11B can be transformed to A' by a single 90° or 180° rotation, although both screw pairs cannot be distinguished from the preceding pairs. So, two codes give rise to four options.

Case 3 deals with two screws that merely share the screw axis. Then, their codes cue two 90° rotations around the common screw axis. One is forward and one is backward. For instance, they cue the backward x-rotation of Figure 11.11B to C and the forward x-rotation of Figure 11.11A to D. After all, these pairs of screws are indistinguishable. So, two codes simultaneously give rise to two options.

Case 4 deals with two screws that do not share any component. Then, their codes cue two 90° rotations around the third axis, for instance, the forward y-rotation of Figure 11.11A towards C″ and the backward y-rotation of Figure 11.11A towards D″. Figure 11.11B neither can be transformed to C″ nor to D″ by single 90° or 180° rotations, but both pairs of screws cannot be distinguished from the preceding two pairs. So, two codes simultaneously give rise to four options.

All in all, there are many 180° rotations cued by the codes but all of them are already cued by 90° rotations. Indeed, the H-codes constrain the rotations to be tested during mental rotation but they do not sufficiently constrain them towards unique rotation cues. The general argument is that there are twelve versions of a certain screw but there are only six distinguishable codes. All in all, the difference between α and β screws is determined by different combinations of code components which supply handedness cues, whereas the variety of versions within the α or the β screw category is determined by different permutations of code components which do not supply rotation cues.

The symmetry-sensitive system

The symmetry or mirror sensitive system, briefly M-system, does not use particular labels for left and right turns and is, therefore, insensitive to handedness. Instead, its codes are sensitive to the bilateral symmetries shown in Figure 11.13. It represents a hill shape by **M** and a valley shape by **W**. Like the coding of the H-system, this coding approach represents a line pattern in a simplified fashion. Only its turns are represented, namely, by the above single labels. Their exact magnitudes are disregarded. Besides, like the H-codes, the M-codes describe left and right positions of pattern elements not explicitly but merely stimulus analogously.

M-cues for handedness A crucial feature of M-codes is that they lack the symmetry-inversion which H-codes exhibit. That is, in the M-system, symmetrical patterns have symmetrical codes and asymmetrical patterns have asymmetrical codes. For instance, if an image is described by **MW**, its mirror-image is described by **WM**. As a consequence, M-codes do not supply 2-D handedness cues. Notice again that the

M-system

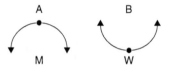

Figure 11.13 The symmetry sensitive system represents a hill shape A by **M** and a valley shape B by **W**.

stimulus-analogous order of code elements as such does not yet give rise to any conclusion. This implies that an image and a mirror-image can only be discriminated by a mental rotation applied to one image and by matching the result with the other image.

The M-system represents screws in about the same way as the H-system. Each screw has one central component and two outer components. The central component, also called the screw axis, either agrees with the **x, y,** or **z** axis and is indicated that way. One outer component describes a 3-D aspect of the screw. If this outer component is oriented forward it is indicated by **f,** and if it is oriented backward it is indicated by **b**. The other outer component refers to a 2-D aspect of a screw and is specific for the M-system. If this component makes a hill turn it is represented by **M** and if this component makes a valley turn it is represented by **W**.

To illustrate the screw codes, we make use of Figure 11.14 which presents all possible screw versions in exactly the same way as Figure 11.11. Only the codes are different. In contrast to the H-codes, the M-codes of the α screw do not exclude particular combinations of outer component symbols. In other words, any specific α screw is fixated by a unique combination of components. The same holds for the β screw. However, the difference between the α and β codes is merely determined by permutations of code symbols and as permutations are not identifiable they do not supply 3-D handedness cues. Therefore, mental rotation is needed for the mirror-image discrimination of objects.

M-cues for rotation M-codes describe an α or a β screw by unique combinations of code components and we claim that these codes supply, therefore, unique minimal rotation cues. As all these cues equally apply to α and β screws we will illustrate our claim only for the pairs of α screws in Figure 11.14.

In contrast to H-codes, M-codes supply unique cues for the 180° rotations that cannot be taken as 90° rotations. These cues are provided

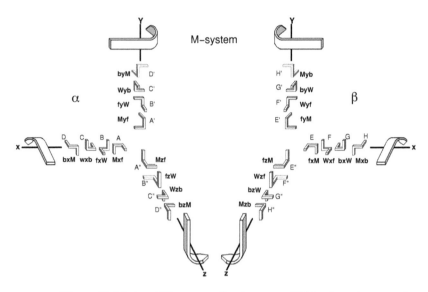

Figure 11.14 A to D″ present all subsequent 90° backward **x**, **y**, and **z** rotations of the α screw. Equally, E to H″ present all subsequent 90° backward **x**, **y**, and **z** rotations of the β screw. These backward rotations are indicated by bended arrows. Each screw is represented by three code components. The central screw leg either agrees with the **x**, **y**, or **z** axis and is indicated that way. The **f** refers to a forward and the **b** to a backward screw leg. The third component either is an **M** turn or a **W** turn (Leeuwenberg and van der Helm, 2000).

by two codes that only share their central components. An instance is the x-rotation from Figure 11.14A to C.

M-codes also supply unique cues for 90° rotations. We first consider screws with common central axes. Then, the series of 90° backward rotated screws is fixated by the sequence of code symbols both of the left and the right outer components of codes. This sequence is: **f** → **W** → **b** → **M** → and is equally present in α and in β codes. In effect, this sequence is twelve times present in the codes in Figure 11.14 of subsequently backward rotated screws. Of course, the reverse sequence deals with forward rotated screws. Notice that in H-codes the symbol sequence of the left outer components differs from the sequence of the right outer components. So, as the positions of these sequences are not identifiable the H-codes do not supply cues for backward versus forward 90° rotations of screws.

For screws with different central axes the story is somewhat more complex. In fact, of pairs of such screws 50 per cent can directly be matched by a single 90° rotation but 50 per cent cannot; that is, they can only be matched by two well chosen 90° rotations. The following schema shows pairs of screw axes and outer components that should be in their codes to ensure that the screw pairs can be matched by a single 90° rotation. Furthermore, it indicates the axis around which one screw should be rotated to match with the other. This rotation axis is not one of the two given screw axes but the third axis.

Screw axes	X–Y	Y–Z	Z–X
Outer components	f–W	f–W	f–W
Outer components	b–M	b–M	b–M
Axis of 90° rotation	Z	X	Y

To illustrate an application of this schema we consider some pairs of screws. The code in Figure 11.14A contains an x-axis and an f component. The code in Figure 11.14B′ contains a y-axis and a W component. Hence, a 90° z-rotation of the first screw matches with the second screw. Another example is as follows. The code in Figure 11.14D″ contains a z-axis and a b component. The code in Figure 11.14A contains an x-axis and an M component. Hence, a 90° y-rotation of the first screw matches with the second screw.

An M-code supplies the following unique cue for rotation direction, that is, for forward versus backward rotation. If the screw axes of the first and the second screw agree with the reading order of screw axes in the above schema, that is, in line with $x \to y \to z \to$, and if the codes of two screws share one component, then the rotation is forward. From this rule the rotation directions in all other conditions can be derived. For instance, if the screw axes of the first and the second screw are reverse the rotation direction is reverse. Also, if the codes of two screws do not share any component or share two components the rotation direction is reversed. For example, the rotation of Figure 11.14D″ towards Figure 11.14A is forward. Instead, the rotation of Figure 11.14A towards Figure 11.1D″ and the rotation of Figure 11.14C″ towards Figure 11.14A are backward.

For an object consisting of three screws, e.g., the ββα series in Figure 11.12A, it is sufficient to attend to the central β screw, e.g., Figure 11.12C, and to test its rotation cues. Generally, the complexity of the cues correlates with the complexity of the objects. The given rotation cues, anyhow, are rather complex. Therefore, we assume that the use of rotation cues requires learning.

All in all, the difference between α and β screws is determined by different permutations of code components which do not supply handedness cues, whereas the variety of versions within the α or the β screw category is determined by different combinations of code components which supply rotation cues. Obviously, what is a combination in the H-system is a permutation in the M-system, and vice versa. Hence a cue in one system is not a cue in the other system, and vice versa. The specific consequences for the M-system are that codes are completely view dependent and that handedness discrimination requires mental rotation.

Finally, we make some concluding remarks. Both the absent and present cues of the M-system are consistent with the outcomes of the handedness discrimination experiments by Shepard and Metzler (1971). The absent handedness cues explain the need for mental rotation of images to judge whether two objects match or mismatch. This mental rotation is plausible because the reaction time is linearly related to the shortest angle between the two stimulus objects. This linear relationship also suggests that the mental rotation does not involve an exhaustive test of all possible rotations. Hence, also the present rotation cues of the M-system are plausible. For these reasons, we reject the H-system and adhere the M-system.

Another question is whether mental rotation is applied to 2-D stimulus-analogous representations of images or to 2-D or 3-D interpretations of images. According to Cooper (1976) and Finke (1980), it is applied to 2-D stimulus-analogous representations. This might hold for images with 2-D interpretations, but not for images with 3-D interpretations. For instance, the 90° backward y-rotation of the literal 2-D picture in Figure 11.14A does not match with the literal 2-D picture in Figure 11.14D″ although both screws are equal. As we already argued in Chapter 1.1, even z-rotations in the picture plane of 2-D stimulus-analogous representations of equal screws do not necessarily lead to a match (Shepard and Metzler, 1971). Another objection is that stimulus analogous representations are insensitive to object complexity whereas mental rotation is sensitive to it (Moran, 1968; Pylyshyn, 1973). Furthermore, Koning and van Lier (2003, 2004) have shown that connected objects are more easily mentally rotated than disconnected objects irrespective of whether their 2-D retinal projections are connected or disconnected. This means that mental rotation is an operation which is applied not to a 2-D stimulus-analogous representation but to a 3-D object-analogous representation, that is, to a 3-D interpretation of the 2-D image.

Of course, this representation presupposes a 3-D object interpretation. Hence, it stems from a classifying code such as an M-code. If so, it is a reconstruction of an M-code. As the complexity of such a code reflects the complexity of an object, an object-analogous representation is affected by object complexity (Pylyshyn, 1973). So, we assume two kinds of codes for handedness discrimination, namely, an M-code and an object-analogous representation stemming from this code.

An M-code is generated in line with the usual perception steps indicated by Marr and Nishihara (1978), namely, from a 2-D viewpoint-dependent retinal image, via a 2.5-D viewer-centred object representation, towards a 3-D object-centred code. In the subsequent imagery stage the process hierarchy is about the reverse, as argued by Pinker and Finke (1980), namely, from concept to pattern. It agrees with what we call code evaluation or pattern reconstruction (see Chapter 1.1). The M-code supplies the rotation cue to guide mental rotation and the object-analogous image representation is mentally rotated to establish the object's handedness.

There is another argument in favour of the M-system. As shown by Freudenthal (1962), the handedness components left and right are not definable and, according to Leibniz (1714), handedness is merely a matter of viewpoint. As is said in the introduction, the views of both authors are generally accepted. The M-system is in line with both views. After all, the M-codes miss labels for left and right. Moreover, they fixate the handedness of shapes merely in a stimulus analogous fashion. In other words, the codes do not explicitly reveal the handedness of shapes.

We end with the conclusion that the H-stem is untenable. It means that the handedness components left and right are not categories of genuine perception. This claim seems to conflict with the everyday life use and experience of left and right, for instance, in traffic. In our view, the solution is the distinction, already made in Chapter 1.1, between perception in the narrow sense and perception in the broad sense. In the same section, we referred to experiments that support this distinction. The first kind of perception is supposed to precede the process that makes use of knowledge. The second kind of perception includes both this autonomous perception and the subsequent recognition process. Our claim merely deals with the first kind of perception. Any learning does not help to incorporate the concepts left and right in this autonomous perception. It only affects judgments at a post-perceptual level.

Summary

Section 11.1 deals with the metrical information of line lengths and angular changes. An attempt is made to develop a load measure that deals with a common feature of line length and turns. This common feature is the amount of 'change' that, in physical terms, is specified by impulse. The proposal is to model metrical load by all impulses exerted on an accelerating object whose motion pattern agrees with the stimulus pattern. An experiment supports this measure. It tests the judged complexity of patterns. Furthermore, the conclusion is that metrical information is subordinate to structural information.

Section 11.2 deals with visual shape codes involved in handedness discrimination. Experiments on this discrimination make it plausible that the task is performed by mental rotation. It is argued that only mirror sensitive and handedness insensitive object codes explain the need for mental rotation. These codes, moreover, supply cues for the rotation to be tested. Indeed, also stimulus-analogous image codes are handedness insensitive and explain the need for mental rotation. However, they do not supply rotation cues. The conclusion is that the codes involved in handedness discrimination are object-centred enriched with viewpoint-dependent information, but do not represent handedness. So, handedness does not belong to a basic perceptual category. It is just a product of learning. In contrast, symmetry belongs to a basic perceptual category.

12 SIT beyond perception

Introduction

Because structural information theory (SIT) is a theory on structure, it can be applied to both perceptual and non-perceptual structures. To illustrate this, this chapter deals with topics which, for different reasons, are usually taken to lie just outside the domain of perception but which yet concern structures.

Section 12.1 attends to structures in series of letters. Because these letters are constrained by alphabetic order, the serial structures presuppose knowledge. Therefore, they do not belong to the prototypic domain of perception. The question is whether their preferred extrapolations are determined by representation or by process attributes (a representation is a process product). The codes to be tested are SIT representations, though with minor adaptations due to their reference to knowledge of the alphabet.

Section 12.2 concerns the role of SIT's I-load in inter-pattern measures of evaluative figural qualities, such as distinctiveness, interestingness, and beauty. These qualities are mediated by perception but are not obvious outcomes of perception. They might belong to a broader domain of cognition that includes task demands.

12.1 Alphabetic letter series

For an experiment to test intelligence, Thurstone and Thurstone (1941) designed fifteen-letter series in which each letter referred not just to itself but also to its position in the Roman alphabet (Baldwin, 1946; Thurstone and Thurstone, 1941). The task was to extrapolate each series by one letter. According to Thurstone and Thurstone, for each series, there was only one correct extrapolation and others were incorrect. The correct extrapolation is supposed to reflect sound logical reasoning. We disagree with this point of view. We claim that extrapolations are not to be evaluated on correctness but on simplicity (Frearson et al., 1990;

Hersh, 1974; Myors *et al.*, 1989; Quereshi and Seitz, 1993a, 1993b; Reber *et al.*, 1991; Stankov and Cregan, 1993). They are the output of inductive or rule finding reasoning (like perception), instead of the output of deductive or rule applying reasoning.

In contrast, the study by Scharroo and Leeuwenberg (2000), discussed in this section, did not aim at testing the subject's intelligence but at testing the hypothesis that the preferred extrapolation is the one that yields the simplest extrapolated series (Colberg *et al.*, 1985; Hofstadter, 1985; Simon, 1972, 1990). Scharroo and Leeuwenberg (2000) too used the task to extrapolate letter series. To ensure a large variety of extrapolations, their series were shorter than those used by Thurstone and Thurstone. Furthermore, the number of extrapolated letters steadily was five instead of one to minimize the ambiguity of extrapolations. The response frequencies, which refer to the numbers of subjects that produce specific extrapolations, were compared to the loads of simplest SIT codes. It was tested whether high frequencies were paired with lower loads. Those SIT codes are slightly different from standard visual SIT codes because they have to include knowledge of the Roman alphabet. This is discussed next.

Coding and complexity

We start dealing with SIT codes and their loads. To establish the structure and the complexity of an extrapolated series, that is, the stimulus plus extrapolation, it seems obvious to consider the actually extrapolated series and to assess its simplest code. However, this code depends on the accidental number of letters that happens to be added according to the task, so that it may not represent a stable underlying concept by which the series could be extrapolated indefinitely. Therefore, the code should deal with the simplest extrapolated series without restriction on the number of letters that may be added. This may be illustrated as follows:

Stimulus + extrapolation (five letters)	Code	
AKUMAK UMAKU	$2*(AKUM) AKU$	
	$I = 8$	
Stimulus + extrapolation (six letters)	Code	Concept
AKUMAK UMAKUM	$3*(AKUM)$	$N*(AKUM)$
	$I = 5$	$I = 5$

At the top, a letter stimulus is presented with an extrapolation by five letters. This number agrees with the number of letters that are to be added in the experiment by Scharroo and Leeuwenberg (2000). The simplest code of this extrapolated series has the load $I = 8$. At the bottom, the same stimulus is presented but with an extrapolation by six letters. Among all possible extrapolations, this one yields the simplest extrapolated series, having load $I = 5$. Therefore, its code is supposed to represent a concrete version of the concept underlying the stimulus extrapolated by five letters. The final concept is represented by a more abstract version which represents the actual threefold repeat by the indefinite N-fold repeat.

In the above illustration, the letters themselves constitute the primitive code and they are the elements at nominal level. However, equally plausible primitives are the numbers that refer to distances in the alphabet taken cyclically. After all, the alphabet is characterized by both the set of letters and the order of the letters (see also melody coding in Chapter 8.2). Such numbers, being the elements at interval level, represent a series independently of their positions in the alphabet and reveal, therefore, a structure underlying actually given letters. Numbers are positive in case of forward and negative in case of backward directions in the alphabet. In fact, each letter is represented by an interval, namely, between this letter and the preceding letter. The letter preceding the first letter is supposed to be the virtual starting letter that fits with the simplest description of the whole series. Next, the steps are illustrated from a series towards its concept code of basic intervals:

Series	Intervals	Code	Concept
KLMN	1,1,1,1	4*(1)	N*(1)
I-load: 4	4	1	1

The four letters of the series KLMN give rise to three intervals 1, 1, 1. These intervals, however, represent only the last three letters LMN. To represent also the first letter K, an extra interval is inserted at the left. For this extra interval the number 1 is chosen such that it leads to the simplest code of all intervals. This final code represents the concept. It takes the four intervals of the actual letters as a sample of an ever (N) repeated constant interval across the whole cyclic alphabet. In other words, the code neglects the actual starting letter and represents a class of patterns.

Series of letters can also be described at a higher interval level, namely by intervals between intervals. The steps towards the concept code at this level are illustrated as follows:

Series	Intervals	Higher intervals	Code	Concept
ACFJ	1, 2, 3, 4	1, 1, 1, 1	4*(1)	N*(1)
I-load: 4	4	8	2	2

The procedure is analogous to the previous one. The series ACFJ gives rise to three intervals, namely, 2, 3, 4. These intervals only represent the last three letters CFJ. Therefore, an extra interval is inserted at the left to represent also the first letter A. For this extra interval, the number 1 is a proper choice from the perspective of a simple final code. The four intervals 1, 2, 3, 4, in turn, give rise to three higher level intervals, namely, $\underline{1}$, $\underline{1}$, $\underline{1}$, indicated by underlined numbers. These higher level intervals merely represent the last three basic level intervals 2, 3, 4. To represent also the first basic interval an extra high level interval $\underline{1}$ is inserted at the left to obtain the simplest final code. This code represents the concept. It takes the four higher level intervals as a sample of an ever (N) repeated constant higher level interval across the whole cyclic alphabet. In other words, the code neglects the actual starting letter and represents a class of patterns. One unit of information is attributed to the higher interval level as it differs from the basic interval level. So, the load of the $N^*(\underline{1})$ concept is $I = 2$. One unit stems from the actual interval number 1 and one for its higher level, say, for its underlining.

A code may combine subcodes at various levels, namely, at nominal, interval, or higher interval level. To indicate their internal independence, each subcode, except the first, is enclosed within brackets, and to the introduction of each extra subcode, one unit of information is attributed. So, for each pair of brackets holds $I = 1$ extra load. The combining of coding levels is illustrated next:

Series	Subseries	Concepts	I-load
RARBRCRD	(R,R,R,R) (A,B,C,D)	$<N^*((R))>/<\{(1)\}>$	3
RARCRFRJ	(R,R,R,R) (A,C,F,J)	$<N^*((R))>/<\{(\underline{1})\}>$	4
KALCMFNJ	(K,L,M,N) (A,C,F,J)	$<N^*((1))>/<\{(\underline{1})\}>$	4
KRLSTMUNVW	(K,L,M,N) (R,ST,U,VW)	$<N^*((1))>/<\{(1)\ (2^*(1))\}>$	5

The first series alternately combines a nominal and an interval subseries. The second series alternately combines a nominal and a high-level interval subseries. The third series alternately combines an interval subseries and a high-level interval subseries. The fourth series is added to show how an interval subseries of single elements is alternately combined with an interval subseries of single and paired elements. Each subseries is represented by a subcode in the concept representation.

Serial extrapolation

Our goal is to verify whether the preference of serial letter extrapolations is predictable from I-loads. Because these loads characterize pattern representations and not the extrapolation processes towards these representations, we will relate the loads not to responses that reflect aspects of extrapolation processes, such as complexity judgments or reaction times, but to the numbers of subjects that select certain preferred extrapolations. We expect that higher numbers of subjects correspond to lower concept loads.

In their experiment, Scharroo and Leeuwenberg (2000) tested twenty-five letter series (see Table 12.1). These series belonged to two sets. One set comprised new versions of the fifteen-letter series designed by Thurstone and Thurstone (1941). These new versions were about two times shorter and therefore more ambiguous than the original ones. As a consequence, the series gave rise to more different extrapolations. The second set was designed by Scharroo and Leeuwenberg (2000) and contained series that reveal regularities, like symmetries, that were absent in the first set. Forty-eight students participated in the experiment and the series were presented to them in random order. The subjects were asked to extrapolate the letter series by five letters. There was no time pressure and subjects had the opportunity to change their response.

For each series, the Spearman rank correlation was established between the I-loads and the number of subjects who produced the various extrapolations. Twenty of the twenty-five correlations were in line with the expectation and seven were significant ($p < .05$ or $.01$). For ten series, the number of extrapolations was less than 4. This number was too low to give rise to significant correlations. Inspection of Table 12.1 reveals direct support. For all series except no. 11, the most preferred extrapolation is a simplest extrapolation. There are, however, nine more or less ambiguous series. An extreme case is series no. 8. All its four given extrapolations are equally simple simplest extrapolations, so, their loads sustain all four extrapolations.

There are two exceptional series, namely, nos. 9 and 18. Of both series, the lowest load of the given extrapolations is $I = 3$. However, under the theoretical condition that each series is conceived of as a sample of two independent subseries, the load can be still lower. We illustrate this for series AAAB (no. 9). Extrapolated towards AAABBBBBB, it has the code: $3^*(A) \ N^*(B)$. This extrapolation disregards the first subseries AAA. It merely takes the last symbol B as a sample of an extended structure. However, although its load, $I = 2$, is lower than that of any other extrapolation, no subject has given this extrapolation. Apparently,

Table 12.1 Twenty-five alphabetical letter series tested by Scharroo and Leeuwenberg (2000). The first fifteen series stem from Thurstone and Thurstone (1941). The extrapolation of each series deals with five letters. N refers to the number of subjects that produced the given extrapolation. I refers to the structural information load of the extrapolated series (Scharroo and Leeuwenberg, 2000).

Series	Extra	N	I	Series	Extra	N	I	Series	Extra	N	I
(1) URTUST	UTTUU	24	5	(12) PONON	MNMLM	15	3	(20) ABCCBA	ABCCB	12	4
(2) ABMCD	NEFOG	13	4		PONON	3	5		DEFFE	7	5
	MEFMG	11	4		ONOPO	2	5		BCCBA	3	4
(3) CDC	DCDCD	21	3		OPONO	2	5		ABCDD	1	6
	ECFCG	2	4		PPONO	1	6		EFGGF	1	5
	DEDEF	1	3		NOPON	1	6	(21) ABABCD	CDEFE	16	3
(4) WXAXYB	YZCZA	22	4	(13) DEFGE	FGHFG	14	3		ABCDE	5	4
	CYZDZ	1	8		HIJFK	3	4		EFEFG	1	3
	XCZWX	1	8		HIEJK	2	5		CBABC	1	4
(5) RSCDST	DETUE	21	4		EFGFE	2	6		DEDEF	1	5
	CDTUC	2	6		DCBAB	1	4	(22) AABDEE	FHIIJ	11	4
	ABCTU	1	8		IJELM	1	5		GHHJK	5	5
(6) NPAOQA	PRAQS	15	5		FGFEF	1	7		GGHJK	4	5
	RTAQS	7	7	(14) ABYAB	YABYA	14	4		FHIIK	2	5
	RSART	2	9		ZABAA	10	5		GHHIJ	1	6
(7) ATBATAAT	ZATYA	12	5	(15) JKQRK	LRSLM	12	4		FFGIJ	1	5
	BATAA	9	6		YZKGH	3	5		GHIIK	1	6
	BBTAT	2	8		LSTMU	1	7	(23) ABDG	KPVCK	17	2
	CATAT	1	9		QZKHK	1	7		KPVCJ	1	4

Code	n	k		Code	n	k		Code	n	k
(8) MABMB				STKUV	1	6		KPVBI	1	4
CMCDM	21	5		KQRLK	1	6		HJMNP	1	4
MABMB	1	5		LJKQR	1	7		KPBUB	1	5
AMABM	1	5		JRQKJ	1	8		IMOTV	1	6
AMMAB	1	5		STLUV	1	7		GMJRM	1	6
(9) AAAB				XYKFG	1	7		KGDBA	1	5
BBCCC	15	3		BJBJK	1	7		GHJLM	8	4
AAABA	3	3		EEEFG	23	3	(24) AABDFG	IIJLM	3	5
BBAAA	2	3		DDEFG	1	3		HHIKM	3	5
ACADA	2	3	(16) AAABCD	SMTLU	21	4		IIJLN	2	5
BBBAA	2	3		OMPLM	2	5		HJLMM	1	5
(10) QXAPXBQ				OMPQO	1	6		HIJKL	1	5
XCPXD	14	7	(17) PQORN	BCCDD	16	3		GIKMN	1	6
XCRXD	4	8		CCDEE	5	3		GIKLL	1	5
XAPXD	3	8		AACAA	2	4		GFDBA	1	6
XCQXD	2	8	(18) AAB	BBCCC	1	3		HJJKL	1	6
XCOXD	1	8		EEFFF	11	5		GHJKK	1	6
(11) ADUACUAEU				EEEEF	9	5		IIKLN	1	7
ABUAF	9	7		CCBBB	3	5	(25) ABCDHIJ	KOPQR	23	3
ADUAF	9	7		EFFGG	1	6		OPQRV	1	5
ACUAF	3	6	(19) AAAABBBCCD							
AFUAF	2	8								
AGUAF	1	8								

subjects merely accepted extrapolations for which all the stimulus elements play a role as, for instance, in the extrapolation towards AAABBBCCC.

Process versus representation

A main goal of Scharroo and Leeuwenberg (2000) was to show that the preferred extrapolation is not determined by process factors but only by representation properties. To this end, they also derived extrapolation predictions from the model by Klahr and Wallace (1970) which is a pure process approach, and from the model by Simon and Kotovsky (1963) which combines process and representation factors. By applying the Mantel-Haenszel analysis (Fleiss, 1973), Scharroo and Leeuwenberg (2000) showed that, for the twenty-five serial extrapolations above, the predictions by these models are less successful than those by the representation approach presented here. This outcome is an indication against the process role in serial extrapolation. However, it is not a sufficient argument. After all, the three models also differ in other respects, for instance, with respect to the accepted kinds of regularity.

Another indication against the role of process factors is as follows. Without doubt, the higher interval level coding requires more processing effort than the basic interval level coding, and the latter coding requires more processing effort than the nominal level coding. The lowest hierarchical level extrapolation just reveals a periodical repeat of the literal stimulus itself, and requires hardly any processing effort. However, whereas each experimental series could be extrapolated as a periodical repeat of the literal stimulus series, only in one case (no. 21) is such an extrapolation the simplest and has the highest response frequency. Besides, only 3 of the 116 different extrapolations given in the experiment reflect this literal repeat concept. This supports the idea that the simplest representation is more preferred than the representation that requires the least effort.

A third indication against process factors in the selection of the extrapolation stems from another experiment by Scharroo and Leeuwenberg (2000), designed to experimentally disentangle representation and process complexity. We briefly sketch this study. All stimuli were graphs consisting of a series of four bars. So, without loss of generality, the I-load can be used as an inter-stimulus complexity measure. The experiment dealt with two conditions.

In one condition of the experiment, subjects had to judge the complexity of each extrapolated stimulus. This judgment was not preceded by an extrapolation task. It applied to the given stimulus plus extrapolation. So, the subjects had direct access to the best solution and did not have experience with the mental process towards the solution. The complexity judgments correlated positively with the I-loads of the preferred extrapolations (r = .81; p < .0001) and negatively with their response frequencies (r = −.77; p < .0001). In other words, the judgments reflected the complexity of the representation concept.

As in the first condition, in the second condition the task was to judge the complexity of each extrapolated stimulus, but this time, after having performed the extrapolation task. So, the subjects had experienced the mental processes towards the extrapolation. Like the results for the letter series, the I-loads and N(Ss), or response frequencies, correlated negatively (r = −.84; p < .0001), in line with the expectation. However, the complexity judgments did not correlate with the I-loads of the preferred extrapolations (r = .07). Furthermore, the correlation between the complexity judgments and the response frequencies was even slightly positive (r = .34; p < .05). The latter results suggest that these judgments deal with the extrapolation process and that the most frequent extrapolation rather requires the lengthiest process. Also, according to the analysis of correlations among the reaction time (RT) data, these complexity judgments reflect the complexity of the extrapolation process. So, there is at least a difference between process complexity and representation complexity.

To evaluate the outcomes of this study, we compare extrapolation with problem solving tasks (Newell, 1990) such as in mathematical structure detection (Hofstadter, 1985), the magic cube (Hofstadter, 1985), the mutilated checkerboard (Kaplan and Simon, 1990), and the tower of Hanoi (Kotovsky et al., 1985). A main difference is as follows. The correct response to a task within problem solving is characterized by its logical correctness. As a rule, there is only one correct solution and all other responses are incorrect. In our view, the solution is to a great extent obtained by deductive reasoning, which aims at deriving a concrete instance from abstract propositions.

As suggested in the introduction of this section, Thurstone and Thurstone classified the extrapolation task as one that belongs to problem solving, giving rise to correct or incorrect solutions. According to our analysis of the data, the favoured extrapolations are characterized by their simplest representations and are, therefore, as correct as any other. Besides, the extrapolations mainly deal with inductive reasoning, which aims at inferring an abstract concept from concrete instances. It plays not only a role in serial extrapolation (Holzman et al., 1983; Simon and Kotovsky, 1963), but also in stimulus classification (Medin and Schaffer, 1978; Medin and Smith, 1984), recognition of analogies (Alexander et al., 1989; Sternberg and Gardner, 1983), and analogue thinking (Gick and Holyoak, 1980; Halford, 1992; Spellman and Holyoak, 1996).

According to our observations, the simplest representation of the extrapolated stimulus determines the favoured response. There is no further differentiation of the quality of this representation. Instead, there might be a further differentiation of the quality of a correct solution. A correct solution might be obtained by more or less reasoning steps. Of course, the minimal amount is preferred. Some aesthetic riddles give rise to both a rather complex and a very simple solution. The simple solution is based on a sudden insight that often might be combined with a so-called 'Aha!' experience (Posner, 1973).

All in all, we conclude, as we have argued earlier, that inductive mental processes are involved not only in perception but also in semi-perceptual extrapolation tasks whose solutions are simple or complex but not correct or incorrect. We furthermore claim that the preferred extrapolations reflect the simplest representations of the extrapolated stimuli and not the simplest mental process towards the given extrapolations.

12.2   Evaluative pattern qualities

There are properties such as salience, interestingness, and beauty that deal with evaluative aspects of patterns but that do not belong to the prototypical issues of perception. Here, these concepts will be defined operationally by the tasks. Their common feature is that all of them are supposed to be codetermined by pattern complexity which we have expressed in terms of structural information load.

Distinctiveness

More or less analogous to Mackay's (1950, 1969) distinction between constructive information and selective information (see Chapter 11.1) is Evans' (1967) distinction between constraint salience and distinctive salience. The first kind of salience is supposed to characterize a pattern on the basis of its own merits, like its figural goodness discussed in Chapter 6.2. The second kind of salience deals with a pattern as distinct from its surrounding patterns and is supposed to reflect the ease of detecting this pattern (target) amidst other patterns (distracters). This kind of salience is the topic in this subsection and has been the topic of research by Treisman (Treisman, 1969, 1982, 1986; Treisman and Gelade, 1980).

Salience factors To illustrate some of Treisman's findings, we introduce Figure 12.1 which presents stimuli in a simplified and schematic fashion. In contrast to her stimuli which dealt with a target

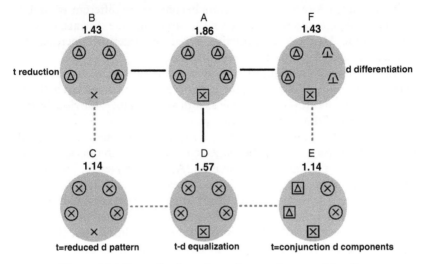

Figure 12.1 Six stylized configurations each comprising five patterns. The pattern at the bottom of each configuration is the target (t) and the four remaining patterns are the distracters (d). The configurations vary along three factors. From A to B, the target loses features (t reduction). From A to D, the target and the distracters become more equal (t-d equalization). From A to F, the distracters become more different (d differentiation). C combines t reduction and t-d equalization. Its target is a reduced d pattern. E combines d differentiation and t-d equalization. Its target is a conjunction of features. The numbers indicate the theoretical distinctiveness measures of targets amid distracters (see text).

(t) among many randomly positioned distracters (d), each configuration in this schema deals with one target, presented at the bottom, and just four distracters. The configurations are embedded in a global structure that reveals three main factors and two combined factors. Next, we describe these factors in combination with the empirical salience effects observed by Treisman (1969, 1982, 1986):

Factor 1: from A to B, the target loses a feature (t reduction). The distinctiveness of the target appears to decrease (see also comments on Figure 2.4 dealing with prototypes based on simplicity). An extreme case deals with a pin in a haystack. Evidently, it is not easy to detect the pin.

Factor 2: from A to D, the target and the distracters gradually share more features (t-d equalization). So, the uniqueness of the target decreases. Hence, its distinctiveness decreases. In an extreme case all five patterns are equal.

Factor 3: from A to F, the distracters become more different (d differentiation). So, the difference between the target and the distracters is no longer unique. Hence, the distinctiveness of the target will decrease. In an extreme case all five patterns are different.

Factors 1 and 2: configuration C is a result of t reduction and t-d equalization. As a consequence, the target is a reduced d pattern without any unique feature. It is only unique as it misses a feature. Obviously, the distinctiveness of the target is extra low.

Factors 2 and 3: configuration E is a result of t-d equalization and d differentiation. As a result, the target comprises no unique feature. It merely comprises a unique combination. As a consequence, its distinctiveness is extra low and its detection requires extra focal attention. After all, the detection presumes a test of each square or each cross to establish their unique combination. Hence, the number of distracters affects the detection of the target. Notice that in all other conditions (A, B, C, D, and F), this number hardly affects the detection of the target.

Segmentation indices Duncan and Humphreys (1989) explained target distinctiveness on the basis of Gestaltist organization principles rather than on specific interactions between separable features (Treisman, 1969, 1982). According to their analysis, pattern segmentation supplies indices for target distinctiveness. Here we present a similar analysis. To this end, we introduce Figure 12.2 in which the components such as the distracters and target in Figure 12.1 are represented by dots. Furthermore, a set of components with common features constitutes a cluster, and each cluster in Figure 12.1 is in Figure 12.2 encircled by a closed curve.

Analogous to Duncan and Humphreys' (1989) approach, we propose the following qualitative indices for target distinctiveness. First, the more the target is exclusively encircled the higher is its distinctiveness. Hence, the target distinctiveness in A is higher than in B. Second, the more the target and the distracters share clusters the lower is the target distinctiveness. Hence, the target distinctiveness in D is lower than in A. Third, the larger is the number of mere distracter clusters the lower is the target distinctiveness. So, the target distinctiveness in F is lower than in A. The low target distinctiveness of C is due to both the first and second indices, and the low target distinctiveness of E is due to both the second and third indices.

A distinctiveness measure All three aforementioned qualitative indices for target distinctiveness deal with the distinctive information of target pattern t amidst surrounding distracters d, and this common

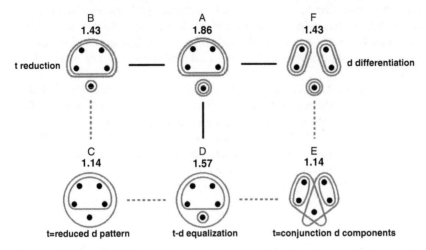

Figure 12.2 The components, such as the distracters and the target, in Figure 12.1 are presented by dots, and clusters of components with identical features in Figure 12.1 are encircled. These clusters supply indices for the target distinctiveness. The theoretical target distinctiveness values are indicated by numbers (see text).

concept inspired a quantitative salience measure in terms of SIT codes. As a step towards this measure, we first consider the load of an imaginary base line configuration in which the target has been replaced by a distracter. Obviously, this limiting case misses a target and cannot evoke any target distinctiveness. It merely deals with distracters. Therefore, the load of its representation is indicated by $I(d)$. This load is contrasted to the load $I(c)$ of the actual configuration comprising the target amid distracters. The ratio of $I(c)$ and $I(d)$ is supposed to express the distinctiveness of the target, that is, the distinctiveness measure S is as follows:

$$S = I(c)/I(d)$$

This ratio might remind one of a perceptual preference measure because it opposes two concepts, namely, an actual and a virtual configuration. However, it is not a purely perceptual preference measure because it does not deal with two interpretations of the same stimulus.

We will apply this measure to the configurations in Figure 12.1. The frequent pattern features, such as the squares, circles, triangles, crosses, U shapes, and T shapes, all contribute to $I = 3$ each. Furthermore, we describe each cluster in Figure 12.2 by a unified representation and a combination of clusters by a dissociated representation. This representation disregards the spatial relationships between the clusters (according to the rules of van Lier *et al.*, 1994, the spatial relationships in the patterns are not coincidental). The actual S values are indicated above the configurations in Figures 12.1 and 12.2 and are assessed as follows:

Figure 12.1A: $I(c) = 13$, namely, for the target (6) and the fourfold repeat (1) of the distracter (6). $I(d) = 7$, namely, for the fivefold repeat (1) of the distracter (6). $S = 1.86$.

Figure 12.1B: $I(c) = 10$, namely, for the target (3) and the fourfold repeat (1) of the distracter (6). $I(d) = 7$, namely, for the fivefold repeat (1) of the distracter (6). $S = 1.43$.

Figure 12.1C: $I(c) = 8$, namely, for the fivefold repeat (1) of the cross (3), and the fourfold repeat (1) of the distracter's circle (3). $I(d) = 7$, namely, for the fivefold repeat (1) of the distracter (6). $S = 1.14$. This outcome just combines the additional effects of the previous and the following figure. In effect, its S value is a city-block distance from the S value of A. So, $S(C) - S(A) = S(B) - S(A) + S(D) - S(A)$. Here, the labels refer to the configurations.

Figure 12.1D: $I(c) = 11$, namely, for the fivefold repeat (1) of the cross (3), the target's square (3), and the fourfold repeat (1) of the distracter's circle (3). $I(d) = 7$, namely, for the fivefold repeat (1) of the distracter (6). $S = 1.57$.

Figure 12.1E: $I(c) = 16$, namely for the threefold repeat (1) of the square (3), the threefold repeat (1) of the cross (3), the twofold repeat (1) of the distracter's triangle (3), and the twofold repeat (1) of the circle (3). $I(d) = 14$, namely for the threefold repeat (1) of one distracter (6) and the twofold repeat (1) of the other distracter (6). $S = 1.14$. Also, this outcome just combines the additional effects of the previous and the following figure. In effect, its S value is a city-block distance from the S value of A. So, $S(E) - S(A) = S(D) - S(A) + S(F) - S(A)$. Here, the labels refer to the configurations.

Figure 12.1F: $I(c) = 20$, namely, for the target (6), the twofold repeat (1) of one distracter (6) and the twofold repeat (1) of the other distracter (6). $I(d) = 14$, namely, for the threefold repeat (1) of one distracter (6) and the twofold repeat (1) of the other distracter (6). $S = 1.43$.

All in all, the order of S measures along each factor roughly agrees with the distinctiveness orders observed by Treisman and Gelade (1980). Besides, the underlying codes reveal that the numbers of equal distracters within a cluster do not affect the target detection, which is more or less in line with observations. After all, the number of equal components within a cluster does not affect the load. In fact, the dissociated representation, which we use to describe the various clusters within a configuration, is in line with Treisman's assumption that clustered features are to be taken as independent separable features of the patterns. In line with the observations by Treisman and Gelade (1980) and Treisman (1969, 1982, 1986), the codes also reveal that the number of equal distracters only affects the target detection if the target combines features from different distracters. Then, this detection requires the extra focal attention needed to find the unique combination.

About one effect we are skeptical. It deals with the decrease of distinctiveness due to the reduction of target features. The visual search studies by Scharroo *et al.* (1994) of complex configurations with large numbers of distracters reveal a distinctiveness increase as a function of target simplicity. In fact, the next topic deals with this ambiguous effect of simplicity.

Interestingness

Here, we attend to the extent in which a pattern triggers a perceiver's interest. This quality, indicated by interestingness, is meant to be a characteristic of a pattern as such, that is, without context and independently of knowledge. We start by considering stimuli that range from regular to irregular patterns. For such patterns, Ruyer (1956) argued that interest is an inverted-U function of this range. He illustrated his claim by the following three serial letter configurations:

No. 1	No. 2	No. 3
EEEEEEEEEEEEE	EFKWBAMABWKFE	EFKWBARPZGMTH

No. 1 is very regular and no. 3 is very random. In Ruyer's view, neither of them evokes interest. Instead, interest is triggered by a deviation from these two extremes. So, series no. 2 evokes interest. It deviates from series no. 1 as it is less regular and it deviates from series no. 3 as it is less irregular. So, a semi-irregular and semi-regular series exhibits the maximum deviation from both extremes and is, therefore, the most interesting pattern. This conclusion was also drawn by Berlyne (1971) for abstract art configurations such as dot patterns (see also later on).

A theoretical measure If the letters are taken as symbols, not defined by alphabetical meaning and order, the irregularity levels of the

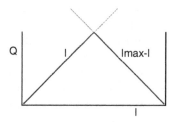

Figure 12.3 The interestingness (Q) of each configuration is assumed to be the minimum of complexity (I) and redundancy (Imax-I).

series are reflected by their structural loads (I). These are 1, 7, and 13 for series nos. 1, 2, and 3, respectively. So, in as far as interestingness (Q) is evoked by a deviation from maximal regularity, it is an increasing function of I-load. Furthermore, in as far as interestingness is evoked by a deviation from maximal irregularity, it is a decreasing function of I-load (see Figure 12.3).

By Ruyer's (1956) suggestion that interestingness (Q) is triggered by deviations from both extremes, maximal interest is supposed to be triggered by series that deviate as much from one extreme as from the other. This can be expressed as follows in terms of I-loads:

$$Q = \text{minimum}(I, \text{Imax} - I)$$

For the three series above, this implies levels of interestingness Q of 1, 6, and 1, respectively. In fact, this Q measure can also be paraphrased as the minimum of complexity (I) and redundancy (Imax − I). The experiment discussed next deals with visual patterns and was set up to verify Ruyer's claim (1956) that the maximal interest is in between regularity and irregularity.

Empirical evidence The visual relevance of the Q measure was tested in an experiment using twenty-five configurations of forty-four dots each (Leeuwenberg, 1973). The regularity of the stimuli was varied and care was taken that this regularity was globally spread across the whole configuration and not concentrated at a local part. The load range of the unified representations was $3 \leq I \leq 85$. The number 85 approximates the load of a random dot configuration whose code is as follows:

subpattern positions(N)

$< (\text{dot}) > / < 1 - - - - 44) >$

The load of the dot is supposed to be $I = 1$. Because the description of the whole pattern is view-independent, like that of any pattern, the

subsets

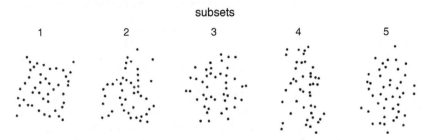

| 1 | 2 | 3 | 4 | 5 |

Figure 12.4 Each configuration of forty-four dots is an exemplar of a subset. The subsets range from regular (1) to irregular (5) configurations. The central configuration in subset 3 is expected to evoke the most interest.

load of the position of the first dot is supposed to be zero. As each next position is determined by two coordinates (e.g., by its orientation and distance with respect to the previous dot) its load is $I = 2$. So, $I_{max} = 1 + 2^* (43) = 87$. Hence, the most interesting configuration is predicted to have the mean load $I = 87/2 = 43.5$.

The twenty-five stimuli were divided into five subsets of five configurations each. One exemplar from each subset is shown in Figure 12.4. The loads of the configurations in these subsets vary within the following ranges:

Subset	1	2	3	4	5
Load	3–45	13–55	23–65	33–75	43–85

Each subset was tested separately. To each subject, five configurations of a subset were presented in random order and the task was to indicate the most 'interesting pattern'. In the experiment, seventy-five subjects were involved, that is, fifteen subjects per subset.

The overall mean load of all patterns that were judged to be most interesting is: $I = 42.2$. This value is close to the expected mean load $I = 43.5$. Besides, the judged interestingness appeared to closely approximate the predicted inverted-U function Q of I-load. This result seems to support the Q measure. It might, however, stem from an artifact, namely, from a response bias towards the pattern with about the mean load per subset. To test if the results reflect the hypothesis and not merely locally biasing context effects of the subsets, we present the data in more detail as follows:

Subset	1	2	3	4	5
Mean loads	24	34	44	54	64
Mean loads of selected patterns	32	37	39	45	58

The first row indicates the five subsets. The second row presents the mean I-loads per subset. The third row presents, per subset, the mean I-loads of the patterns selected by the subjects. So, if row 3 would be identical to row 2, the results could be attributed to a response bias towards selecting the pattern having the mean load per subset. However, for subsets 1 and 2 the loads of the selected patterns are higher than the mean loads per subset and for subsets 4 and 5 the loads of the selected patterns are lower than the mean loads per subset. That is, except for subset 3, the loads of the selected patterns are in between the mean loads per subset and the overall mean load 43.5. So, the data do reveal a local bias towards the mean within each subset, but meanwhile, they also reveal the predicted tendency towards the overall mean.

The middle stimulus in Figure 12.4 is a pattern of which either the irregularity or the regularity is taken as the variable that evokes interest. In this sense, this pattern is ambiguous (Leeuwenberg, 1978). The latter feature of interestingness seems to be in line with Attneave's (1971) claim that 'disjunctive ambiguity' attracts attention and interest. This kind of ambiguity is supposed to deal with two mutually exclusive interpretations, irrespective of their equal strengths, and characterizes illusory phenomena, such as transparent patterns, neon illusions, subjective contours, Poggendorff illusions, Rubin vases, and impossible figures. Without doubt, these phenomena evoke interest. Attneave (1971) distinguished this disjunctive ambiguity from 'conjunctive ambiguity'. The latter kind of ambiguity deals with pattern aspects that do not exclude each other. In his view, it is a characteristic of beauty, which is the next topic.

Beauty

Aesthetics has been mainly a topic of armchair speculation. Its meaning is intriguing but, in principle, highly subjective (for an overview, see Arnheim, 1954; Berlyne, 1971; Gombrich, 1956). Beauty is a matter of taste and, in principle, quite variable. Without doubt, this is especially true among laymen with respect to art. In our view, there is still a surprising concordance among experts of art. They tend to make almost definite claims about who belongs to the few great artists and who belongs to less successful artists. So, the common opinion of experts gives rise to the assumption that beauty is, at some level of cognition, a rather stable concept and this might have inspired scientists of empirical aesthetics to develop quantitative beauty measures (Birkhoff, 1933; Boselie, 1982; Eysenck, 1942). Such a measure does not pretend to be a recipe for art production that prescribes how to paint or to compose music. At best, it is a post-hoc assessment of aesthetics. Moreover, it applies to a very restricted domain, namely, of stimuli whose attributes are measurable. So, it mainly deals with ornamental qualities of geometrical shapes without emotional value.

According to Plato, goodness is the origin of beauty. In our view, however, beauty differs from goodness. Goodness is rather specific. It either applies to a goal or the means to reach a goal. A goal might be good or bad from a moralistic perspective, for instance. The means might be good or bad from an economical perspective, for instance. Even within each perspective, goodness needs further specification. After all, what is good in one respect might be bad in another respect. For instance, large letters are more readable but might cause a too heavy book. In contrast, beauty is less specific and more abstract than goodness. In fact, beauty applies to almost everything. It applies to art but also to furniture, riddles, jokes, games, performances, sounds, colours, thoughts, tutorials, landscapes, flowers, and stones, for instance. Beauty is evoked spontaneously by an object irrespective of its function. In our view, this is why beauty does not apply to either goals or means but to the relation between goal and means. This relation is reflected, in various forms, by the measures discussed next.

Birkhoff's (1933) measure The mathematician Birkhoff (1933) was the first to attempt to formulate a measure of beauty, and he used goals and means as basic concepts. In his opinion, beauty reflects an economical principle: 'It attains a maximum effect by a minimum of means'. Indeed, in many cases, great effects and minimal means are well recognizable attributes of beauty, for instance, in preventing an inundation by putting a finger in a hole of the dyke, or in drawing a well resembling portrait by means of a few lines. However, in these cases, the effects and means are hardly quantifiable. Instead, geometrical patterns are more suitable for a falsifiable beauty test as their means and effects are measurable once it is clear what they are.

About these two attributes, Birkhoff (1933) made the following proposals. Perception aims at detecting order. Hence, it is likely that pattern order (O) reflects the effect of perception. Then, it is plausible that the information involved in the perception of a pattern corresponds with the means. So, pattern complexity (C) is supposed to stand for the means.

The ratio of order and complexity reflects the economy of beauty (β). So, his formula is:

$$\beta = O/C$$

Birkhoff (1933) specified order and complexity in terms of selective information (H) as follows:

$$O = (Hmax - H)/(Hmax) \quad \text{and} \quad C = H$$

He designed fifty figures and established their β measures. For whatever reason, he did not test these measures against beauty judgments. However, without calculation, it is clear that according to his β measure, beauty just agrees with pattern redundancy or pattern goodness (see Chapter 6.2). In our view, this equivalence is implausible. Later on, Eysenck and Castle (1970) tested Birkhoff's β measures of the fifty figures against their seven-point-scale aesthetic pleasantness judgments stemming from 100 artists and 1,000 non-artists. The outcomes, however, hardly supported his measure. The correlation between the beauty measure and these judgments was: r = .28 (for artists) and r = .40 (for non-artists). Nevertheless, Birkhoff's underlying economy concept of beauty is intriguing and seems relevant for a broad domain of phenomena.

Eysenck's (1942) measure A second attempt was made by Eysenck (1942). His expression of beauty shares the two components (**O**) and (**C**) of Birkhoff, but his guiding principle is different. He refers to the ancient Greek saying: 'Beauty is unity in variety' (Bosanquet, 1892). Unity is supposed to refer to order and variety is supposed to refer to complexity. Beauty (β) just is their product. So, his formula is:

$$\beta = O^*C$$

Obviously, this measure is quite different from Birkhoff's formula. Eysenck's measure does not attribute a highest value to a most regular pattern. Instead, Eysenck's formula is one way to achieve the inverted-U shape of aesthetics as a function of pattern complexity, which was established by Berlyne (1971). This function implies that intermediate levels of complexity or regularity are more appreciated than low and high levels. Yet, there are some objections to make against Eysenck's formula:

(1) In Eysenck's approach, the quantifications of O and C are not *a-priori* specified but are derived from experiments. As a consequence, his actual measure varies from experiment to experiment (Zusne, 1970).

(2) Eysenck's formula rather reflects unity and variety instead of unity in variety. According to his formula unity and variety are separate factors and not simultaneously present pattern aspects. In effect, his formula agrees more with interestingness than with aesthetics (Boselie, 1982). After all, if $O = Imax - I$, and $C = I$, his formula is equivalent to $\beta = (Imax - I)^*(I)$, which predicts the same values as the measure of interestingness (see previous subsection).

Boselie's (1982) measure Boselie (1982) returned to Birkhoff's economy principle, according to which beauty is characterized by a maximal effect attained by minimal means. Furthermore, also Boselie assumed that effect deals with order and that means deal with complexity. Thus, beauty is a positive function of order and a negative function of complexity. However, there is a crucial difference with respect to Birkhoff's approach. Boselie's measure reflects the idea that 'Beauty is hidden order' (Arnheim, 1954; Gombrich, 1956). As a consequence, beauty deals with an improbable maximal effect attained by minimal means or a maximal effect attained by improbable and surprising means. The concrete implementation of this idea is elaborated next.

According to Birkhoff, complexity deals with all irregularities and order deals with all regularities in a stimulus. In Boselie's approach this is not the case. In line with Goethe's saying 'Durch die beschränkung zeigt sich der meister' ('Self-restriction characterizes the master'), Boselie proposed that a good result is a surprising effect in spite of restricted means, and he determined effect and means on the basis of the simplest code of the stimulus. The negative means component simply is the complexity I of this simplest code. A simplest code, however, does not necessarily describe all regularities in a stimulus, but it describes one specific interpretation which may leave some regularities unaccounted for. Boselie took these 'hidden regularities' as the effect R. More specifically, a simplest code specifies a stimulus as belonging to a certain class, and Boselie quantified the positive effect component R by the number of parameters (in the simplest code) that need additional specification to pin-point the 'hidden order' in the stimulus.

Here, we formalize Boselie's (1982) idea by way of a slightly different formula than the one proposed by Boselie and Leeuwenberg (1985). We formalize Boselie's (1982) idea by:

$$\beta = (1 + R)/I$$

where the constant 1 merely establishes that the beauty measure is positively affected by simplicity (i.e., by a lower I), even if there is no effect at all (i.e., if $R = 0$).

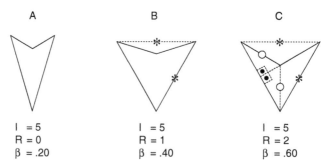

A   B   C

A	B	C
I = 5	I = 5	I = 5
R = 0	R = 1	R = 2
β = .20	β = .40	β = .60

Figure 12.5 An illustration of the beauty measure $\beta = (1 + R)/I$. The I stands for the load of the simplest code and R for the number of independent pattern regularities that are not described by the simplest code. From A to C the β measure increases (Boselie and Leeuwenberg, 1985).

An application of this beauty measure is illustrated by way of the patterns in Figure 12.5. Their descriptions determine the I components of their beauty values. In fact, all patterns in this figure share the same simplest code: $S[(K)(a)(L),(b)]c$ with load $I = 5$. Figure 12.5A reveals no hidden order. So, $\beta = (1 + 0)/5 = .20$. Figure 12.5B reveals a regularity that is not described by the simplest code, namely, the distance between the two top turns is equal to a lateral line-segment. It is important to note that we do not assert that this additional regularity, like any other, actually will be perceived by everyone. Our only contention is that the impression of beauty a pattern makes is related to the sensing of these regularities. So, $\beta = (1 + 1)/5 = .40$. Figure 12.5C shares this regularity, but reveals extra hidden order. The pattern consists of two adjacent equilateral triangles. The pattern also consists of two overlapping rectangular triangles. However, as this regularity is derivable from the previous ones, it does not count extra. So, $\beta = (1 + 2)/5 = .60$.

To test Boselie's beauty measure, Boselie and Leeuwenberg (1985) made use of the beauty judgments established by Eysenck and Castle (1970) for the patterns designed by Birkhoff (1933). From the fifty Birkhoff patterns, thirteen polygons were excluded because they revealed hardly noticeable length and angular differences (beyond the human 3 bit information transmission per dimension, see Chapter 11.1). The Spearman rank correlation between β and judged beauty is: $r = .78$; $p < .001$ (100 artists) and $r = .69$; $p < .001$ (1,000 non-artists). In the remaining part of this subsection, we present various illustrations.

Boselie (1997) focused on rectangles with length-width proportions (L-W proportions) of 1.41:1, 1.50:1, and 1.62:1. Such rectangles are

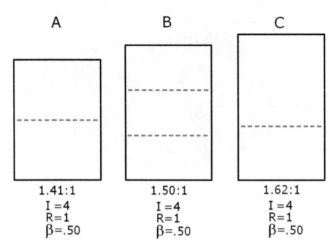

Figure 12.6 A, B, C are rectangles with the length-width proportions 1.41:1, 1.50:1, and 1.62:1, respectively. The latter rectangle reveals the proportion of the golden section (Boselie, 1997).

presented in Figure 12.6. In the first proportion, L is defined by the length of the diagonal of a square with side W. The third proportion deals with the golden section and is characterized by $L/W = W/(L - W)$ (Fechner, 1876; McManus, 1980). The rectangles share the same load $I = 4$. The hidden order in these rectangles becomes clear by subdividing them into two equal parts or in a square plus a remaining part. For instance, if the rectangle in Figure 12.6A is subdivided in two equal parts, then each part has the same length-width proportion as the total rectangle. So, $R = 1$. Furthermore, if the rectangle in Figure 12.6B is subdivided in a square plus a remaining part and this square is again subdivided in two equal parts, then all three parts are equal. So, $R = 1$. Finally, if the rectangle in Figure 12.6C is subdivided in a square plus a remaining part, then this remaining part has the same length-width proportion as the total rectangle. So, $R = 1$. Hence, for each rectangle holds $\beta = (1 + 1)/4 = .50$. In other words, the three proportions have the same predicted beauty values. This prediction is supported by an experiment by Piaget (1961) who showed that all three rectangles are about equally well appreciated though more appreciated than arbitrary rectangles.

A prominent natural instance of beauty is a peacock's feather. Figure 12.7 illustrates an exemplar. It shows patterns of colours that are quite unrelated to the form of the feather. Here, the separately coloured feather strips are taken as the means and the global envelopes of the

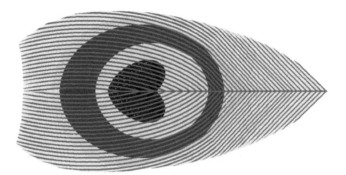

Figure 12.7 The beauty of a peacock's feather is explainable under the assumption that the separately coloured feather strips belong to the means and that the envelopes of the colours belong to the effect. The fact that the feather shape is quite unrelated to the circular colour patterns explains the beauty of a peacock's feather. The coloured version of this figure is presented in the separate colour section of this book.

colours are supposed to constitute the effect. The means are improbable with respect to the effect.

To explain the beauty of the peacock's feather by means of Boselie's beauty measure, we consider Figures 12.8A and D which present two simple stylized feathers, with D corresponding to a peacock's feather. The patterns below these figures are introduced next to illustrate the I and R assessments. The code, $I = 4$, of the common grid structure we do not expose here (see neon illusion, Chapter 8.1). We merely attend to the subordinate cream-blue strips. Each blue strip in Figure 12.8A can be described by the two coordinates of its two ends. The five blue strips in this figure can be described by a five times repeat of the same two coordinates. So, $I = 3$. This description, however, merely establishes that all blue strips start at same positions and end at same positions. So, their envelope just is a rectangle such as the one in Figure 12.8B. Figure 12.8C illustrates the equalization of the height (M) and width (N) of this rectangle to obtain the square envelope in Figure 12.8A. So, $R = 1$. Thus, for Figure 12.8A holds $\beta = (1 + 1)/(4 + 3) = .28$.

The code of the six blue lines in Figure 12.8D describes their twelve coordinates. So, the load of the grid plus that of the coordinates is $I = 4 + 12$. In fact, the code just describes twelve arbitrary coordinates like those in Figure 12.8E. Figure 12.8F shows the extra equalizations needed to obtain the square envelope in Figure 12.8D. These equalizations apply to the angles between the horizontals and the local orientations of the square contour ($a2 = a1$, $a3 = a2$, $a4 = a3$, $b1 = 270\text{-}a1$, $b2 = b1$, $b3 = b2$, $c1 = 180\text{-}a1$, $c2 = c1$, $c3 = c2$, $d1 = 180\text{-}b1$, $d2 = d1$). Their

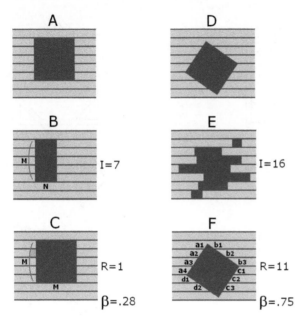

Figure 12.8 Patterns A and D present simplified feathers. In A, the blue square is related and in D the blue square is unrelated to the grid structure. The configurations below these patterns, namely BC and EF, illustrate the assessments of the loads I and the additional regularity R. The β of D appears to be higher than the β of A. The argument for the beauty of D explains the beauty of the peacock's feather (see Figure 12.7). The coloured version of this figure is presented in the separate colour section of this book.

total number equals the additional regularity being $R = 11$. Thus, for Figure 12.8D holds $\beta = (1 + 11)/(4 + 12) = .75$. We claim that this quantitative argument for the beauty of Figure 12.8D also explains the beauty of a peacock's feather.

To give a further example, consider the patterns in Figures 12.9A and F, which have been topic of study by Boselie (1983). These patterns belong to the most frequently used ornamental designs (Gombrich, 1956; Hardonk, 1999) and give rise to a clear distinction between means and effect. Both patterns evoke interlace effects of two intertwined squares brought about a mosaic of pieces. So, the 2-D mosaic parts can be taken as the means.

Figure 12.9A is rated as less beautiful than Figure 12.9F (Boselie, 1983) and next we check whether this outcome agrees with Boselie's beauty measure. The derivation of the I and R values is illustrated by the patterns below these figures. We assume that the suggestion of two

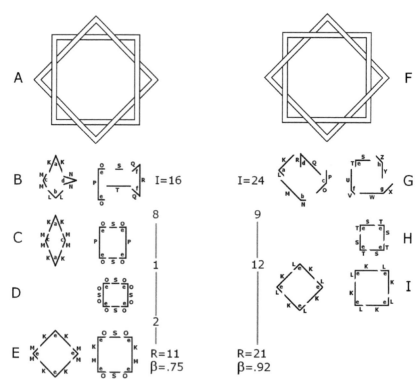

Figure 12.9 The eight mosaic parts in A and in F evoke 3-D inter-lace effects. The configurations below these patterns, namely BCDE and GHI, illustrate the assessments of the loads I and the additional regularity R. A is rated as less beautiful than F.

intertwined squares is due to the mutual context of the separate mosaic parts. Therefore, the separate mosaic parts, without their mutual context, are taken as the means. So, the means component of the beauty value for each figure is given by the sum of the complexities of the codes of the separate mosaic parts.

We first consider the codes of the mosaic parts in Figure 12.9A. The classes of the parts described by these codes are indicated in Figure 12.9B. In fact, this figure presents arbitrary exemplars of these classes. Only the V and U shapes give rise to code reduction, namely, due to their symmetries. Their descriptions reveal two and three information units, respectively. The total load is $I = 16$ (it equals the number of different symbols in Figure 12.9B). The subsequent Figures 12.9C, D, and E illustrate stepwise the extra pair-wise equalizations that are needed to obtain the two squares in Figure 12.9A. As the unique global structure of the intertwining squares furthermore fixates the actual shapes of the mosaic parts, the pair-wise equalizations of symbols sufficiently determine the additional regularity. Their total number equals $R = 11$. Hence, $\beta = (1 + 11)/16 = .75$.

For Figure 12.9F, the same analysis applies. Figure 12.9G presents arbitrary exemplars of the classes described by the codes of the mosaic parts. These parts are eight equal asymmetrical hook shapes represented by three parameters each. Their total load is $I = 24$ (which equals the number of different symbols in Figure 12.9G). Figures 12.9H and I show the extra identities being present in the two squares of Figure 12.9F. As the unique global structure of the intertwining squares furthermore fixates the actual shapes of the mosaic parts, the pair-wise equalizations between symbols sufficiently determine the additional regularity. Their number equals $R = 21$. Hence, $\beta = (1 + 21)/24 = .92$. Thus, in agreement with the data, the beauty value of Figure 12.9A is lower than that of Figure 12.9F.

In the foregoing example, different effects are obtained by different means. Clearly, at least in our view, in case the effects are equal, only the simplicity of the means is decisive. Here, we present an illustration stemming from a quite different domain, namely, that of chess-playing. Margulies (1977) asked expert chess-players to select the most aesthetic one of two moves that both lead to checkmate. Figure 12.10 illustrates the two options. The white horse is on move. Move 1 captures the black tower and move 2 does not take any piece. As it is generally profitable to capture as many pieces as possible, the move 1 is plausible and the move 2 is improbable. Nevertheless, the latter move was judged to be more aesthetic than the first move. This illustrates that aesthetic value stems from the improbability of the means used to reach the goal.

Boselie and Leeuwenberg (1985) also dealt with series of patterns. The patterns on which we focus varied with respect to their shapes and colours. Figure 12.11 illustrates two series. From the first pattern to the second pattern in Figure 12.11A, both shape and colour change, whereas from the second pattern to the third pattern, there is no change. The transitions between the patterns in Figure 12.11B are gradual: from the first pattern to the second pattern, only the colour changes, and from the second pattern to the third pattern, only the shape changes. Here, we explore how such abrupt and smooth transitions affect the beauty measure. Notice that the series are not necessarily temporally ordered, that is, they do not impose a specific scanning order.

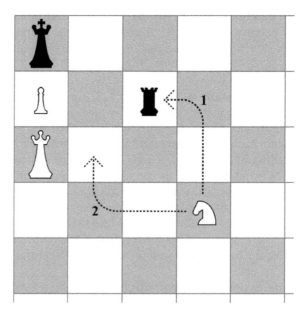

Figure 12.10 Two moves, that equally lead to checkmate, are compared. Move 1 takes a piece and seems therefore more safe. Move 2 takes no piece and seems therefore less plausible. Yet, the latter move is judged to be more aesthetic than the first move (Margulies, 1977).

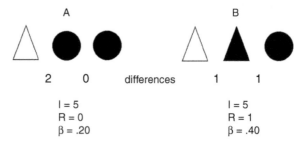

Figure 12.11 The subpatterns A and B vary with respect to shape and colour. Each transition in A reveals either all differences or all similarities whereas each transition in B reveals one difference or one similarity. Due to these distributions, the simplest code of A describes all regularity whereas the simplest code of B does not describe all regularity. Therefore, the β measure for B is higher than that for A.

Triangle shapes are indicated by T, circle shapes by C, white colours by w and black colours by b. The next schema presents the various codes of the two series:

Patterns	A	B
Primitive codes	Tw, Cb, Cb	Tw, Tb, Cb
Simplest codes	Tw, 2*(Cb)	<(T)>/<(w)(b)>,Cb or Tw, <(T)(C)>/<(b)>

The code of Figure 12.11A, with $I = 5$, covers all the regularity of the stimulus. So, $R = 0$ and $\beta = .20$. Figure 12.11B does not give rise to one single code but to two codes, both with $I = 5$. Neither one describes all regularity. One code does not identify the repeat of black colours and the other does not identify the repeat of identical triangular shapes. So, for each code holds $R = 1$ and $\beta = .40$.

Boselie and Leeuwenberg (1985) found that these predictions agree with judged beauty. That is, the abrupt colour plus shape transition in Figure 12.11A is appreciated less than the partial colour and shape transitions in Figure 12.11B. In fact, the beauty of the peacock's feather in Figure 12.7 can indirectly be explained along this line. Its colour transitions around the pens do not go together with changes of shape. Transitions with respect to colour alone are, in our view, rather prominent in art. For instance, in paintings by Rembrandt, brightness contrasts are rarely combined with hue and saturation contrasts. If a bright part is gold-like, an adjacent dark part is equally gold-like. Furthermore, in paintings of Claude Monet, hue transitions are rarely combined with brightness and saturation transitions. If orange refers to a sunny part, an equally bright and equally pastel-like blue-violet might refer to a shadow part. In our view, this strategy reflects economy. After all, an unnecessary usage of tools at one transition restricts the options at other transitions (Leeuwenberg, 1985).

Finally, we attend to serial patterns in the auditory domain. This time, we focus on series of tones that may give rise to a high contrast between expectation and reality. Such patterns may contain so-called tension tones evoking dissonances, and among musicians there is widespread conviction that such tones contribute to beauty in case the dissonance is resolved into consonance at a later stage. To illustrate this idea, we consider the melodies in Figures 12.12A and B. Notice that the series of tones in B is the reverse of the series of tones in A. High tones are represented by high numbers and low tones by low numbers. The clusters based on their codes, which ignore accent, rhythm, modularity, and other musical attributes, are as follows:

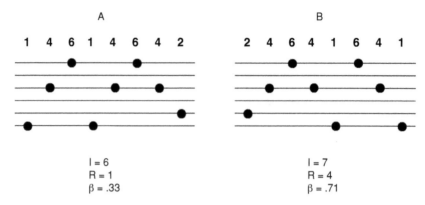

Figure 12.12 Two tone series A and B. Series B is the reverse of series A. The numbers refer to the pitch of the tones. A reveals a repeat structure within the first six tones. The seventh tone is unexpected. At a later stage, it appears to fit in a local symmetry of three tones (R = 1). The first four tones of B evoke a symmetry structure. The fifth tone distorts this structure but, at a later stage, this tone appears to be well embedded, together with the following three tones (R = 4), in the repeat structure of the last six tones. The beauty measure of B is therefore higher than that of A.

Melody	A		B	
Primary clusters	(1 4 6)(1 4 6) 4 2	I = 6	2 (4 6 4) 1 6 4 1	I = 7
Secondary clusters	1 4 6 1 (4 6 4) 2	R = 1	2 4 (6 4 1)(6 4 1)	R = 4

We start by discussing how the tones in Figure 12.12A are interpreted one after another. Without doubt, the first six tones are taken as the elements of a twofold repeat structure. The seventh tone (4) distorts this expectation and the eighth tone is a dummy, that is, it does not fit in a regular structure. This first online impression determines the load (I = 6). At a slightly later moment, when the whole series of tones might be accessible from echoic memory and open for reconsideration, the seventh tone (4) may appear to take part in a symmetry structure (4–6–4). Thus, the seventh tone contributes to additional regularity (R = 1). In other words, the initially dissonant seventh tone is resolved into a consonant. However, in our view, this change is not considerable and even questionable. After all, this symmetrical structure is too weak to cause a revision of the initial code, because such a revision would increase the complexity from I = 6 to I = 7.

For Figure 12.12B the story is different. The first four tones give rise to expect a large symmetrical pattern of five tones (2–4–6–4–2). The fifth tone (1), however, distorts this expectation, leaving merely a small symmetry structure of three tones (4–6–4). The remaining tones, namely, the first and the last four tones, then are dummies. This first online impression contributes to the load ($I = 7$). At a later stage, when there is more simultaneous access to all tones, the last six tones appear to fit in a code containing a twofold repeat structure which, due to its simplicity ($I = 6$), overrules the initial, more complex, code containing the local symmetry structure ($I = 7$). Notice that the new code changes the initially dissonant fifth tone into a consonant that fits in the repeat structure. Furthermore, in this new code, the last four tones are embedded in a repeat structure, so that the additional regularity is $R = 4$. Hence, in line with judgments, the beauty value is higher for series B than for series A.

The fact that the beauty values differ for the two series explains the preference for one specific order of tones over another. So, it explains the irreversibility of music. Notice that code revision not only is a characteristic of the most beautiful order. As we have argued in Chapter 9.1, it also is a cue for temporal order. In fact, the most beautiful order agrees with the cued order. In our view, this explains why art products that are considered to be beautiful might be experienced as impressive, unique, compelling, and recognizable (Arnheim, 1987; Boselie, 1982; Gombrich, 1956).

To conclude, we make a final comment on art. Art aims at beauty which, as we have argued, is characterized by an interplay of effect and means. Ideally, the challenge of art is to obtain an effect by improbable means. In our view, without both components, art is experienced as arbitrary and empty. For instance, a photograph that only supplies one component by presenting a silk robe, is not taken as a piece of art. Instead, a silk robe painted by Gerard Terborg is intriguing: it deals with both paint and suggested silk. Sometimes, in case of a painted snow landscape by Monet, for instance, a painting is so impressive that an actual snow landscape reminds us of the painting rather than that the painting reminds of a real snow landscape. Notice that a real snow landscape lacks the mentioned interplay of effect and means in a painting.

Summary

Section 12.1 deals with alphabetic letter series and the question is whether highly preferred extrapolations of these series can be derived from the loads of the simplest codes. As the structure of a letter series comes across by its extrapolation, the simplest code of this structure describes a given letter series plus its extrapolation. A test of twenty-five letter series reveals a negative correlation between extrapolation preference and I-load. Furthermore, there are indications that the preference for extrapolations is hardly affected by the process of detecting the underlying structure of a given letter series. In other words, the preferred solution may require more effort than a less preferred solution. Due to the use of knowledge about the alphabet, the letter extrapolation is not supposed to belong to the prototypical domain of perception. Nevertheless, this extrapolation shares features of perception in as far as it is an inductive inference process.

Section 12.2 deals with evaluative aspects of patterns such as distinctiveness, interestingness, and beauty. All their measures make use of I-loads as indices of information content. The distinctiveness applies to a target amidst distracters, and its measure reflects the distortion of the distracters by the target. Interestingness is approximated by the minimum of complexity and redundancy. Beauty is supposed to deal with an economy principle, namely, a maximal effect attained by a minimum of means. Besides, it expresses a surprise component of 'hidden order', that is, of attaining a maximal effect attained by improbable means. The negative component of the beauty measure is the complexity of the simplest code. The positive component is the additional regularity, that is, the regularity in the pattern that is not described by the simplest code. Various demonstrations show that both components are determinants of aesthetics.

Overview

Here, we highlight a number of global characteristics of structural information theory (SIT) as applied to visual form perception. Because we focus on global characteristics, we do not include technical details, illustrations, experiments, and literature references. We merely refer to the chapters and sections where these specifics have been elaborated.

On codes

Within the domain of visual form perception, the simplicity principle is SIT's selection criterion for preferred stimulus interpretations. This principle holds that the visual system prefers the interpretation with the simplest descriptive code, that is, the code that requires a minimum number of descriptive parameters to reconstruct the stimulus.

In SIT's formal coding model, this selection criterion is applied to symbol strings, using a formal syntax comprising coding rules for the description of visual regularities in strings. Visual regularity refers to configurations of identical stimulus parts and is characterized by two properties which specify highly accessible information, namely, holography and hierarchical transparency. A regularity is holographic if all its substructures reflect the same kind of regularity. This implies that its code can be built easily by going step-wise from small to large substructures. Furthermore, a stimulus regularity is hierarchically transparent if regularities nested in its code are stimulus regularities; this ensures that codes specify hierarchical organizations with properly nested wholes and parts. Only three kinds of regularity share both properties, namely, iteration, symmetry, and alternation (Chapter 5.3), and these are the ones SIT uses to obtain simplest codes.

The application of SIT's formal coding model in the empirical practice involves a semantic mapping between visual stimuli and symbol strings (Chapter 7). This mapping implies that the symbols in a string refer to visual elements in such a way that the string can be read as a reconstruction recipe of a stimulus according to some interpretation. SIT's formal coding model can then be applied to the strings to see which interpretation has the simplest descriptive code. Notice that this does not mean that SIT assumes that the visual system converts visual stimuli into symbol strings (Chapter 5.2). Instead, a perceptually plausible semantic mapping merely serves to supply experimenters with testable quantitative predictions.

On information loads

The structural information load, or complexity, of a code is taken to be the number of different constituents it specifies in the resulting hierarchical organization (Chapters 5.3 and 6.1). These constituents are the arguments of the regularity extracting operations in a code. Hence, the load is determined by the arguments and not by the operations as is the case in the transformational approach (Chapter 2.3). Furthermore, we distinguish two kinds of representations, namely, unified and dissociated representations (Chapter 7.1).

A unified representation describes all elements in a stimulus in relation to each other, that is, as belonging to one whole. For a unified representation simply holds: the more regularity it captures, the simpler it is.

A dissociated representation takes a stimulus as a composition of independent objects. This representation deals with two or three structures. The objects constitute the internal structure and are described separately by unified representations. Hence, the more regular the objects as such are, the simpler the internal structure is. The relative positions of the objects constitute the external structure, which has a complexity that reflects the effort to bring the objects in the given position starting from a 'general-viewpoint' position. This incorporates the avoidance-of-coincidences assumption, that is, the complexity of the external structure roughly equals the number of coincidences one would count intuitively in the relative position of the objects. In case of occlusion, also the virtual structure is relevant (Chapter 7.2). It is constituted by the occluded part, and its complexity is measured by the number of elements in this occluded part. Hence, the internal structure deals with view-independent aspects of objects, and the external and virtual structures deal with view-dependent aspects of objects. So-called local effects, being alleged falsifications of the global minimum principle, are explained by such globally simplest dissociated representations (Chapter 8.1).

While structural information deals with identical and non-identical elements, that is, with categories, metrical information deals with gradual aspects of dimensions, that is, with quantities (Chapter 11.1). There is ample evidence that metrical information is subordinate to structural information, but in case structural load does not favour one interpretation over another, metrical load may be decisive (Chapter 3.2). It is quantified by the sum of changes or impulses involved in scanning a pattern. For instance, an acute turn appears to be more complex than an obtuse turn and a long line appears to be more complex than a short line.

On rivalry

By the simplicity principle, the preferred interpretation of a stimulus is supposed to be selected from among all possible interpretations of this stimulus. The number of possible interpretations, however, can be very large. In SIT's formal model for strings, this selection problem has been solved by employing a special form of processing, called transparallel processing, allowed by special distributed representations, called hyper-strings. This method implies that a simplest code of a string can be selected by judging all possible codes without generating each and every possible code separately. SIT assumes that the visual system applies the same processing principle to visual stimuli (Chapter 5.3).

In our view, there are no reliable cues that, in whatever arrange-ment, straightforwardly fixate the simplest representation (Chapters 2.4 and 3.1). Instead, this representation rather is the outcome of a competi-tion between rivaling interpretations, and there is experimental evidence that even suppressed rivaling pattern codes are generated (Chapter 8.3). In fact, this evidence also is given by the visual relevance of the preference strength measure (Chapter 8). This measure captures the prominence of a target interpretation relative to the prominence of an alternative inter-pretation. It is defined by the load of the alternative code divided by the load of the target code. The visual relevance of the preference strength measure has been shown for phenomena such as pattern occlusion, subjective contours (Chapter 8.1), transparency, brightness contrast, assimilation, and the neon illusion (Chapter 8.2). Even for the task to extrapolate alphabetic letter series, which certainly is not a prototypical visual task, we showed that the preferred extrapolation depends on its simplicity (Chapter 12.1).

On hierarchy

The simplest code of a pattern may reveal an asymmetrical, hierarchical, relationship between superstructures and subordinate structures. Super-structures can be taken as frames that qualify properties of subordinate structures (i.e., not inversely). Therefore, the superstructure dominance hypothesis is proposed, stating that superstructures play a visually more dominant role than subordinate structures (Chapter 3.2).

In a hierarchical code of a string, the superstructure agrees with the most extended regularity at the basic code level, and the subordinate structure agrees with the information at hierarchically deeper nested code levels. In case of a 2-D pattern, the superstructure also always coincides with the most extended or global pattern component, but in case of a 3-D object, the superstructure might refer just as well to smaller components. Therefore, 3-D objects are used in experiments to test the superstructure dominance hypothesis. In fact, this hypothesis is supported by various experiments (Chapter 10).

An alternative is the global precedence hypothesis which claims that processing of global components precedes that of details. This hypothesis is commonly tested for patterns with parallel oriented subpatterns. In fact, such a pattern is structurally ambiguous. This means that the code which describes such a pattern as having a reversed hierarchy has the same structural complexity, in which case metrical properties become decisive (Chapters 3.1 and 3.2). Even so, also for other patterns, the global precedence hypothesis is plausible but only if it applies to top-down attention-driven scrutiny of already-coded percepts, which, just as art production, goes from code to pattern. That is, in our view, global precedence in attentional processing is a consequence of global dominance resulting from the bottom-up perceptual process from pattern to code.

On asymmetrical coding

Another asymmetrical relationship is that between prototypes and non-prototypes. In such a case, the prototype is the common component and the non-prototype has a distinctive component (Chapter 2.2). For instance, the non-prototype may be a more complex version of the prototype, or it may be a fairly ambiguous pattern, that is, it may have two nearly equally strong interpretations, one of which agrees with the interpretation of an unambiguous prototype. In general, the non-prototype is perceptually more similar to the prototype than the prototype is to the non-prototype, and in coding terms, coding the non-prototype starting from the prototype is simpler than coding them in the reversed order.

We discussed two experiments using unambiguous prototypes and ambiguous non-prototypes. One experiment showed that two simultaneously presented patterns induce a perceived temporal order from non-prototype to prototype (Chapter 9.1). Our explanation is that this perceived temporal order is triggered by a code revision, that is, the patterns may be coded in either order, but only this order triggers a recoding of the first pattern (because it yields a simpler global interpretation). Hence, only this order has an identifiable cue, and this may bias participants' judgments towards this order. The other experiment showed a reversed effect, namely, that subsequently presented patterns induce a percept of simultaneously presented patterns (Chapter 9.2). The data of this experiment yielded an estimation of the temporal integration span being the period within which backward context effect may take place.

On pattern qualities

Inter-stimulus comparisons of pattern qualities are assumed to start from the simplest codes of the stimuli involved. In such comparisons, not only the complexities of these codes but also other properties of these codes may play a role. We discussed this for two qualities dealing with pattern salience, namely, figural goodness and distinctiveness, and for two qualities dealing with pattern attractiveness, namely, interestingness and beauty.

Figural goodness refers to the detectability of a regularity in a stimulus (Chapter 6.2). It is measured according to the concept of weight of evidence, that is, by the number of non-redundant identity relationships specified by the simplest code divided by the total number of elements in the stimulus. In contrast to the traditionally considered transformational approach, this goodness measure accounts for many phenomena regarding the detectability of single and combined regularities, whether or not perturbed by noise.

Distinctiveness deals with the ease of detecting a target item among distracter items (Chapter 12.2). Various search effects can be explained by a distinctiveness measure which reflects the distortion of the distracters by the target, that is, by the complexity of the simplest code of the given configuration divided by the complexity of the simplest code of the configuration without the target.

Interestingness is a quality that applies to patterns in the range from completely regular ones to completely irregular ones (Chapter 12.2). Interest appears to be focused on irregularity when a pattern contains more regularity than irregularity and on regularity when it contains more irregularity than regularity. The most interesting pattern is in the middle of the range, where regularity rivals with irregularity. Accordingly, interestingness is measured by the minimum of complexity and redundancy.

Beauty is a pattern quality that is supposed to reflect an economy principle, namely, a maximal effect attained by a minimum of means. Besides, it is supposed to have a surprise component, that is, of attaining a maximal effect reached by improbable means (Chapter 12.2). This suggests that a crucial role is played by 'hidden order', that is, by regularities that are present in a pattern but that are not described by the simplest code of the pattern. Various effects can be explained by measuring beauty by the amount of hidden order in a pattern divided by the complexity of the simplest code of the pattern.

On classification

The foregoing sketches a picture of perception as being governed by the simplicity principle. That is, for an incoming stimulus, perception is assumed to select the interpretation with the simplest descriptive code, and this code is taken to underlie perceived pattern qualities. A central point herein is that codes specify organizations of stimuli in terms of wholes and parts. In other words, a simplest code classifies a stimulus by subdividing it into segments and these segments are supposed to refer to perceived objects (Chapter 4.1 and 5.2). In this sense, objects are not the input of perception but they are the output.

Classification by descriptive codes differs fundamentally from classification by sets of features. The class of objects represented by a feature set is larger as this set is simpler, that is, as it contains fewer features (Chapter 2.1). In contrast, the class of objects represented by a descriptive code is smaller as this code is simpler, that is, as it contains fewer parameters. In other words, a simpler descriptive code gives a more accurate account of an object in the sense that it is classified as belonging to a smaller class (Chapter 4.1).

Furthermore, classification by codes results from the description of regularities in individual stimuli. These regularities are taken to be transparent and holographic, which refers to the intrinsic nature of these regularities (Chapter 5.3). That is, they are not based on an external factor like their frequencies of occurrence in the world. Indeed, there is empirical evidence for an autonomous perception stage that precedes recognition and that is not affected by knowledge (Chapter 1.2). Any effect of knowledge should be attributed to a post-perceptual stage of perception. This is in line with the Gestaltist observation of the restricted effect of context, for instance, and also with the visual insensitivity for the learned concepts left and right (Chapter 11.2).

On simplicity

From the foregoing, it may be clear that the simplicity paradigm aims at predicting the outcomes of perception, irrespective of whether such an outcome reflects the situation in the world that is most likely to have caused the stimulus (Chapter 4.2). The likelihood principle is an alternative which does assume that the outcome of perception reflects the situation in the world that is most likely to have caused the stimulus. We cannot exclude that, either phylogenetically or ontogenetically, the visual system has adapted gradually to the world. However, scientific models of the likelihood principle suffer from the problem that the required probabilities in terms of frequencies of occurrence of objects in the world cannot be assessed without presupposing a perceptual classification of objects in the world. This implies that such models may be fine to model outcomes of perception but not to explain them, because such an explanation would be circular in that it assumes to be an explained perceptual classification (Chapter 4.2 and 5.1). The simplicity paradigm does not suffer from this problem because it assumes an autonomous visual system using an intrinsically based selection criterion which, in models, relies on descriptive codes yielding classification.

The aforementioned argument against the likelihood paradigm applies not only to objects as such but also to the spatial arrangements in which two or more objects may appear in a proximal stimulus (this distinction between objects as such and their proximal arrangements complies with the distinction between priors and conditionals in Bayesian models). That is, a specific spatial arrangement can be said to be unlikely or coincidental only if it is taken as an exemplar of some class of spatial arrangements (Chapter 1.1 and 4.2). Again, likelihood models have to assume such classes, whereas simplicity models can rely on descriptive coding to obtain such classes, implying that more coincidental arrangements are more complex (Chapter 7.1). This implication means that simplicity models incorporate the general assumption, which holds that the visual system tends to avoid interpretations that require coincidental proximal arrangements.

Finally, the focus of the simplicity paradigm on likely outcomes of perception rather than on likely situations in the world may raise doubts about its veridicality, that is, about its reliability in guiding us through the world. However, as sustained by theoretical considerations from the mathematical domain of algorithmic information theory, the simplicity principle does seem to yield fairly veridical perception in many imaginable worlds, possibly including this world (Chapter 5.3). This suggests that the simplicity principle is a general purpose principle in that it promises to be fairly adaptive to many different worlds. This contrasts with the likelihood principle which is a special purpose principle in that it is highly adapted to one specific world. In our view, the simplicity principle is evolutionarily more appealing because it seems to yield better survival chances in changing environments.

Conclusion

Here, we highlight distinctive features of perception as discerned from the perspective of structural information theory (SIT). This conclusion about perception overlaps with the foregoing overview of SIT but also differs from it as it puts SIT in the historical context of some related and alternative approaches.

According to Plato (428–347 BC), the sensory stimulus supplies insufficient information about the world. He illustrated this in *The Republic* by way of the following well-known metaphor. Imagine a prisoner who, since birth, is held captive in a cave (see Figure C.1). He sits on a bench and cannot look backward to see the fire and objects behind him. He merely sees a picture of flickering shadows on a wall. Actually, just that is his sensory input. Obviously, based on this information only, the prisoner is unable to obtain an adequate picture of the objects behind him. Because a human gains sure knowledge about the world, Plato argued that he must have inborn ideas as compensation. For instance, a human knows that an elephant cannot hide in a matchbox. Generally, he knows what is possible or impossible. In the domain of mathematics, in particular, he arrives at definite conclusions. For instance, the sum of angles within a triangle amounts to 180 degrees. A general proof of this is convincing without having to demonstrate it for every imaginable triangle.

With respect to visual form perception, our approach shares Plato's position insofar as it holds that the sensory stimulus underdetermines the actual scene and that there must be compensatory inborn qualities. In our approach, however, these inborn qualities are not given by knowledge about the world but they are given by properties of the visual system. More specifically, we assume an inborn sensitivity for only three kinds of regularity and an inborn tendency to select simplest view-independent stimulus representations. These inborn qualities are syntactic frames which enable a structuring of stimuli (Neisser, 1967) and which are appealing for intrinsic reasons. First, as we argued, those three kinds of regularity reflect highly accessible visual information, which guarantees a fast and flexible process. Second, simplest stimulus representations are

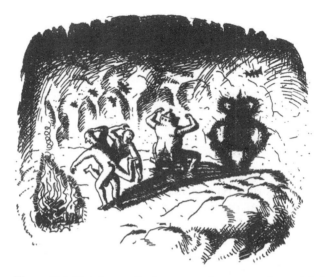

Figure C.1 Plato's cave. In the centre of a cave, a prisoner is held captive since birth. He sits on a bench and cannot see what happens behind him. He only sees flickering shadows on a wall. Therefore, it is improbable that he can infer the actual scene behind him from these shadows (in this illustration, some shadows even stem from the prisoner himself). So, more information is needed to gain sure knowledge about this scene.

highly accurate in the sense that they account maximally for stimulus regularity. Notice that such inborn properties of the visual system imply that regular patterns are more noticeable than irregular patterns, which might explain that regular patterns seem to occur more frequently in the world. That is, in our approach, this subjective impression is a consequence of the visual relevance of regularity, which contrasts with the often expressed idea that the frequency of occurrence of things in the world is the cause of their visual relevance.

Historically, the ideas incorporated in SIT arose in around 1960, when many studies of perception dealt with applications of Shannon's (1948) selective information theory (see Quastler, 1955). These studies did not focus on pattern representation, but this topic gradually became more interesting, and to that topic, the distinction between structural and metrical information appeared to be relevant (van Soest, 1952). Structural information deals with identical and non-identical elements, that is, with categories, and metrical information deals with gradual aspects of dimensions, that is, with quantities. In fact, visually, the structural content of a pattern appeared to be more crucial than its metrical content. Slightly

later, Garner (1966) focused on the abstract character of visual structures. He argued that visually relevant alternative patterns of a stimulus
are not actually given alternative stimuli, as commonly supposed within
the selective information approach, but that they are patterns induced
by the stimulus itself. These alternative patterns share the structure of
the stimulus and vary merely in a metrical sense. SIT incorporated Garner's idea and showed that an induced class of alternative patterns can
be derived from a structural representation of a stimulus (Collard and
Buffart, 1983). In line with Garner's motto that 'good patterns have few
alternatives', the preferred stimulus interpretation then is taken to be
given by the simplest structural representation, that is, by the one that
is most accurate in the sense that it yields the smallest induced class of
alternative patterns.

Notice that the latter idea contrasts with pattern descriptions in terms
of sets of separate features: a smaller set of separate features corresponds
to a larger induced set of alternative patterns, that is, it stems from
a more complex pattern representation. Small sets of separate features
may be convenient in pattern recognition, but pattern perception seems
to focus on small sets of alternative patterns as induced by simplest
pattern representations.

Furthermore, in line with Hochberg and McAlister (1953), SIT quantifies the complexity of a stimulus interpretation in terms of the amount
of structural information needed to specify the interpretation such that
the stimulus can be reproduced. In case of view-independent representations of the internal structure of objects, structural information is related
inversely to regularity, so, an object with more internal regularity is less
complex. Before 1970, this internal structure of objects was the main
topic of research in perception. After 1970, the focus shifted to effects
of spatial arrangements of two or more objects, in particular to so-called
local effects. Local effects are due to coincidental proximal arrangements
of objects and seem to go against the idea that perception aims for interpretations involving simplest objects. To deal with such local effects, van
Lier et al. (1994) quantified not only view-independent aspects but also
view-dependent aspects of interpretations in terms of structural information. This quantification implies that a coincidental proximal arrangement, though reflecting a spatial regularity, is yet more complex than a
non-coincidental proximal arrangement. The rationale for this quantification can be stated in reproduction terms: the total complexity of an
interpretation reflects the sum of (a) the effort to construct the hypothesized objects (more regular objects require less effort), and (b) the effort
to bring the hypothesized objects in the given proximal arrangement
(more regular arrangements require more effort). This way, van Lier

et al. (1994) were able to show that also local effects comply with the tendency of the visual system to arrive at simplest interpretations.

In fact, the distinction between view-independent and view-dependent pattern aspects within the domain of the simplicity principle is analogous to the distinction between Bayesian priors and conditionals within the domain of the likelihood principle. The latter principle was proposed by von Helmholtz (1962/1909). It holds that the preferred stimulus representation is the one most likely to be true (based on objective frequencies of occurrence of things in this world). These two principles have been compared to each other in SIT as well as in the mathematical domain of algorithmic information theory (AIT; Li and Vitányi, 1997). Like SIT, AIT got off the ground in the 1960s as an alternative to Shannon's (1948) selective information theory, but until the 1990s, AIT and SIT developed independently of each other. In the 1990s, however, their interaction led to the conclusion that the simplicity principle yields fairly veridical perception in many imaginable worlds, possibly including this world. This suggests that this principle is a general purpose principle in that it promises to be fairly adaptive to many different worlds. This contrasts with the likelihood principle which is a special purpose principle in that it is highly adapted to one specific world.

Our stance that human perception is guided by the simplicity principle instead of the likelihood principle agrees with Bolk's (1926) argument in biology. With respect to the evolution of perception, he argued that a tendency towards an open-minded *tabula rasa* (blank sheet) that is adaptive to new circumstances is more plausible than a tendency towards an expert system that is adapted to one specific world. He concluded this on the basis of observations which suggest that, in animals, the adults of a next generation adopt features of the young of the preceding generation rather than that the young of a next generation adopt features of the adults of the preceding generation. For instance, over generations, monkeys show a decrease in hair growth. Furthermore, over species, the newborns of higher organisms are generally more helpless than the newborns of lower organisms.

Though perception is hardly time consuming, it does seem to give rise to temporal effects. At least, according to Navon (1977), the visual system processes global stimulus features before local features. Within SIT, however, this so-called global precedence is conceived of as a post-perceptual side-effect of the visual dominance of superstructures over subordinate structures. Both kinds of structure are specified by the simplest hierarchical representation of a stimulus, which is a static representation yielded by a dynamic interaction between global and local features rather than by some linear stage process. In our view, Navon's idea rather seems to apply in imagination or art production, which is the inverse of perception (Marr and Nishihara, 1978). In that case, a hierarchical mental representation is evaluated into a stimulus, which involves serial effects from superstructures to subordinate structures. In effect, the hierarchical nature of a mental representation allows a large amount of information to be stored efficiently in a static way (Palmer, 1977), whereas its evaluation may be a time-consuming serial process (Collard and Povel, 1982). This clarifies why Mozart could say to his father: 'I am ready with symphony no. 36; I only have to write it down'.

Generally, in contrast to perception, conscious reasoning is time consuming and mainly guided by the likelihood principle. Besides, conscious decisions often are goal oriented because they are based on imagination which, as said, is inverse to perception. For instance, when people organize their holidays, they usually first imagine a destination with favourite conditions such as a cool climate, good food, and sport facilities. The conclusion might be to go to the Alps and to climb mountains. The top-down actions that meet this plan are executed subsequently. In SIT, the simplicity principle may suggest that perception is also some sort of goal-oriented process, namely, in that it aims at simplest representations. However, to be clear, in SIT, such simple interpretations are assumed to result from an autonomous unconscious process that proceeds bottom-up from stimuli to interpretations. In line with Herbart (1816), SIT also assumes a competition between rivaling representations. This suggests that the selection of simplest interpretations is cumbersome and time consuming but, at least in SIT's formal model for strings, this problem has been solved by employing a special form of processing called transparallel processing, as allowed by special distributed representations called hyperstrings. This method implies that a simplest hierarchical representation of a string can be selected by judging all possible representations without having to consider each of them separately.

Finally, as said, our approach to perception differs from Plato's stance insofar as we do not assume that perception relies on knowledge about the world. As we argued, not even left and right are perceptual categories. We assume that perception is a *tabula rasa* which structures incoming stimuli by way of automatic internal mechanisms yielding perceived objects. Hence, we do not specify knowledge as a resource of perception, but we specify perception as an autonomous source of knowledge. First, there is no indication that knowledge acquired during preceding generations is hereditary. Second, knowledge acquired during one's life may affect perception (Pomerantz and Kubovy, 1986), but this seems to apply only in case of ambiguous patterns (Rock, 1985) and only under marginal temporal conditions (Mens, 1988).

All in all, we think there is an autonomous stage of visual information processing that precedes recognition (Bachmann and Allik, 1976). This stage is what we prefer to call perception. Instead of using knowledge, it yields knowledge. Whereas reasoning at higher cognitive levels starts from knowledge about objects to establish their properties, perception starts from proximal properties to establish knowledge about objects. In other words, perception is like a witness who gives, as accurately as possible, an account of events. Subsequently, this account is evaluated by a judge who may include information from other sources. The roles of judges and witnesses are fundamentally different, which is similar to the fundamentally different roles of conscious reasoning and unconscious perception.

References

Ahissar, M. and Hochstein, S. (2004). The reverse hierarchy theory of visual perceptual learning. *Trends in Cognitive Science*, **8**, 457–64.

Alexander, P. A., Willson, V. L., White, C. S., Fuqua, J. D., Clark, G. D., Wilson, A. F., and Kulikowich, J. M. (1989). Development of analogical reasoning in four- and five-year-old children. *Cognitive Development*, **4**, 65–88.

Anderson, N. S. and Fitts, P. M. (1958). Amount of information gained during brief exposures of numerals and colors. *Journal of Experimental Psychology*, **56**, 362–9.

Aristotle (1957). *On the Soul, Parva Naturalia, On Breath* (W. S. Hett, trans.). London: Heinemann (original work published *c*. 350 BC).

Arnheim, R. (1954). *Art and Visual Perception*. Berkeley and Los Angeles: University of California Press.

(1987). Prägnanz and its discontents. *Gestalt Theory*, **9**, 102–7.

Attneave, F. (1971). Multistability in perception. *Scientific American*, **225**, 62–71.

(1982). Prägnanz and soap-bubble systems: a theoretical exploration. In J. Beck (ed.), *Organization and Representation in Perception* (pp. 11–29). Hillsdale, NJ: Lawrence Erlbaum.

Bachmann, T. and Allik, J. (1976). Integration and interruption in the masking of form by form. *Perception*, **5**, 79–97.

Baldwin, G. W. (1946). *Inductive Reasoning Test*. Philadelphia: Educational Test Bureau.

Barlow, H. B. and Reeves, B. C. (1979). The versatility and absolute efficiency of detecting mirror symmetry in random dot displays. *Vision Research*, **19**, 783–93.

Barrow, H. G. and Tenenbaum, J. M. (1981). Computational vision. *Proceedings of the Institute of Electrical Engeneers*, **69**, 572–95.

Baylis, G. C. and Driver, J. (1994). Parallel computation of symmetry but not repetition within single visual shapes. *Visual Cognition*, **1**, 377–400.

Beck, J. (1966). Contrast and assimilation in lightness judgments. *Perception and Psychophysics*, **1**, 342–4.

(1982). Textural segmentation. In J. Beck (ed.), *Organization and Representation in Perception* (pp. 285–318). Hillsdale, NJ: Lawrence Erlbaum.

Beller, H. (1971). Priming: effects of advance information on matching. *Journal of Experimental Psychology*, **87**, 176–82.

Berkeley, G. (1710). The principles of human knowledge. In G. J. Warnock (ed.), *The Fontana Library Phylosophy*. London and Glasgow: Collins Clear-Type Press.

Berlyne, D. E. (1971). *Aesthetics and Psychobiology*. New York: Appleton.

Biederman, I. (1987). Recognition-by-components: a theory of human image understanding. *Psychological Review*, **94**, 115–47.

Binford, T. (1981). Inferring surfaces from images. *Artificial Intelligence*, **17**, 205–44.

Birkhoff, G. D. (1933). *Aesthetic Measure*. Cambridge, MA: Harvard University Press.

Blum, H. and Nagel, R. N. (1978). Shape description using weighted symmetry axis features. *Pattern Recognition*, **10**, 167–80.

Bolk, L. (1926). Das problem der menschwerdung [The problem of human evolution]. University paper, University of Jena, Germany.

Bosanquet, B. (1892). *A History of Aesthetic*. New York: Macmillan.

Boselie, F. (1982). Over visuele schoonheidservaring [On visual aesthetic sensation]. PhD thesis, University of Nijmegen, Netherlands.

  (1983). Ambiguity, beauty, and interestingness of line drawings. *Canadian Journal of Psychology*, **37**, 287–92.

  (1984). The aesthetic attractivity of the golden section. *Psychological Research*, **45**, 367–75.

  (1988). Local versus global minima in visual pattern completion. *Perception and Psychophysics*, **43**, 431–45.

  (1994). Local and global factors in visual occlusion. *Perception*, **23**, 517–28.

  (1997). The golden section and the shape of objects. *Empirical Studies of the Arts*, **15**, 131–41.

Boselie, F. and Leeuwenberg, E. L. J. (1985). Birkhoff revisited: beauty as a function of effect and means. *American Journal of Psychology*, **98**, 1–39.

  (1986). A test of the minimum principle requires a perceptual coding system. *Perception*, **15**, 331–54.

Boselie, F. and Wouterlood, D. (1989). The minimum principle and visual pattern completion. *Psychological Research*, **51**, 93–101.

  (1992). A critical discussion of Kellman and Shipley's (1991) theory of occlusion phenomena. *Psychological Research*, **54**, 278–85.

Brigner, W. L. and Gallagher, M. B. (1974). Subjective contour: apparent depth or simultaneous brightness contrast? *Perceptual and Motor Skills*, **38**, 1047–53.

Brunswick, E. (1956). *Perception and the Representative Design of Psychological Experiments*. Berkeley, CA: University of California Press.

Buffart, H. F. J. M. and Leeuwenberg, E. L. J. (1983). Structural information theory. In H. Geissler, H. Buffart, E. Leeuwenberg, and V. Sarris (eds.), *Modern Issues in Perception* (pp. 48–72). Berlin: VEB Deutscher Verlag der Wissenschaften.

Buffart, H. F. J. M., Leeuwenberg, E. L. J., and Restle, F. (1981). Coding theory of visual pattern completion. *Journal of Experimental Psychology: Human Perception and Performance*, **7**, 241–74.

Calis, G., Sterenborg, J., and Maarse, F. (1984). Initial microgenetic steps in single glance face recognition. *Acta Psychologica*, **55**, 215–30.

Chaitin, G. J. (1969). On the length of programs for computing finite binary sequences: statistical considerations. *Journal of the Association for Computing Machinery*, **16**, 145–59.

Chapanis, A. and McCleary, R. (1953). Interposition as a cue for the perception of relative distance. *Journal of General Psychology*, **48**, 113–32.

Chater, N. (1996). Reconciling simplicity and likelihood principles in perceptual organization. *Psychological Review*, **103**, 566–81.

Cherry, C. (1961). *On Human Communication*. New York: Science Editions.

Churchland, P. S. (1986). *Neurophilosophy*. Cambridge, MA: MIT Press.

(2002). *Brain-Wise: Studies in Neurophilosophy*. Cambridge, MA: MIT Press.

Churchland, P. S. and Sejnowsky, T. J. (1990). Neural representation and neural computation. In W. G. Lycan (ed.), *Mind and Cognition: A Reader* (pp. 224–52). Oxford: Blackwell.

(1992). *The Computational Brain*. Cambridge, MA: MIT Press.

Cohen, D. and Kubovy, M. (1993). Mental rotation, mental representation, and flat slopes. *Cognitive Psychology*, **25**, 351–82.

Colberg, M., Nester, M. A., and Trattner, M. H. (1985). Convergence of the inductive and deductive models in the measurement of reasoning abilities. *Journal of Applied Psychology*, **70**, 681–94.

Collard, R. F. A. and Buffart, H. F. J. M. (1983). Minimization of structural information: a set-theoretical approach. *Pattern Recognition*, **16**, 231–42.

Collard, R. F. A. and Leeuwenberg, E. (1981). Judged temporal order of visual patterns. *Canadian Journal of Psychology*, **35**, 323–9.

Collard, R. F. A. and Povel, D. J. (1982). Theory of serial pattern production: tree traversals. *Psychological Review*, **89**, 693–707.

Cooper, L. A. (1976). Demonstration of a mental analog of an external rotation. *Perception and Psychophysics*, **19**, 296–302.

Corballis, M. (1988). Recognition of disoriented shapes. *Psychological Review*, **95**, 115–23.

Corballis, M. C. and Roldan, C. E. (1974). On the perception of symmetrical and repeated patterns. *Perception and Psychophysics*, **16**, 136–42.

Coren, S. (1972). Subjective contours and apparent depth. *Psychological Review*, **79**, 359–67.

Csathó, Á. (2004). The versality of visual regularity. PhD thesis, Radboud University, Nijmegen, Netherlands.

Csathó, Á., van der Vloed, G., and van der Helm, P. A. (2003). Blobs strengthen repetition but weaken symmetry. *Vision Research*, **43**, 993–1007.

(2004). The force of symmetry revisited: symmetry-to-noise ratios regulate (a)symmetry effects. *Acta Psychologica*, **117**, 233–50.

de Boer, L. and Keuss, P. (1981). Global precedence as a postperceptual effect: an analysis of speed-accuracy tradeoff functions. *Perception and Psychophysics*, **31**, 358–66.

de Wit, T. (2004). Disoccluding completions. PhD thesis, Radboud University, Nijmegen, Netherlands.

de Wit, T. and van Lier, R. (2002). Global visual completion of quasi-regular shapes. *Perception*, **31**, 969–84.

Dember, W. N. (1965). *Psychology of Perception*. New York: Holt, Rinehart, and Winston.

Descartes, R. (1644). Les principes de la philosophy [Principles of philosophy]. In A. Bridoux (1953). *Oeuvres et Lettres [Works and Letters]*. Paris: Gallimard.

Deutsch, J. A. (1955). A theory of shape recognition. *British Journal of Psychology*, **46**, 30–7.

Dijkstra, E. W. (1959). A note on two problems in connexion with graphs. *Numerische Mathematik*, **1**, 269–71.

Dinnerstein, D. and Wertheimer, M. (1957). Some determinants of phenomenal overlapping. *American Journal of Psychology*, **70**, 21–37.

Donderi, D. C. (2006). Visual complexity: a review. *Psychological Bulletin*, **132**, 73–97.

Dumais, S. T. and Bradley, D. R. (1976). Effects of illumination level and retinal size on the apparent strength of subjective contours. *Perception and Psychophysics*, **19**, 339–45.

Duncan, J. and Humphreys, G. (1989). Visual search and stimulus similarity. *Psychological Review*, **96**, 433–58.

Edelman, G. M. (1987). *Neural Darwinism: The Theory of Neuronal Group Selection*. New York: Basic Books.

Ehrenstein, W. (1941). Ueber abwandlungen der L. Hermannschen helligkeitserscheinung [On changes of L. Hermann brightness sensations]. *Zeitschrift für Psychologie*, **150**, 83–91.

Enquist, M. and Arak, A. (1994). Symmetry, beauty and evolution. *Nature*, **372**, 169–72.

Erikson, C. W. and Hake, H. W. (1955). Multidimensional stimulus differences and accuracy of discrimination. *Journal of Experimental Psychology*, **50**, 155–60.

Evans, S. (1967). Redundancy as a variable in pattern perception. *Psychological Bulletin*, **67**, 104–13.

Eysenck, H. J. (1942). The experimental study of the 'Good Gestalt' – a new approach. *Psychological Review*, **49**, 344–64.

Eysenck, H. J. and Castle, M. (1970). Training in art as a factor in the determination of preference judgments for polygons. *British Journal of Psychology*, **61**, 65–81.

Farah, M. J. (1995). The neural basis of mental imagery. In M. Gazzaniga (ed.), *The Cognitive Neurosciences* (pp. 963–75). Cambridge, London: MIT Press.

Fechner (1876). *Vorschule der Ästhetik*. Leipzig: Breitkopf and Härtel.

Felleman, D. J. and van Essen, D. C. (1991). Distributed hierarchical processing in the primate cerebral cortex. *Cerebral Cortex*, **1**, 1–47.

Finke, R. A. (1980). Levels of equivalence in imagery and perception. *Psychological Review*, **87**, 113–32.

Finkel, L. H., Yen, S-C., and Menschik, E. D. (1998). Synchronization: the computational currency of cognition. In L. Niklasson, M. Boden, and T. Ziemke (eds.), *ICANN 98: Proceedings of the 8th International Conference on*

Artificial Neural Networks (Skövde, Sweden, 2–4 September). New York: Springer-Verlag.

Fleiss, J. L. (1973). *Statistical Methods for Rates and Proportions*. New York: John Wiley.

Fodor, J. A. (1983). *The Modularity of Mind*. Cambridge, MA: MIT Press.

Fodor, J. A. and Pylyshyn, Z. W. (1988). Connectionism and cognitive architecture, a critical analysis. *Cognition*, **28**, 3–71.

Frearson, W., Eysenck, H. J., and Barrett, P. T. (1990). The Furneaux model of human problem solving: its relationship to reaction time and intelligence. *Personality and Individual Differences*, **11** (3), 239–57.

Freudenthal, H. (1962). *Lincos: Design of a Language for Cosmic Intercourse*. Amsterdam: North-Holland.

Frisby, J. and Clatworthy, J. (1975). Illusory contours: curious cases of simultaneous brightness contrast? *Perception*, **4**, 349–57.

Gabor, D. (1946). Theory of communication. *Journal of the Institution of Electrical Engineers*, **93**, 429–57.

Gardner, M. (1964). *The Ambidextrous Universe: Mirror Asymmetry and Time-reversed Worlds*. New York: Basic Books.

Garner, W. R. (1962). *Uncertainty and Structure as Psychological Concepts*. New York: Wiley.

(1966). To perceive is to know. *American Psychologist*, **21**, 11–19.

(1970). Good patterns have few alternatives. *American Scientist*, **58**, 34–42.

(1974). *The Processing of Information and Structure*. Potomac, MD: Lawrence Erlbaum.

Gerbino, W. and Salmaso, D. (1987). The effect of amodal completion on visual matching. *Acta Psychologica*, **65**, 25–46.

Gibson, J. (1966). *The Senses Considered as Perceptual Systems*. Boston, MA: Houghton Mifflin.

Gick, F. and Holyoak, K. J. (1980). Analogical problem solving. *Cognitive Psychology*, **12**, 306–55.

Gigerenzer, G. and Murray, D. J. (1987). *Cognition as Intuitive Statistics*. Hillsdale, NJ: Lawrence Erlbaum.

Gilbert, C. D. (1992). Horizontal integration and cortical dynamics. *Neuron*, **9**, 1–13.

Goldmeier, E. (1972). Similarity in visually perceived forms. *Psychological Issues*, **8** (1), Monograph 29 (originally published in German, 1937).

Gombrich, E. (1956). *Art and Illusion*. Princeton University Press.

Goodman, N. (1972). *Problems and Projects*. Indiana: Bobbs Merrill.

Gottschaldt, K. (1929). Über den Einfluss der Erfahrung auf die Wahrnehmung von Figuren [On the influence of experience on the perception of form]. *Psychologischen Forschungen*, **129**, 1–87.

Gray, C. M. (1999). The temporal correlation hypothesis of visual feature integration: still alive and well. *Neuron*, **24**, 31–47.

Gregory, R. L. (1972). Cognitive contours. *Nature*, **238**, 51–2.

(1980). Perceptions as hypotheses. *Philosophical Transactions of the Royal Society of London*, **290**, 181–97.

Gregory, R. L. and Gombrich, E. H. (1973). *Illusion in Nature and Art*. London: Duckworth.

Halford, G. S. (1992). Analogical reasoning and conceptual complexity in cognitive development. *Human Development*, **35**, 193–217.

Hanssen, A., Leeuwenberg, E., and van der Helm, P. (1993). Metrical information load of lines and angles in line patterns. *Psychological Research*, **55**, 191–9.

Hardonk, M. (1999). Cross-cultural universals of aesthetic appreciation in decorative band patterns. PhD thesis, Radboud University, Nijmegen, Netherlands

Hatfield, G. C. and Epstein, W. (1985). The status of the minimum principle in the theoretical analysis of visual perception. *Psychological Bulletin*, **97**, 155–86.

Hawking, S. (1988). *Brief History of Time*. New York: Bantam Dell.

Hebb, D. O. (1949). *The Organization of Behavior: A Neurophysiological Theory*. New York: Wiley.

Helson, H. (1964). *Adaptation-level Theory*. New York: Harper and Row.

Herbart, J. H. (1816). *Lehrbuch zur Psychologie [Introduction to Psychology]*. Königsberg, Germany: August Wilhelm Unzer.

Hermens, F. and Herzog, M. H. (2007). The effects of the global structure of the mask in visual backward masking. *Vision Research*, **47** (1), 790–7.

Hersh, H. M. (1974). The effects of irrelevant relations on the processing of sequential patterns. *Memory and Cognition*, **24**, 771–4.

Hinton, G. and Parsons, L. (1981). Frames of reference and mental imagery. In J. Long and A. Baddeley (eds.), *Attention and Performance, Vol. 9* (pp. 261–77). Hillsdale, NJ: Lawrence Erlbaum.

Hochberg, J. E. (1968). *Perception*. Englewood Cliffs, NJ: Prentice-Hall.
    1982). How big is a stimulus? In J. Beck (ed.), *Organization and Representation in Perception* (pp. 191–217). Hillsdale, NJ: Lawrence Erlbaum.

Hochberg, L. and Gellman, L. (1977). The effect of landmark features on mental rotation times. *Memory and Cognition*, **5** (16), 23–6.

Hochberg, J. E. and McAlister, E. (1953). A quantitative approach to figural 'goodness'. *Journal of Experimental Psychology*, **46**, 361–4.

Hochstein, S. and Ahissar, M. (2002). View from the top: hierarchies and reverse hierarchies in the visual system. *Neuron*, **36**, 791–804.

Høffding, H. (1891). *Outlines of Psychology*. New York: Macmillan.

Hoffman, D. D. (1996). What do we mean by 'The structure of the world'? In D. K. Knill and W. Richards (eds.), *Perception as Bayesian Inference* (pp. 219–21). Cambridge University Press.

Hoffman, D. D. and Richards, W. A. (1984). Parts of recognition. *Cognition*, **18**, 65–96.

Hoffman, J. (1975). Hierarchical stages in the processing of visual information. *Perception and Psychophysics*, **18**, 348–54.

Hofstadter, D. R. (1985). *Metamagical Themas: Questing for the Essence of Mind and Pattern*. New York: Basic Books.

Holzman, T. G., Pellegrino, J. W., and Glazer, R. (1983). Cognitive variables in series completion. *Journal of Educational Psychology*, **75**, 603–18.

Hubel, D. H. and Wiesel, T. N. (1968). Receptive fields and functional architecture of monkey striate cortex. *Journal of Physiology (London)*, **195**, 215–43.

Hulleman, J. and Boselie, F. (1999). Perceived shape regularity does not depend on regularities along the contour. *Perception*, **28**, 711–24.

Johansson, G. (1975). Visual motion perception. *Scientific American*, **232** (6), 76–88.

Julesz, B. (1971). *Foundations of Cyclopean Perception*. University of Chicago Press.

Kanizsa, G. (1975). The role of regularity in perceptual organization. In F. D'Arcais (ed.), *Studies in Perception* (pp. 48–66). Florence, Italy: Martello.

(1976). Subjective contours. *Scientific American*, **234** (4), 48–52.

(1979). *Organization in Vision. Essay on Gestalt Perception*. New York: Praeger Publishers.

(1985). Seeing and thinking. *Acta Psychologica*, **59**, 23–33.

Kant, I. (1783). *Prolegomena zu einer Jeden Kunftigen Metaphysic [Prolegomena to any Future Metaphysics]*. Available from Project Gutenberg (www.gutenberg.org).

Kaplan, C. A. and Simon, H. A. (1990). In search of insight. *Cognitive Psychology*, **22**, 374–419.

Kellman, P. and Shipley, T. (1991). A theory of visual pattern interpolation in object perception. *Cognitive Psychology*, **23**, 141–221.

Kennedy, J. M. (1978). Illusory contours not due to completion. *Perception*, **7**, 187–9.

Kimchi, R. and Palmer, S. (1982). Form and texture in hierarchically constructed patterns. *Journal of Experimental Psychology: Human Perception and Performance*, **8**, 521–35.

Kinchla, R. (1977). The role of structural redundancy in the perception of visual targets. *Perception and Psychophysics*, **22**, 19–30.

Klahr, D. and Wallace, J. G. (1970). The development of serial completion strategies: an information processing analysis. *British Journal of Psychology*, **61**, 243–57.

Koenderink, J. and van Doorn, A. (1976). The singularities of the visual mapping. *Biological Cybernetics*, **24**, 51–9.

Köhler, W. (1920). *Die Physischen Gestalten in Ruhe und im station¨aren Zustand [Static and Stationary Physical Shapes]*. Braunschweig, Germany: Vieweg.

Koffka, K. (1935). *Principles of Gestalt Psychology*. London: Routledge and Kegan Paul.

Kolmogorov, A. N. (1965). Three approaches to the quantitative definition of information. *Problems in Information Transmission*, **1**, 1–7.

Koning, A. and van Lier, R. (2003). Object-based connectedness facilitates matching. *Perception and Psychophysics*, **65**, 1094–102.

(2004). Mental rotation depends on the number of objects rather than on the number of image fragments. *Acta Psychologica*, **117**, 65–77.

Kopfermann, H. (1930). Psychologische untersuchungen über die wirkung zweidimensionaler darstellung körperlicher gebilde. *Psychologische Forschung*, **13**, 292–364.

Kosslyn, S. M. (1975). Information representation in visual images. *Cognitive Psychology*, **7**, 341–70.

(1981). The medium of the message in mental imagery: a theory. *Psychological Review*, **88**, 46–66.

Kotovsky, K., Hayes, J. R., and Simon, H. (1985). Why are some problems hard? Evidence from tower of Hanoi. *Cognitive Psychology*, **17**, 248–94.

Kruskal, J. B. (1964). Nonmetric multidimensional scaling: a numerical method. *Psychometrika*, **29**, 115–29.

Kurbat, M. A. (1994). Structural description theories: is RBC/JIM a general-purpose theory of human entry-level object recognition? *Perception*, **23**, 1339–68.

Lamme, V. A. F., Supèr, H., and Spekreijse, H. (1998). Feedforward, horizontal, and feedback processing in the visual cortex. *Current Opinion in Neurobiology*, **8**, 529–35.

Leeuwenberg, E. (1968). *Structural Information of Visual Patterns*. The Hague and Paris: Mouton and Co.

(1969). Quantitative specification of information in sequential patterns. *Psychological Review*, **76**, 216–20.

(1971). A perceptual coding language for visual and auditory patterns. *American Journal of Psychology*, **84**, 307–49.

(1973). Meaning of perceptual complexity. In D. E. Berline and O. O. Madsen (eds.), *Pleasure, Reward, Preference* (pp. 100–14). New York: Academic Press.

(1974). Een statisch criterium voor perceptieve tijdrichting [Later-earlier illusion versus the coding of asymmetry]. *Nederlands Tijdschrift voor de Psychologie*, **28**, 533–48.

(1976). Figure-ground specification in terms of structural information. The rivalry between different pattern codings. In H. Geissler and Y. Zabrodin (eds.), *Advances in Psychophysics* (pp. 325–37). Berlin: VEB Deutscher Verlag der Wissenschaften.

(1978). Quantification of certain visual pattern properties: salience, transparency, similarity. In E. Leeuwenberg and H. Buffart (eds.), *Formal Theories of Visual Perception* (pp. 299–314). Chichester, New York, Brisbane, and Toronto: John Wiley.

(1982a). Metrical aspects of patterns and structural information theory. In J. Beck (ed.), *Organization and Representation in Perception* (pp. 57–72). Hillsdale, NJ: Lawrence Erlbaum.

(1982b). The perception of assimilation and brightness contrast as derived from code theory. *Perception and Psychophysics*, **32**, 345–52.

(1985). Paradoxale kenmerken van creatieve prestaties [Paradoxical properties of creative achievements]. In *Kreativiteit en Wetenschap, Studium Generale [Creativity and Science, General Studies]* (pp. 52–71). University paper: University of Delft, Netherlands.

(2003a). Miracles of perception. *Acta Psychologica* (Special Issue), **114**, 379–96.

(2003b). Structural information theory and visual form. In C. Kaernbach, E. Schroeger, and H. Mueller (eds.), *Psychophysics Beyond Sensation: Laws and Invariants of Human Cognition* (pp. 481–505). Mahwah, NJ: Lawrence Erlbaum.

Leeuwenberg, E. L. J. and Boselie, F. (1988a). Against the likelihood principle in visual form perception. *Psychological Review*, **95**, 485–91.

(1988b). How good a bet is the likelihood principle? In B. A. G. Elsendoorn and H. Bouma (eds.), *Working Models of Human Perception* (pp. 363–79). London: Academic Press.

Leeuwenberg, E. L. J. and Buffart, H. F. J. M. (1983). An outline of coding theory: a summary of related experiments. In H.-G. Geissler, H. F. J. M. Buffart, E. L. J. Leeuwenberg, and V. Sarris (eds.), *Modern Issues in Perception* (pp. 1–47). Berlin: VEB Deutscher Verlag der Wissenschaften.

Leeuwenberg, E. L. J., Mens, L., and Calis, G. (1985). Knowledge within perception: masking caused by incompatible interpretation. *Acta Psychologica*, **59**, 91–102.

Leeuwenberg, E. L. J. and van der Helm, P. A. (1991). Unity and variety in visual form. *Perception*, **20**, 595–622.

(2000). A code-theoretic note on object handedness. *Perception*, **29**, 5–29.

Leeuwenberg, E., van der Helm, P., and van Lier, R. (1994). From geons to structure. A note on object representation. *Perception*, **23**, 505–15.

Leeuwenberg, E. and van Lier, R. (2005). Symmetry cues for matching mirrored objects. *Spatial Vision*, **18** (1), 1–24.

Leibniz, G. W. (1714/1979). *Monadologie [Monadology]*. Stuttgart, Germany: Reclam.

Levelt, W. J. M. (1996). Perspective taking and ellipsis in spatial descriptions. In P. Bloom, M. A. Peterson, M. F. Garret, and L. Nadel (eds.), *Language and Space* (pp. 77–107). Cambridge, MA: MIT Press.

Leyton, M. (1992). *Symmetry, Causality, Mind*. Cambridge, MA: MIT press.

Li, M. and Vitányi, P. (1997). *An Introduction to Kolmogorov Complexity and its Applications* (2nd edn.). New York: Springer-Verlag.

Locke, J. (1690/1968). *An Essay Concerning Human Understanding*. Cambridge, MA: Harvard University Press.

Mach, E. (1886). *Beiträge zur Analyse der Empfindungen [Contributions to the Analysis of Sensations]*. Jena, Germany: Gustav Fisher.

MacKay, D. (1950). Quantal aspects of scientific information. *Philosophical Magazine*, **41**, 289–301.

(1969). *Information, Mechanism and Meaning*. Boston, MA: MIT Press.

Margulies, S. (1977). Principles of beauty. *Psychological Reports*, **41**, 3–11.

Marr, D. (1982). *Vision*. San Fransisco, CA: Freeman.

Marr, D. and Nishihara, H. K. (1978). Artificial intelligence and the sensorium of sight. *Technology Review*, **81**, 2–23.

Martin, M. (1979). The role of sparsity. *Memory and Cognition*, **7**, 476–84.

McManus, I. C. (1980). The aesthetics of simple figures. *British Journal of Psychology*, **71**, 505–24.

Medin, D. L. and Schaffer, M. M. (1978). Context theory of classification learning. *Psychological Review*, **85**, 207–38.

Medin, D. L. and Smith, E. E. (1984). Concepts and concept formation. *Annual Review Psychology*, **35**, 113–38.

Mens, L. (1988). Primary perception of stimulus structure. PhD thesis, Radboud University, Nijmegen, Netherlands.

Mens, L. and Leeuwenberg, E. L. J. (1988). Hidden figures are ever present. *Journal of Experimental Psychology: Human Perception and Performance*, **14**, 561–71.

(1994). Can perceived shape be primed? The autonomy of organization. *Giornale Italiano di Psicologia*, **20**, 821–36.

Metelli, F. (1974). The perception of transparency. *Scientific American*, **230** (4), 91–8.

Michels, C. F. and Turvey, M. T. (1979). Central sources of visual masking: indexing structures supporting seeing at a single brief glance. *Psychological Research*, **41**, 1–61.

Milner, P. (1974). A model for visual shape recognition. *Psychological Review*, **81**, 521–35.

Monod, J. (1970). *Le Hazard et la Nécessité [Chance and Necessity]*. Paris: Editions du Seuil, Institut Pasteur.

Moran, T. (1968). The grammar of visual imagery. University paper, Carnegie-Mellon University, Pittsburgh.

Moore, C. M., Mordkoff, J. T., and Enns, J. T. (2007). The path of least persistence: evidence of object-mediated visual updating. *Vision Research*, **47**, 1624–30.

Moyer, R. S. (1973). Comparing objects in memory: evidence suggesting an internal psychophysics. *Perception and Psychophysics*, **13**, 180–4.

Myors, B., Stankov, L., and Oliphant, G. (1989). Competing tasks, working memory, and intelligence. *Australian Journal of Psychology*, **41**, 1–16.

Navon, D. (1977). Forest before trees: the precedence of global features in visual perception. *Cognitive Psychology*, **9**, 353–83.

Neisser, U. (1967). *Cognitive Psychology*. New York: Appleton-Century-Crofts.

(1976). *Cognition and Reality*. San Francisco, CA: Freeman.

Newell, A. (1990). *Unified Theory of Cognition*. Cambridge, MA: Harvard University Press.

Newton, I. (1687/1960). *Philosophiae Naturalis Principia Mathematica [Mathematical Principles of Natural Philosophy and his System of the World]*. Berkeley, CA: University of California Press.

Nucci, M. and Wagemans, J. (2007). Goodness of regularity in dot patterns: global symmetry, local symmetry, and their interactions. *Perception*, **36**, 1305–19.

Palmer, S. (1977). Hierarchical structure in perceptual representation. *Cognitive Psychology*, **9**, 441–74.

(1983). The psychology of perceptual organization: a transformational approach. In J. Beck, B. Hope, and A. Rosenfeld (eds.), *Human and Machine Vision* (pp. 269–339). New York: Academic Press.

(1999). *Vision Science: Photons to Phenomenology*. Cambridge, MA: MIT Press.

Palmer, S. E. and Bucher, N. M. (1982). Textual effects in perceived pointing of ambiguous triangles. *Journal of Experimental Psychology: Human Perception and Performance*, **8**, 693–708.

Palmer, S. E. and Rock, I. (1994). Rethinking perceptual organization: the role of uniform connectedness. *Psychonomic Bulletin and Review*, **1**, 29–55.

Palmer, S. E., Brooks, J. L., and Nelson, R. (2003). When does grouping happen? *Acta Psychologica*, **114**, 311–30.

Pani, J. R., Jeffres, J. A., Shippey, G. T., and Schwartz, K. J. (1996). Imagining projective transformations: aligned orientations in spatial organization. *Cognitive Psychology*, **31**, 125–67.

Perkins, D. (1976). How good a bet is a good form? *Perception*, **5**, 393–406.

(1983). Why the human perceiver is a bad machine. In J. Beck, B. Hope, and A. Rosenfeld (eds.), *Human and Machine Vision* (pp. 341–64). New York: Academic Press.

Petersen, M. J. (1975). The retention of imagined and seen spatial matrices. *Cognitive Psychology*, **7**, 181–93.

Petter, G. (1956). Nuove ricerche sperimentali sulla totalizzazione percettiva [New experimental studies on perceptual organization]. *Rivista di Psicologia*, **50**, 213–27.

Piaget, J. (1961). *Les Méchanismes Perceptifs*. Paris: Presses Universitaires de France.

Pinker, S. and Finke, R. A. (1980). Emergent two-dimensional patterns in images rotated in depth. *Journal of Experimental Psychology: Human Perception and Human Performance*, **6** (2), 244–64.

Pollack, I. and Klemmer, E. T. (1954). The assimilation of visual information from linear dot patterns. *Air Force Cambridge Research Center, Technical Report*, July, 54–66.

Pomerantz, J. R. and Kubovy, M. (1986). Theoretical approaches to perceptual organization: simplicity and likelihood principles. In K. R. Boff, L. Kaufman, and J. P. Thomas (eds.), *Handbook of Perception and Human Performance. Vol. 12* (pp. 1–46). New York: Wiley.

Pomerantz, J. R., Agrawal, A., Jewell, S. W., Jeong, M., Kahn, H., and Lozano, S. C. (2003). Contour grouping inside and outside of facial contexts. *Acta Psychologica* (Special Issue), **114**, 245–72.

Posner, M. I. (1973). *Cognition: An Introduction*. Glenview, IL: Scott, Foresman and Co.

Prigogine, I. and Stengers, I. (1984). *Order Out of Chaos: Man's New Dialogue with Nature*. New York: Bantam Books.

Pylyshyn, Z. W. (1973). What the mind's eye tells the mind's brain: a critique of mental imagery. *Psychological Bulletin*, **80**, 1–24.

(1999). Is vision continuous with cognition? The case of impenetrability of visual perception. *Behavioral and Brain Sciences*, **22**, 341–423.

Quastler, H. (ed.) (1955). *Information Theory in Psychology: Problems and Methods*. Glencoe, IL: Free Press.

Quereshi, M. Y. and Seitz, R. (1993a). Identical rules do not make letter and number series equivalent. *Intelligence*, **17** (3), 399–405.

(1993b). Gender differences in reasoning ability measured by letter series items. *Current Psychology Developmental, Learning, Personality, Social*, **12**, 268–72.

Quinlan, P. T. (1995). Evidence for the use of scene-based frames of reference in two-dimensional shape recognition. *Spatial Vision*, **9**, 101–25.

Reber, A. S., Walkenfeld, F. F., and Hernstadt, R. (1991). Implicit and explicit learning: individual differences and IQ. *Journal of Experimental Psychology: Learning, Memory, and Cognition*, 17, 888–96.

Reed, S. K. (1972). Pattern recognition and categorization. *Cognitive Psychology*, 3, 382–407.

Reed, S. K. and Johnsen, J. A. (1975). Detection of parts in patterns and images. *Memory and Cognition*, 3, 569–75.

Reichenbach, H. (1956). *The Direction of Time*. Berkeley, CA: University of California Press.

Restle, F. (1979). Coding theory of the perception of motion configurations. *Psychological Review*, 86, 1–24.

   (1982). Coding theory as an integration of Gestalt psychology and information processing theory. In J. Beck (ed.), *Organization and Representation in Perception* (pp. 31–56). Hillsdale, NJ: Lawrence Erlbaum.

Restle, F. and Decker, J. (1977). Size and the Müller-Lyer illusion as a function of its dimensions. *Perception and Psychophysics*, 21, 489–503.

Rock, I. (1973). *Orientation and Form*. New York: Academic Press.

   (1983). *The Logic of Perception*. Cambridge, MA: MIT Press.

   (1985). Perception and knowledge. *Acta Psychologica*, 59, 3–22.

Rosch, E. (1975). Cognitive representations of semantic categories. *Journal of Experimental Psychology: General*, 104, 192–233.

Runeson, S. and Frickholm, G. (1981). Visual perception of lifted weight. *Journal of Experimental Psychology: Human Perception and Performance*, 7, 733–40.

Ruyer, R. (1956). *La Cybernetique et l'Origine de l'Information [Cybernetics and Origin of Information]*. Paris: Flammarion.

Scharroo, J. and Leeuwenberg, E. (2000). Representation versus process in simplicity of serial pattern completion. *Cognitive Psychology*, 40, 39–86.

Scharroo, J., Stalmeier, P., and Boselie, F. (1994). Visual search and segregation as a function of display complexity. *Journal of General Psychology*, 121, 5–18.

Schumann, F. (1900). Beiträge zur analyse der gesichtswahrnemungen: einige beobachtungen über die zusammenfassung von Gesichtseindrücken zu Einheiten [Contributions to visual perception research: some observations on the integration of visual sensations toward perceptual components]. *Zeitschrift fur Psychologie*, 23, 1–32.

Sekuler, A. and Palmer, S. (1992). Perception of partly occluded objects: a microgenetic analysis. *Journal of Experimental Psychology, General*, 121, 95–111.

Sekuler, A., Palmer, S., and Flinn, C. (1994). Local and global processes in visual completion. *Psychological Science*, 5, 260–7.

Shannon, C. E. (1948). A mathematical theory of communication. *Bell System Technical Journal*, 27, 379–423, 623–56.

Shannon, C. E. and Weaver, W. (1949). *The Mathematical Theory of Communication*. Urbana, IL: University of Illinois Press.

Shepard, R. N. (1962a). The analysis of proximities: multidimensional scaling with an unknown distance function I. *Psychometrika*, 27, 125–40.

   (1962b). The analysis of proximities: multidimensional scaling with an unknown distance function II. *Psychometrika*, 27, 219–46.

(1980). Multidimensional scaling, tree-fitting, and clustering. *Science*, **210**, 390–8.

Shepard, R. N. and Metzler, J. (1971). Mental rotation of three-dimensional objects. *Science*, **171**, 701–3.

Shimaya, A. (1994). A perceptual model of figure segregation and amodal completion. *Investigative Ophtalmology and Visual Science, Supplement*, **35**, 16–44.

Simon, H. A. (1969). *The Science of the Artificial*. Cambridge, MA: MIT Press.

(1972). Complexity and the representation of patterned sequences of symbols. *Psychological Review*, **79**, 369–82.

(1990). Invariants of human behavior. *Annual Review of Psychology*, **41**, 1–19.

Simon, H. A. and Kotovsky, K. (1963). Human acquisition of concepts for sequential patterns. *Psychological Review*, **70**, 534–46.

Singer, W. and Gray, C. M. (1995). Visual feature integration and the temporal correlation hypothesis. *Annual Review of Neuroscience*, **18**, 555–86.

Smolensky, P. (1988). On the proper treatment of connectionism. *Behavioral and Brain Sciences*, **11**, 1–23.

Sober, E. (1975). *Simplicity*. London: Oxford University Press.

Solomonoff, R. J. (1964a). A formal theory of inductive inference, part 1. *Information and Control*, **7**, 1–22.

(1964b). A formal theory of inductive inference, part 2. *Information and Control*, **7**, 224–54.

Spellman, B. A. and Holyoak, K. J. (1996). Pragmatics in analogical mappings. *Cognitive Psychology*, **31**, 307–46.

Stankov, L. and Cregan, A. (1993). Quantitative and qualitative properties of an intelligence test: series completion. *Learning and Individual Differences*, **5** (2), 137–69.

Sternberg, R. J. and Gardner, M. K. (1983). Unities in inductive reasoning. *Journal of Experimental Psychology: General*, **112** (1), 80–116.

Sundqvist, F. (2003). *Perceptual Dynamics: Theoretical Foundations and Philosophical Implications of Gestalt Psychology*. Göteborg, Sweden: Gothenburg University.

Takano, Y. (1989). Perception of rotated forms: a theory of information types. *Cognitive Psychology*, **21**, 1–59.

Tarr, M. J. (1995). Rotating objects to recognize them: a case study on the role of viewpoint dependency in the recognition of three-dimensional objects. *Psychonomic Bulletin and Review*, **2**, 55–82.

Thurstone, L. L. and Thurstone, T. G. (1941). *Factorial Atudies of Intelligence*. University of Chicago Press.

Tippett, L. J. (1992). The generation of visual images: a review of neuropsychological research and theory. *Psychological Bulletin*, **112**, 415–32.

Treder, M. S. and van der Helm, P. A. (2007). Symmetry versus repetition in cyclopean vision: a microgenetic analysis. *Vision Research*, **47**, 2956–67.

Treder, M. S., van der Vloed, G., and van der Helm, P. A. (2011). Interactions between constituent single symmetries in multiple symmetry. *Attention, Perception, and Psychophysics*, **73**, 1487–502.

Treisman, A. (1969). Strategies and models of selective attention. *Psychologica Review*, **76**, 282–99.

(1982). Perceptual grouping and attention in visual search for features and for objects. *Journal of Experimental Psychology: Human Perception and Performance*, **8**, 194–214.

(1986). Properties, parts, and objects. In K. R. Boff, L. Kaufman, and J. P. Thomas (eds.), *Handbook of Perception and Human Performance: Vol. 1. Cognitive Processes and Performance* (pp. 1–70). New York: Wiley.

Treisman, A. and Gelade, G. (1980). A feature integration theory of attention. *Cognitive Psychology*, **12**, 97–136.

Tversky, A. (1977). Features of similarity. *Psychological Review*, **84**, 327–52.

Ungerleider, L. G. and Mishkin, M. (1982). Two cortical visual systems. In D. J. Ingle, M. A. Goodale, and R. J. W. Mansfield (eds.), *Analysis of Visual Behavior* (pp. 549–86). Cambridge, MA: MIT Press.

van Bakel, A. (1989). Perceived unity and duality as determined by superstructure components of pattern codes. Masters thesis, Nijmegen Institute for Information and Cognition (NICI), University of Nijmegen, Netherlands.

van der Helm, P. A. (1988). Accessibility and simplicity of visual structures. PhD thesis, Radboud University, Nijmegen, Netherlands.

(1994). The dynamics of Prägnanz. *Psychological Research*, **56**, 224–36.

(2000). Simplicity versus likelihood in visual perception: from surprisals to precisals. *Psychological Bulletin*, **126**, 770–800.

(2004). Transparallel processing by hyperstrings. *Proceedings of the National Academy of Sciences USA*, **101**, 10862–7.

(2010). Weber-Fechner behaviour in symmetry perception? *Attention, Perception, and Psychophysics*, **72**, 1854–64.

(2011). Bayesian confusions surrounding simplicity and likelihood in perceptual organization. *Acta Psychologica*, **138**, 337–46.

(2012). Cognitive architecture of perceptual organization: from neurons to gnosons. *Cognitive Processing*, **13**, 13–40.

(2013). *Simplicity in Vision: a Multidisciplinary Account of Perceptual Organization*. Cambridge University Press (in press).

van der Helm, P. A. and Leeuwenberg, E. L. J. (1986). Avoiding explosive search in automatic selection of simplest pattern codes. *Pattern Recognition*, **19**, 181–91.

(1991). Accessibility: a criterion for regularity and hierarchy in visual pattern codes. *Journal of Mathematical psychology*, **35**, 151–213.

(1996). Goodness of visual regularities: a nontransformational approach. *Psychological Review*, **103**, 429–56.

(1999). A better approach to goodness: reply to Wagemans (1999). *Psychological Review*, **106**, 622–30.

(2004). Holographic goodness is not that bad: reply to Olivers, Chater, and Watson (2004). *Psychological Review*, **111**, 261–73.

van der Helm, P. A. and Treder, M. S. (2009). Detection of (anti)symmetry and (anti)repetition: perceptual mechanisms versus cognitive strategies. *Vision Research*, **49**, 2754–63.

van der Helm, P. A., van Lier, R. J., and Leeuwenberg, E. L. J. (1992). Serial pattern complexity: irregularity and hierarchy. *Perception*, **21**, 517–44.

van der Vloed, G. (2005). The structure of visual regularities. PhD thesis, Radboud University, Nijmegen, Netherlands.

van der Vloed, G., Csathó, Á., and van der Helm, P. A. (2005). Symmetry and repetition in perspective. *Acta Psychologica*, **120**, 74–92.

(2007). Effects of asynchrony on symmetry perception. *Psychological Research*, **71**, 170–7.

van Leeuwen, C. (2007). What needs to emerge to make you conscious? *Journal of Consciousness Studies*, **14**, 115–36.

van Leeuwen, C., Steyvers, M., and Nooter, M. (1997). Stability and intermittency in large-scale coupled oscillator models for perceptual segmentation. *Journal of Mathematical Psychology*, **41**, 319–44.

van Lier, R. J. (1996). Simplicity of visual shape: a structural information approach. PhD thesis, Radboud University, Nijmegen, Netherlands.

(1999). Investigating global effects in visual occlusion: from a partly occluded square to a tree-trunk's rear. *Acta Psychologica*, **102**, 203–20.

(2000). Separate features versus one principle: comment on Shimaya (1997). *Journal of Experimental Psychology: Human Perception and Performance*, **26**, 412–17.

(2001). Simplicity, regularity, and perceptual interpretations: a structural information approach. In T. Shipley and P. Kellman (eds.), *From Fragments to Objects: Segmentation in Vision* (pp. 331–52). New York: Elsevier.

(2003). Differential effects of object orientation on imaginary object/viewer transformations. *Psychonomic Bulletin and Review*, **10**, 455–61.

van Lier, R. and Wagemans, J. (1999). From images to objects: global and local completions of self-occluded parts. *Journal of Experimental Psychology: Human Perception and Performance*, **25**, 1721–41.

van Lier, R. J., Leeuwenberg, E. L. J., and van der Helm, P. A. (1995). Multiple completions primed by occlusion patterns. *Perception*, **24**, 727–40.

(1997). In support of structural hierarchy in object representations. *Psychological Research*, **60**, 134–43.

van Lier, R. J., van der Helm, P. A., and Leeuwenberg, E. L. J. (1994). Integrating global and local aspects of visual occlusion. *Perception*, **23**, 883–903.

van Noorden, L. (1975). Temporal coherence in the perception of tone sequences. PhD thesis, Eindhoven University of Technology.

van Soest, J. L. (1952). *Informatie en Communicatie Theorie*. University paper, Department of Electronics, University of Delft, Netherlands.

van Tuijl, H. (1975). A new visual illusion: neonlike colour spreading and complementary colour induction between subjective contours. *Acta Psychologica*, **39**, 441–5.

(1979). Perceptual interpretation of line patterns. PhD thesis, Radboud University, Nijmegen, Netherlands.

van Tuijl, H. and de Weert, C. (1979). Sensory conditions for the occurence of the neon spreading illusion. *Perception*, **8**, 211–15.

van Tuijl, H. and Leeuwenberg, E. L. J. (1979). Neon color spreading and structural information measures. *Perception and Psychophysics*, **25**, 269–84.

(1980). Perceptual interpretation of complex line patterns. *Journal of Experimental Psychology: Human Perception and Performance*, **6**, 197–221.

(1982). Peripheral and central determinants of subjective contour strength. In H. G. Geissler, H. F. J. M. Buffart, P. Petzoldt, and Y. M. Zabrodin (eds.), *Psychophysical Judgement and the Process of Perception* (pp. 114–31). Amsterdam: North-Holland.

Varin, D. (1971). Fenomeni di contrasto e diffusione cromatica nell' organiz-zazione spaziale del campo percettivo [Contrast and colour spreading phe-nomena in the spatial organization of the visual field]. *Rivista di Psicologia*, **65**, 101–28.

von Bezold, W. (1874). *Die Farbenlehre im Hinblick auf Kunst und Kunstgewerbe [Colour Theory for Art and Art Products]*. Braunschweig, Germany: Wester-man.

von der Malsburg, C. (1981). *The Correlation Theory of Brain Function*. Göttingen, Germany: Max Planck Institute for Biophysical Chemistry, Internal Report 81–2.

von Helmholtz, H. L. F. (1962). *Treatise on Physiological Optics* (J. P. C. Southall, trans.). New York: Dover (original work published 1909).

Wagemans, J., van Gool, L., and d'Ydewalle, G. (1991). Detection of symmetry in tachistoscopically presented dot patterns: effects of multiple axes and skewing. *Perception and Psychophysics*, **50**, 413–27.

Wagemans, J., van Gool, L., Swinnen, V., and van Horebeek, J. (1993). Higher-order structure in regularity detection. *Vision Research*, **33**, 1067–88.

Watanabe, S. (1969). *Methodologies of Pattern Recognition*. New York: Academic Press.

Wenderoth, P. and Welsh, S. (1998). Effects of pattern orientation and number of symmetry axes on the detection of mirror symmetry in dot and solid patterns. *Perception*, **27**, 965–76.

Wertheimer, M. (1923). Untersuchungen zur lehre von der Gestalt [On Gestalt theory]. *Psychologische Forschung*, **4**, 301–50.

Weyl, H. (1952). *Symmetry*. Princeton University Press.

Wiener, N. (1948). *Cybernetics*. New York: Wiley.

Wouterlood, D. and Boselie, F. (1993). Shape decomposition as a function of concave discontinuity. Report, Nijmegen Institute for Information and Cog-nition (NICI), University of Nijmegen, Netherlands.

Zusne, L. (1970). *Visual Perception of Form*. New York: Academic Press.

Author index

313

Subject index

aesthetics 268, 269, 270, 282
algorithmic information theory (AIT) 5, 6, 92, 94, 96, 294
algorithmic level 6
alignment axis 205, 207, 208
alternation 98, 101, 109, 110, 118, 283
ambiguity 20, 25, 29, 31, 35, 57, 134, 238, 268
amodal completion (completion, occlusion) 15, 95
analogue thinking 259
asymmetrical coding 286
attention 22, 32, 262, 265, 268, 286

backward masking 194, 195, 196
backward rotation 247
backward scanning 122
Bayes rule 75, 77, 78, 92, 95, 150
beauty (aesthetics) 260, 268, 269, 270, 271, 277, 288
bit 225, 272
bootstrap model 101
branching pattern 122
broken symmetry 98, 110

chunk 98, 99, 110, 111
class code 73, 74
classification 5, 14, 24, 70, 72, 74, 80, 111, 253, 271, 276, 289
cluster 39, 46, 47, 50, 110, 115, 262
code argument 38, 41, 42, 44, 46, 99, 284
code evaluation 249, 295
code hierarchy 31, 32, 43, 63, 107, 115, 203, 216
colour assimilation 147, 154, 166, 168, 169, 170, 172
colour contrast 154, 171
colour filling-in 127
complementary code 114
computational level 6, 83
concurrent presence 179, 203, 204
conditional likelihood 80, 81

conjunction 261
conjunctive ambiguity 86, 268
connectionism 6, 103, 172
conscious reasoning 18, 21, 52, 295
constraint salience 260
context effect 19, 21, 183, 189, 193, 267, 287
corkscrew rule 135, 236
cut-off operation 142, 143, 145, 146

deductive reasoning 22, 259
descriptive simplicity 81, 83
dimensional scaling 27, 28, 31, 33, 35, 43
disjunctive ambiguity 268
dissociated representation 121, 124, 126, 130, 134, 145, 149, 151, 156
distal stimulus 75, 84, 86, 87, 90, 120
distinctive salience 260
distracter 31, 32, 260, 262, 263, 264, 265, 282
dynamic system theory 6, 86

entropy 181, 182, 183
external structure 125, 132, 145, 166, 284
extrapolation 223, 251, 252, 255, 258, 259

familiarity cue 4, 18, 19, 20
feed-forward connection 104
figural goodness 113, 115, 116, 117, 118, 119, 234, 260, 287
forward masking 195
forward rotation 243

general viewpoint 75, 125, 126, 284, 289
geon 64, 65, 68, 70, 78, 212
Gestalt cue 4, 20, 38, 39, 41, 226
global completion 175, 176
global precedence 48, 49, 50, 51, 55, 56, 63, 286
global structure 48, 54, 58
golden section 273

317

9 781107 531758